The Remarkable Story of Copaxone®

An Approach to the Treatment of Multiple Sclerosis

To Cindy

Regards

K. Johnson

COPAXONE® (glatiramer acetate injection) is indicated for the reduction of the frequency of relapses in relapsing-remitting multiple sclerosis, including patients who have experienced a first clinical episode and have MRI features consistent with multiple sclerosis.

Important Safety Information about COPAXONE®

- The most common side effects of COPAXONE® are redness, pain, swelling, itching, or a lump at the site of injection, flushing, rash, shortness of breath, and chest pain. These reactions are usually mild and seldom require professional treatment. Patients should tell their doctor about any side effects.
- Some patients report a short-term reaction right after injecting COPAXONE®. This reaction can involve flushing (feeling of warmth and/or redness), chest tightness or pain with heart palpitations, anxiety, and trouble breathing. These symptoms generally appear within minutes of an injection, last about 15 minutes, and go away by themselves without further problems.
- A permanent indentation under the skin at the injection site may occur, due to a local destruction of fat tissue. Patients should follow proper injection technique and inform their doctor of any skin changes.
- After injecting COPAXONE®, patients should call their doctor right away if they develop hives, skin rash with irritation, dizziness, sweating, chest pain, trouble breathing, severe pain at the injection site or other uncomfortable changes in their general health. Patients should not give themselves any more injections until their doctor tells them to begin again.

You are encouraged to report negative side effects of prescription drugs to the FDA. Visit www.fda.gov/medwatch, or call 1-800-FDA-1088.

Please see enclosed additional important information.

COPAXONE® is a registered trademark of Teva Pharmaceutical Industries Ltd.

COP101039705/100279

The Remarkable Story of Copaxone®

An Approach to the Treatment of Multiple Sclerosis

Kenneth P. Johnson, M.D.
Professor Emeritus
Department of Neurology
University of Maryland School of Medicine
Baltimore, Maryland

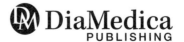 **DiaMedica** PUBLISHING

DiaMedica Publishing, 150 East 61st Street, New York, NY 10065
Visit our website at www.diamedicapub.com

Library of Congress Cataloging-In-Publication Data is available upon request.

ISBN: 978-0-9823219-4-2 (softcover)
       978-0-9823219-5-9 (hardbound)

To Jackie

About the Author

Dr. Kenneth P. Johnson has been involved in and in a leadership position in the development of new treatments for benefiting multiple sclerosis (MS) for the past 25 years. He is an academic neurologist with special expertise in viral and immunologic disorders of the nervous system and has authored or co-authored over 175 scientific articles in leading worldwide medical journals.

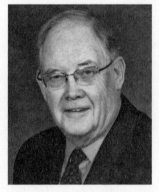

Dr. Kenneth P. Johnson

After graduating from Jefferson University School of Medicine in Philadelphia, he held faculty positions at Case Western Reserve University, Cleveland, the University of California, San Francisco, and, beginning in 1981, as Chair of the Department of Neurology at the University of Maryland School of Medicine in Baltimore. He is currently Professor Emeritus in the Department.

Among other achievements he founded the Americas Committee for Treatment and Research in Multiple Sclerosis (ACTRIMS), which has become a leading North American organization for advancing MS science and patient care; the annual meeting in Montreal of September 2008 attracted 5,500 attendees. In 2000, he was awarded the Dystel Prize by the National MS Society and the American Academy of Neurology for his pioneering work on developing new treatments for MS.

Contents

Contents

PART III: Teva Pharmaceuticals

Foreword

Desperate patients, international geopolitics, pharmaceutical competition, governmental secrecy, a race against time—sounds like the stuff of a best-selling novel. But, no. It is "The Remarkable Story of Copaxone®." In this book, Dr. Kenneth P. Johnson, a highly respected scientist and world-renowned expert on multiple sclerosis, recounts the fascinating tale of the development and rise to prominence of the drug Copaxone®, one of the first agents to significantly impact the course of multiple sclerosis, an often devastating disease of the brain, spinal cord, and optic nerves.

What is multiple sclerosis or MS, as it is commonly known? It is not muscular dystrophy, the group of diseases for which Jerry Lewis has raised so much money over the years in his annual telethon. Rather, it is a disease whose cause is unknown, in which the body's immune system, which is critically important in protecting us from "foreign invaders" such as bacteria, viruses, and malignant (cancer-causing) cells, goes haywire and attacks the body's own central nervous system (CNS). The process is highly unpredictable and seemingly random. Because the CNS consists of the brain, spinal cord, and optic nerves, these assaults, which often appear to come "out of the blue," can cause a wide range of neurologic symptoms. Patients may experience loss of vision in one eye, double vision, or vertigo. They may notice strange numbness and tingling in various parts of the body, most commonly the legs, or, worse yet, weakness or even paralysis of one or more limbs.

The disease, tragically, most often strikes young adults—much more commonly women than men—in the prime of life. Typically, the disease initially follows a relapsing-remitting course with periods of stability punctuated by attacks (also known as relapses or exacerbations). The unpredictability of the occurrence of these episodes creates an incredible emotional challenge for those affected, just as they are trying to establish their careers and their families. Sadly, as the years go on, people with MS often become disabled, most typically by problems in walking, by severe and inexplicable fatigue, and by difficulty controlling their urinary and bowel functions. In the United States, an estimated 400,000 people have the disease, and there are millions more worldwide. But the disease does not only affect an individual; it also impacts their entire sphere of family and friends.

Given the dramatic and often devastating effects that MS has on patients and their loved ones, it is no surprise that medical scientists for years have deliberately, thoughtfully, and purposefully sought effective treatments to control and—hopefully—halt its damage. But the development of Copaxone as an effective and ultimately widely prescribed treatment for MS, actually begins with serendipity, an accidental stroke of good fortune. Scientists at the Weizmann Institute, a highly respected basic science research facility in Israel, were actually seeking a new compound that would mimic the action of a naturally-occurring protein (known as myelin basic protein, a component of myelin, the fatty covering of nerve fibers that is a principal site of damage in MS), in producing an animal model of MS known as experimental autoimmune encephalomyelitis or EAE. The investigators failed in this quest. But, in the course of their work, the scientists recognized that one of the compounds they generated, known originally as Copolymer 1 (or Cop 1) and subsequently as Copaxone®, actually seemed to prevent or lessen the effects of EAE in their rats and mice. Eureka! As the brilliant scientist Louis Pasteur noted, "Chance favors the prepared mind." And, indeed, these astute scientists at the Weizmann Institute recognized the potential to use their compound to treat

MS, a disease for which no effective therapy was available at that time, and thus began the fascinating development of Copaxone.

And, as they say, "The rest is history." But, what a history! And no one is in a better position to recount it than Dr. Johnson. Medically trained as a neurologist and eventually rising to the position he held for many years as Chairman of the Neurology Department at the University of Maryland, Dr. Johnson began his scientific career as a neurovirologist. He undoubtedly became particularly interested in MS because of the theory, unproved to this day, that the disease was caused by a viral infection. He became one of the leading investigators of interferon treatment of MS, undertaken because one of the principal effects of this class of biologicals is interference with viral infection. Honed by lessons learned from the clinical trials of interferon beta-1b or Betaseron® (which actually became the first drug marketed for the treatment of MS), he became the lead investigator in the pivotal trial of Copaxone, whose success led to its commercial introduction, first to the U.S. market, in 1997.

My own personal involvement in the Copaxone story dates back to the very late 1970s, when, as a young neurologist and investigator at Albert Einstein College of Medicine, I was asked by Prof. Murray Bornstein to join him in designing and conducting the first trials of Copaxone (then Cop 1) in the U.S. I did so with some trepidation, for the words of H. Houston Merritt, "dean" of neurology in the U.S. rang in my ears. Dr. Merritt allegedly had said, "The best way I know to ruin a good career in neurology is to advocate a treatment for MS." Fortunately, my skepticism was dispelled, as the results of those early trials were positive and the subsequent testing confirmed those successes, leading to the commercialization of Copaxone.

In this volume, Dr. Johnson details the fascinating development of Copaxone, leading to its approval by the U.S. Food and Drug Administration and subsequently by other regulatory agencies. However, the story does not end there. Dr. Johnson goes on to relate the high-stakes battles that have taken place in the marketplace and provides a professional's glimpse into the backrooms of the pharmaceutical industry.

Copaxone is not the end of story of the treatment for MS. Indeed, it is an intriguing and important part of the beginning. Subsequent to the introduction of Copaxone, administered as a daily injection under the skin, we have seen other medicines for MS introduced. We are now on the threshold of a new era of MS treatment, in which the options may be many, including oral medications that are easier to take. It is unlikely, though, that any of these stories will take such twists and turns as the road Copaxone has traversed. Dr. Johnson's insightful recounting of this journey will make exciting reading even for those without a direct connection to MS.

Aaron Miller, MD
Medical Director,
Corinne Goldsmith Dickinson Center for Multiple Sclerosis
and
Professor of Neurology
Mount Sinai School of Medicine
New York, NY

Preface

Multiple sclerosis (MS) is, after trauma, the most common crippling neurologic disease of young adults. Over 400,000 people with MS live in the United States, and the worldwide population exceeds 1.2 million. For good reason, it has been termed the "disease that shatters dreams." Within 15 years after the first symptoms appear, half (50%) of MS patients require some type of walking aid, and most have life-long problems with vision, lack of coordination, poor bladder control and—most concerning—some decline in cognitive function. The course is unpredictable; the patient never knows when new symptoms may appear or if improvement will follow. In the period between 15 and 45 years of age, when MS symptoms most commonly first appear, people with MS are likely to be completing their education, choosing a career path, entering the job market, and considering marriage or starting a family. Because 65% to 70% of people with MS are women, the impact on their young families is often devastating. The concern and constant fear of when the next symptoms of MS will surface has understandably made the desperate search for a treatment vitally important, and any claim of benefit generates compelling interest to both patients and doctors.

Over the last 80 to 100 years, virtually every therapy for any human disease has been considered and tried for MS, without finding a useful treatment. From antibiotics to anticoagulants, from radiation to acupuncture, numerous diets, and physical therapy programs, none was shown to be useful. Practically every patent medicine and herbal supplement has been claimed to improve the disease, and a number of potentially dangerous procedures, like injections of snake venom, multiple bee stings, and repeated hyperbaric oxygen exposures, have all had their day, but nothing was found to be useful in altering the downhill course of MS. The situation understandably led to despair for MS patients and to frustration and disappointment for clinicians and the MS research community.

The August 13, 1987, issue of the *New England Journal of Medicine* contained an article describing the results from a clinical trial of an MS treatment comparing daily injections of a drug then called Cop 1 (copolymer one) with placebo. The trial, 2 years in length, was small; in fact it was called a pilot trial. It contrasted the experience of 25 very active MS patients receiving daily injections under the skin of Cop 1 with a well matched group of 24 patients who received daily injections of a placebo. It was a classic double-blind, placebo-controlled trial, called *double-blind* because neither patients nor physicians knew during the study which group each patient was in. This method is often called the "gold standard" in clinical trials, and is usually demanded of most drugs seeking approval by the U.S. Food and Drug Administration (FDA) as a commercial prescription treatment. When the trial was completed and the degree of MS disease activity was compared between the two groups, it was clear and statistically proven that Cop 1 controlled MS much better than placebo. It was the first treatment ever that had been clearly shown to control or benefit MS.

This trial was carried out at the Albert Einstein School of Medicine in the Bronx, New York. However, Cop 1 came from the Weizmann Institute of Science in Rehovot, Israel, where it had been developed and extensively studied for over 20 years by three Israeli immunochemists: Michael Sela, Ruth Arnon, and Dvora Teitelbaum.

The story of the development of Cop 1 is among the most unique of modern drug discoveries that are now in everyday use in the pharmacologic armamentarium. Not only is it the enduring legacy of three brilliant and determined scientists working on this project over decades; it is also the story of two organizations working in partnership in Israel during very trying times. The Weizmann Institute was named for talented scientist and statesman Chaim Weizmann, who would one day become the first President of Israel at the time of its creation in 1948. The Institute has, since its founding, been recognized as a world-class center for scientific discovery and development. Teva Pharmaceutical Industries Ltd., now the number-one producer of generic drugs in the world, was formed in 1938, but in fact traces its origins to a drug distribution company established in 1901, in Jerusalem. The remarkable and most unlikely history is that these two organizations, now recognized as pinnacles of science and commerce worldwide, grew and prospered in spite of a most chaotic and dangerous environment during the early years of the State of Israel's creation and founding. Courage, focus, and dedication to high ideals, as well as excellent science, are the essence of this story.

To fully grasp the impact of this story, this book describes the nature and course of MS and how it changes its victims in a desperate, life-defining way. In addition, two volunteers who participated in a major MS trial of Cop 1 are followed for over 15 or more years. Cop 1 and how it was developed can be better understood by a brief description of the central nervous system and how it is damaged by MS. The long, sometimes discouraging, and often unpredictable road from the first idea that Cop 1 could be an MS treatment to the thrilling day when the FDA Expert Panel voted to recommend approval of Cop 1 provides an exciting tale. Now, after almost 15 years of worldwide use, the value of the drug and its long, unique development has become ever more compelling as it has become recognized as the most prescribed treatment for MS.

Anxiety and despair for hundreds of thousands of people with MS has been replaced by hope and reassurance that the disease, while not curable, can now be managed for many patients by this first treatment shown by research to improve the lifetime course of MS.

Acknowledgments

I am grateful to Michael Sela and Ruth Arnon of the Weizmann Institute of Science for invaluable personal information and useful publications, and for reviewing and correcting the manuscript. Larry Downey, Executive Vice President, North America Brand Pharmaceuticals, provided long-term encouragement and support for this effort. Judy Katterhenrich, formerly of Teva Neuroscience, and David Ladkani of Teva Pharmaceuticals gave frequent useful input. Dan Suesskind, former CFO of Teva Pharmaceuticals, reviewed the manuscript to improve historical and accurate information of Teva's development.

At the University of Maryland, David Trisler was the source of important information on the early development of protein structure and discovery of the genetic code. Suhayl Dhib-Jalbut, at the Robert Wood Johnson Medical School, gave me many useful publications on current immunology underpinning the mechanism of action of glatiramer acetate (Copaxone) and then reviewed that section of the manuscript.

I am forever indebted to Mary Rose, who worked on every aspect of this project, searching the Internet for information and putting the manuscript into a beautiful format.

Finally, Dr. Diana M. Schneider of DiaMedica, my publisher, gave freely of her deep knowledge of neurology and particularly multiple sclerosis, in combination with her extensive experience of medical publishing to make this a successful effort.

PART I

Multiple Sclerosis:
The Disease

What Is Multiple Sclerosis?

When did multiple sclerosis (MS) first appear? Few human diseases can be charted with any certainty as to when they first surfaced to torment us, but there must have been an index or first case for all diseases, as human genetics evolved and individuals reacted to their environments. Some conditions are easier to identify historically than others. Individuals described in the Bible probably suffered from epilepsy, and tomb paintings from ancient Egypt show individuals with withered or atrophic limbs that could well have been caused by polio. Skeletal remains prove the existence of various bone diseases in early humans. Thus, for some conditions, at least minimal evidence exists for their presence in early recorded history or even human prehistory.

Multiple sclerosis is different, however, because it affects only the central nervous system (CNS)—the brain and spinal cord—which decay soon after death. Multiple sclerosis is also a relatively uncommon, highly variable, and unpredictable illness that probably would not have been recognized as a specific disease and described with precision in ancient writings. While MS could have afflicted early humans even in their migration out of Africa, it is more likely that the condition first appeared in Northern Europe, such as in the villages of the Vikings in Scandinavia, since MS is most commonly noted in descendants of these populations. It is seldom identified in Asians or in modern Africans.

As noted by Dr. T. Jock Murray in *Multiple Sclerosis: The History of a Disease*, useful information and descriptions about cases which may have been MS can only be traced back to the 14th century AD, where there are records of cases that conform to our modern concepts of MS. One early case thought to be MS is that of Lidwina of Schiedam, Holland, born on April 18, 1380. As a teenager, she developed various acute neurologic symptoms that gradually improved, and as a young adult, she was said to have violent shooting pains in her teeth. These could have been symptoms of trigeminal neuralgia, a condition now commonly recognized in people with MS. She later became blind in one eye, developed difficulty walking, and had paralysis of the right arm. Her disease attracted considerable public notice, and many physicians and nobles were consulted. Over time, her condition progressed, and she became bedridden and had difficulty swallowing. However, she experienced occasional periods of improvement.

As a young adult, she began to describe supernatural visits, and visions that had religious overtones. Finally, she became blind and paralyzed, but continued to attract great public attention, giving rise to numerous myths that obviously are beyond belief. She was said to have subsisted only on Holy Communion and to have had nothing to drink for a period of 7 years. Because of her pious acceptance of pain and increasing paralysis, she was described as saintly and was eventually beatified by the church; she was said to be a prodigy of human suffering and heroic patience. Due to this ecclesiastical interest, several biographies were written while she was still alive or within a few years after her death. Saint Lidwina was canonized by Pope Leo XIII in 1890. Modern neurologists and historians have, in spite of the religious coloring to her history, felt that adequate information is available to say that she most likely suffered from MS.

Another well-documented story of a young man who almost certainly had MS was that of Augustus d'Este, who lived from 1794 to 1848. He was the illegitimate grandson of King George III of England and a cousin of Queen Victoria. He joined the British Army, attained the rank of lieutenant colonel, and served in America, where he was present at the defeat of the British near New Orleans in 1815. He first acquired symptoms of a strange illness at the age of 28, which began with transient blurring of vision that improved, but returned a year later. Other neurologic symptoms followed over the next 10 years. In his detailed diary, he describes multiple therapies recommended by numerous physicians both in England and on the continent. Over time, he developed weakness of both legs, along with impotence. He died in 1848, after an illness of 26 years that was characterized by several bouts of visual loss, double vision, sensory change, and intermittent and progressive paralysis, all being typical characteristics of MS. His story is valuable because of the interesting detail contained in his daily diary and because of the large number of dangerous and often painful therapies that were used at the time, without any reasonable scientific basis and without benefit. These and numerous other well-characterized examples make it clear that MS was present in England and Northern Europe in the 17th and 18th centuries, but was not recognized as a specific illness.

By the mid-19th century, medicine in general, but especially neurology, began to develop a more scientific foundation for classifying disease, with careful observation of changes in a patient's function (weakness, blindness, incoordination, pain, etc.) followed by detailed study of pathologic changes found at autopsy. This process became known as *clinico-pathologic correlation*. Physicians throughout Europe and North America, but especially in Paris, began to describe in detail the characteristics of patients with chronic illnesses, the tempo of change, and—in the case of neurologic conditions—specific abnormalities of gait, weakness, incoordination, vision, sensory loss, and even cognitive change. Following the patients' death, postmortem examinations provided the opportunity to link or correlate the patients' symptoms during life with pathologic changes in the nervous system. Improvements in the microscope and better methods to preserve and stain tissue were indispensable. With this came an increasing and fundamental awareness that the nervous system, unlike any other body organ, was anatomically arranged to control specific functions, such that discrete regions of the brain were responsible for movement or sensory perception or vision or even speech. These localized areas of the brain were found to be linked to specific tracks or bundles of nerve fibers that traveled through the brainstem into the spinal cord and passed on to peripheral nerves in the limbs to facilitate specific functions; for instance, for fine motor movements, coordinated movements required for walking, speech, language, or vision.

Throughout the British Isles and continental Europe, but especially in Paris, physicians began to adopt the new concept of clinic-pathologic correlation and soon made essential contributions to the understanding of human disease based on its underlying brain or spinal cord pathology. This new scientific movement fundamentally changed the nature of observing and then classifying human illness. Many scientists and physicians from that period made valuable contributions, but few came close to those of the towering figure of Paris physician Jean-Martin Charcot, especially when it came to differentiating neurologic diseases based on their underlying pathology.

Charcot was born in Paris in 1825, and studied medicine at the University of Paris. Early on, he was guided by Professor Rayer, who emphasized that a clinician's ability must be based on his skill as a pathologist who could recognize changes in tissues such as the brain. Charcot, who displayed great curiosity and ability as a student, was awarded a professorship in 1860, and soon was appointed to the staff of the Salpetriere. This unique hospital was to become the focal point of his professional activity for the rest of his life. It was an extremely fortunate location, for it was there that he found the singular environment in which to observe, study, and classify clinical conditions.

La Salpetriere, originally a munitions factory and arsenal, was converted by King Louis XIII into a hospice for the care of sick women. Over time, it grew to more than 100 buildings that housed over 5,000 poor, insane, epileptic, sick, elderly, and demented people who could no longer be accommodated in the community. Here was a virtual living museum of women with a vast variety of chronic human illnesses who were likely to live out their days and die within the walls of the institution. A large number of the Salpetriere inmates suffered from neurologic conditions.

Charcot became increasingly attracted to neurologic disease as a field of observation and study. He and his colleague, Edme Vulpian, recognized the unique resource available to them and soon set out to identify and classify neurologic diseases. They made extensive notes, covering years or decades of the lives of individual patients who displayed special patterns of neurologic change. Ultimately, many of these patients died and were then available for postmortem evaluation. A gifted artist with great skill with the microscope, Charcot was able to make unique correlations between these patients' functional abnormalities and behavior during life and the resulting neuropathology, and thus he was able to differentiate and classify a variety of neurologic diseases.

While he made contributions to many conditions, Charcot is best known for his descriptions of MS and amyotrophic lateral sclerosis (ALS or Lou Gehrig's disease) which have, from time to time, been considered as "Charcot's disease." As Charcot's observations and his fame grew, he was invited to give regular lectures that were extremely well received and attracted large medical audiences. In 1868, he gave a series of landmark lectures that described both the clinical features and the pathology of MS, which at the time was often termed *disseminated sclerosis*. These lectures were soon published, along with illustrations of the brain and spinal cord pathology, first in French and then, in 1881, in English translations. They continue to be recognized as an important time point during which MS emerged as a separate and defined human disease with a specific neuropathologic basis.

His illustrations, especially of the pathology of the spinal cord, remain typical of the disease as it is pathologically described even now. Charcot died in 1893, having published 462 medical articles on many diseases. His MS studies remain the foundation for his enduring fame and cherished place in neurologic history. Later in his life, when asked about the treatment of disseminated sclerosis, his bleak conclusion was "the time has not yet come when such a subject can be seriously considered. I can only tell you of some experiments which I have

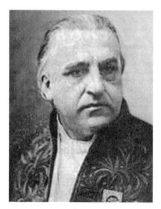

Jean-Martin Charcot, 1825–1893

tried, the results of which unfortunately have not been very encouraging." In fact, there was a lapse of 119 years between Charcot's lucid description of the disease and its pathology in his lectures of 1868, and the first report, in 1987, of a treatment which would significantly change the course of MS relapses. In the intervening decades, virtually every treatment for any human disease was given to people with MS without benefit.

The Relapse in Multiple Sclerosis

Most young adults, unless they have other family members who have experienced MS, have no inkling when the first MS symptoms appear that they are destined to live with this life-long disease. A relapse, also called an attack, exacerbation, or flare, is their first experience with MS. It usually starts with some neurologic symptom that evolves quite abruptly over a matter of hours to 2 or 3 days. Almost any neurologic symptom might announce the beginning of MS, but most commonly the symptoms have features that affect the spinal cord, such as numbness or tingling in a foot or leg. This then fairly rapidly begins to ascend the leg, and may cover a portion of the trunk on the same side of the body up to the level of the waist or even the nipple line. Occasionally, the symptoms will move to the other limb, with a similar progression. Some patients recognize some weakness and difficulty walking in addition to sensory changes. Rarely, patients describe unusual and even bizarre symptoms. One patient, evaluated over several years, developed the sensation of a band-like area of numbness around the waist that included the sense of a large mass the size of a football attached to her trunk. This peculiar feeling, while not painful, never disappeared. It is not unusual for patients with spinal cord lesions to have urinary symptoms in addition to their sensory disturbance, and some patients complain of poorly localized aching pain in the limbs as well.

The second most common area to be affected is the optic nerve, a thin nerve approximately the size of the lead of a pencil that connects the back of the eyeball to the brain. When this nerve is affected, patients usually describe a central area of blurring or even blindness in one eye. This symptom also progresses quite rapidly over a matter of 1 or 2 days and, not uncommonly, is accompanied by pain in the orbit on that side, which is often increased with movement of the eyeball.

Other relapses give rise to a sense of unsteadiness or dizziness, which may include an actual sense of spinning (vertigo). Nausea or even vomiting may complicate such an attack. Incoordination and tremor can also appear. Whatever group of symptoms the patient describes, they rarely expand beyond 4 or 5 days, and then stabilize for an indefinite period that lasts from a few days to 3 or 4 months before fading, often clearing completely. Unfortunately, some abnormalities persist and become part of the signature of chronic MS.

Disturbed and frightened by such symptoms, most patients seek medical attention and are often given a tentative diagnosis of some type of back sprain or injury, a ruptured disc, an inner ear infection, or even some type of meningitis. This of course frequently leads to an extensive medical evaluation, often including a computed tomography (CT) scan, a variety of blood studies, and even, in some cases, examination of the spinal fluid. Numerous medical specialists may be consulted, including orthopedists, neurosurgeons, ophthalmologists, ear-nose-and-throat (ENT) doctors, and others. A magnetic resonance imaging (MRI) test will, in many cases, bring MS to the head of the list as a possible diagnosis, although it is not unusual for the initial MRI to be negative, especially if only the spinal column is imaged. The central importance of MRI in the diagnosis and management of MS is discussed later.

The initial symptoms of the relapse may fade within a matter of days or may persist for a number of weeks or even months, but most of the time they slowly resolve. The patient breathes a sigh of relief and considers that the entire process is over for good. However, as many as 40% of patients do not experience complete relief from their first attack and are left with some residual neurologic problem, perhaps slight weakness of a limb or a decrease in vision in the affected eye.

Some MS relapses come on with a vengeance, appearing as a major neurologic catastrophe. As an example, a woman in her mid-20s with an established diagnosis of MS that had been mild and who was using a standard immunomodulatory drug, became engaged to be married one day in November. The following morning, she awoke with almost complete paralysis of her left side, and she could barely move either her arm or her leg. An immediate MRI scan showed a very large lesion or area of damage in the deep right brain hemisphere which, had she not had an established diagnosis of MS, might have been considered a rapidly growing brain tumor or perhaps a stroke. She pleaded that she be treated aggressively so that in June, 6 months later, she would be able to walk down the aisle at her wedding. With steroids and other drugs, and with physical therapy and exercise, she slowly improved. Although still exhibiting some left arm weakness and a limp, she was able to begin her married life with a beautiful wedding.

Perceiving improvement or even complete recovery from the first attack, patients are typically relieved, their sense of anxiety declines, and they probably begin to feel that they're lucky and the doctor's concern about a serious diagnosis such as MS was probably incorrect. Their family and friends remark that they look well, and life begins to resume its normal routine, and the demands of getting an education or maintaining a household or caring for children thankfully lays claim to the patient's attention. Life is good.

As the patient recovers from the first attack and the neurologic symptoms continue to fade, the patient's improved self-image is readily evident. Natural history studies of MS however, show that new relapses will occur at approximately one per year. Some patients may have a second relapse within a few months, others may experience 3 or 4 years free of symptoms, and—rarely—patients may have a decade or more without any evidence of ongoing MS activity. The pattern of relapse activity is highly unpredictable, and there are no clinical or laboratory indicators that help to prepare the patient for the future. Needing a wheelchair within 3 years of running a marathon is one extreme, while living to old age without ever experiencing neurologic symptoms yet having MS lesions in the brain at autopsy is another, testifying to the vast clinical and pathologic variability of MS.

CIS: Clinically Isolated Syndrome

The first episode of neurologic symptoms in the life of an individual destined to have MS has been termed by physicians as the *clinically isolated syndrome* (CIS). At this time, without a history of repeated relapses or other neurologic problems, it is impossible to know for sure if the patient really suffers from MS. The presence of characteristic abnormalities in the brain MRI give a strong signal that MS is in fact the correct diagnosis. As of 2010, several carefully constructed placebo-controlled clinical trials using currently available MS treatments have shown that active therapy during the recovery period from CIS will delay the occurrence of the next MS relapse in most cases. While the scientific data are clear and the medical recommendation to start therapy is sound, it is often difficult for a CIS patient who is clearly improving or has returned to normal to accept the physician's advice to start treatment with a medication that must be injected frequently, daily to weekly, often with side effects, for the indefinite future.

The Second Clinical Attack or Relapse

The second clinical attack, whenever it occurs, may be perceived by the patient as similar to the first. More likely, because the disease typically reappears in another part of the nervous system, the symptoms will be new; for instance, trouble with unilateral vision if the previous attack had been in the spinal cord. For most patients, the second attack is a life-defining event with serious psychological repercussions, regardless of how mild or serious the neurologic signs are.

Dr. Rosalind Kalb, a psychologist and head of the Professional Resource Center at the National Multiple Sclerosis Society in New York, has written perceptively about the emotionally devastating nature of the second attack:

"I guess I really do have MS."
"The doctor was right after all."
"I'm going to end up in a wheelchair."
"Life will never be the same."
"No one will want me."
"There go my dreams for . . . . "

People begin to acknowledge the end of life as they knew it and the beginning of life with a chronic illness. This requires a change in self-image—from that of an able-bodied person to someone with a chronic disease. For some, the leap from denial to hopelessness may be quick and powerful. Even for those who navigate this change more comfortably, a grieving process is needed; it is impossible to begin planning and problem-solving for a new life with MS without first grieving over the loss of the old one. For many young adults, the diagnosis of MS is the very first threat to their feelings of strength and invincibility.

Patients now must deal with the emotional turmoil that the second relapse engenders. There also are serious implications for others. Family members, especially a spouse, must also begin to adapt or perhaps plan for a different future. What is the risk to a wife being able to function as a homemaker and mother? For instance, will she be able to maintain her career or education? For a man, what will happen to his role as a breadwinner and father? For children, there of course is the chance that the affected parent will, at some time in the future, be unable to participate in parenting to the full extent expected. Of interest, it has been reported that children even blame themselves for their parent's illness, wondering if something that they did played a part in bringing on their parent's condition.

As Dr. Kalb has written, "the patient is faced with the need to redefine *self*:

1. "Who am I now that I can no longer do what I've always done?"
2. "What is my value, what do I still have to contribute to my world?"
3. "What is my role, what can I do for my family, friends, colleagues?"

As the sequence of relapses continues, whether frequently or only occasionally and with serious neurologic consequences or not, the unpredictability and variability of relapsing MS confronts the patient every day. It is as if the person with MS is always aware of a small black storm cloud off on the horizon: it never disappears, but carries the potential of suddenly enlarging and becoming a severe, all-encompassing storm during which he or she is at risk of new and serious symptoms and their consequences as an alarming new relapse develops. Mild or severe, the relapse always raises the image of a life of increasing disability and a blemished future.

The Primary or Secondary Progressive Stages of Multiple Sclerosis

As new relapses occur, as an increased level of fixed disability becomes ever more challenging, and as the patient's self-image is forced to readjust, the unpredictable tempo of MS goes on.

When the natural history evaluation of large populations is followed over several decades, it shows that, within 15 years of onset, almost 50% of MS patients will require a full-time walking aid (cane or crutch) and may have to contend with other impairments as well: decreased vision; distressing problems of poor bowel and bladder control; muscle tightness (termed *spasticity*); poorly understood but common fatigue, weakness, clumsiness, or tremor in an arm; and, possibly a decline in intellectual function (partial dementia). Understandably, patients develop various levels of depression as their loss of function becomes evident and then increases.

The relapsing phase of MS, during which patients experience relapses followed by some recovery, separated by unpredictable intervals, sooner or later disappears. Patients now begin a new, even more ominous stage of their disease, the so-called secondary progressive phase. As the course and pattern of the illness changes, patients experience an increase or progression in neurologic disability, which may advance quite rapidly or may come on slowly over several years, interrupted by plateaus of relative neurologic stability. The term "secondary progressive phase" is used because it is progressive (increasing disability) but is *secondary* to the preceding relapsing-remitting phase.

Patients describe how one year they were able to walk up the stairs to the second floor of their home without difficulty; a year later they needed to grasp the banister to pull themselves up, and a few years later they had great difficulty climbing stairs at all, prompting a family discussion about the need for different housing, without the challenge of stairs.

A valuable scale to measure this increasing disability is called the Expanded Disability Status Scale (EDSS). The EDSS was invented by a creative neurologist, Dr. John Kurtzke, of the Veterans Administration Medical Center in Washington, D.C. It has become an essential tool in measuring the effectiveness of experimental therapies being tested for the treatment of MS. A major component of the EDSS is an analysis of the patient's ability to walk unaided, starting with what is considered normal—the ability to walk for 500 meters (five football fields) without stopping and without aid. As the illness progresses, the patient's walking ability often declines; for example, at EDSS 5, the patient can walk without aid or rest for only 200 meters. A pivotal point in this scale is EDSS 6, which is reached when the patient must use a walking aid, such as a cane or crutch, to ambulate safely. At EDSS 7, the patient is unable to walk more than 5 meters, even with aid, and is essentially restricted to a wheelchair. The full EDSS is divided into 10 steps, each divided into half steps. EDSS 0 signifies normal neurologic function, whereas EDSS 10 is death as a result of MS.

Kurtzke Expanded Disability Status Scale

0.0 Normal neurological examination

1.0 No disability, minimal signs in one FS

1.5 No disability, minimal signs in more than one FS

2.0 Minimal disability in one FS

2.5 Mild disability in one FS or minimal disability in two FS

3.0 Moderate disability in one FS, or mild disability in three or four FS; fully ambulatory

3.5 Fully ambulatory but with moderate disability in one FS and more than minimal disability in several others

4.0 Fully ambulatory without aid, self-sufficient, up and about some 12 hours a day despite relatively severe disability; able to walk without aid or rest some 500 meters

4.5 Fully ambulatory without aid, up and about much of the day, able to work a full day, may otherwise have some limitation of full activity or require minimal assistance; characterized by relatively severe disability; able to walk without aid or rest some 300 meters.

5.0 Ambulatory without aid or rest for about 200 meters; disability severe enough to impair full daily activities (work a full day without special provisions)

5.5 Ambulatory without aid or rest for about 100 meters; disability severe enough to preclude full daily activities

6.0 Intermittent or unilateral constant assistance (cane, crutch, brace) required to walk about 100 meters with or without resting

6.5 Constant bilateral assistance (canes, crutches, braces) required to walk about 20 meters without resting

7.0 Unable to walk beyond approximately five meters even with aid, essentially restricted to wheelchair; wheels self in standard wheelchair and transfers alone; up and about in wheelchair some 12 hours a day

7.5 Unable to take more than a few steps; restricted to wheelchair; may need aid in transfer; wheels self but cannot carry on in standard wheelchair a full day; may require motorized wheelchair

8.0 Essentially restricted to bed or chair or perambulated in wheelchair, but may be out of bed itself much of the day; retains many self-care functions; generally has effective use of arms

8.5 Essentially restricted to bed much of day; has some effective use of arms; retains some self care functions

9.0 Confined to bed; can still communicate and eat.

9.5 Totally helpless bed patient; unable to communicate effectively or eat/swallow

10.0 Death due to MS

The lower steps of the EDSS are derived from the neurologic examination, which is divided into eight functional systems (FS): pyramidal (motor), cerebellar, brainstem, sensory, bowel and bladder, visual, cerebral (mental), and other. These FS are scored 1 to 5.

People with MS must deal with a variety of other impairments that are not well measured by the EDSS scale. While the scale includes components to measure vision, tremor, incoordination, or sensory change, these are not given the same emphasis as walking. Also, the scale does not include a measurement of intellectual or cognitive decline, although this is unfortunately an often-noted component of progressive MS, interfering with employment or normal family relationships.

Natural history studies carried out before 1993, when the new U.S. Food and Drug Administration (FDA)-approved treatments became available, showed that, as a rule, patients began to convert from the relapsing phase to the secondary progressive phase about 10 years after diagnosis, although there was great variability in when this will occur in each individual. By 15 years after the onset of MS, 50% of patients will have declined to the level of EDSS 6, requiring a walking aid. While it is impossible to predict when an individual patient will progress to these levels, nevertheless, in discussion with patients and their support persons, these general guidelines have some value in preparing for the future and underlining the need for therapy.

A small group of patients (10+%) never experience a relapse, but instead display the progressive stage as their only experience with MS. These patients have what is termed the *primary progressive* type of MS, in that they only experience a progressive course from onset. Their symptoms most commonly arise from spinal cord disease, and primarily affect gait and poor bladder control.

The term "life-threatening" has often been attached to descriptions of MS. However, this term, while true, implies a special meaning for MS, quite different from other diseases called life-threatening, such as cancer or full-blown HIV/AIDS. In such diseases, survival without treatment may be short, less than 5 years, and any treatment fostering life beyond that may be considered a success. In contrast, people with MS live for decades after a definite diagnosis. In a recent study from the Mayo Clinic, three out of four patients lived at least 25 years after the onset of MS, which is not too different from the general population in the United States. The likelihood of MS survival, not surprisingly, is closely associated with the level of disability. MS more often destroys the *quality* of life, not life itself.

People with MS are likely to die from one of four causes:

- There are well-recognized but rare cases of death directly from MS, usually from respiratory failure without pneumonia.
- Much more common, however, is death from a complication of MS in a severely disabled person: pneumonia, pulmonary embolism, decubiti (bed sores) leading to generalized infection, aspiration, and dehydration.
- Some people with MS obviously die from totally unrelated causes, such as cancer, heart attacks, stroke, or other diseases in middle or late life.
- Finally, there is a recognized risk from suicide. While not common, suicide occurs more frequently than would be expected in a similar normal population. It is seen more often in men, in patients with the onset of MS before the age of 30, and in individuals with significant early disability. Suicide most often occurs within 5 years of a diagnosis of MS, and is most commonly seen in patients who have poor social support systems or who display a sense of hopelessness.

Although these facts clearly portray MS as life-threatening, it may be more accurately considered as *life-defining*. Patients do survive for decades after their diagnosis, but the unpredictability, the fear of new attacks, the irregular but relentless progression of disability all paint the somber portrait of MS as a disease that shatters life's dreams.

One must conclude that, without effective therapy, the grim implications become evident at several levels. For the individual, the increasing impairment due to abnormalities of gait, decreased vision, incoordination, poor bladder and bowel control, and other symptoms, has a serious negative impact on the activities of daily living. As these symptoms increase, the patient must rely on walking aids, a wheelchair, or even assistance in transferring from bed to chair. The increasing handicap suffered by the patient reduces the chance for employment and necessary income, the joy of homemaking, normal parenting, and the gratification of usual social interaction.

Psychologically, there is the well-recognized negative interaction between increasing disability and depression. Disability leads to personal isolation (inability to work, attend religious services, go shopping, or participate in other social activities) and, as this isolation increases, a bleak future and increasing depression ensues. However, recognition of this downward spiral can be mitigated by various therapeutic interventions by family, friends, churches, voluntary organizations such as the National Multiple Sclerosis Society, or governmental social programs, leading to improved outcomes and quality of life. People fortunate enough to have strong and adaptable personalities and exceptional personal support systems often function well in the face of increasing disability, but it is undoubtedly a daily ongoing struggle.

The impact of progressive MS falls not only on the individual but also on many others, most importantly, the family. For young adults with MS, new unexpected and unwanted roles must be assumed by their parents, who may be called upon to aid the patient directly in terms of finances, housing, or providing social activity. Most commonly, a spouse is confronted with an entirely new set of roles, taking over the responsibilities for the increasingly disabled partner, including housekeeping and caring for children, as well as giving direct hands-on nursing aid to the MS patient. Even children must assume new roles, such as helping with the activities of daily living for the parent. This may even extend to helping with transfers from bed to chair or other activities that interfere with the joys that are natural for children or teenagers. Multiple sclerosis, in a perverse way, even alters the interaction with friends. Being confined to a wheelchair requires that the patient look up to communicate with friends or others standing next to them. This difference in eye level has unfortunate and often unintended consequences. For example, one wheelchair-using MS patient was invited to attend an art show with several of her friends from high school. All were in their mid-20s and had been close for many years. To the patient's distress, however, her friends often spoke over her head to each other, even though they were standing right next to her. They said things such as, "Do you think she would like to have coffee, or do you think she is becoming fatigued?" rather than speaking directly to her. This lack of normal and informal communication brought on simply by the need to sit in a wheelchair indicates the profound isolation which disability may cause.

Who Gets Multiple Sclerosis?

Multiple sclerosis is considered a disease of young adults because most patients note their first symptoms between the ages of 15 and 45, with a peak age of onset of 29. Rarely, children as early as 3 or 4 years of age develop MS, and the disease occasionally appears in people in their 50s and even 60s. Numerous studies confirm that approximately 70% of people who develop MS are women. The reason for this is unknown but is under active investigation.

The native Japanese population is the most thoroughly studied of various Asian groups, and MS is found only rarely there, as it is throughout Southeast Asia. In contrast, MS is common in Australia and New Zealand, where the population is largely of Caucasian background. Similarly, MS is rare in native African populations, although it is regularly seen in Caucasians living in Africa, for instance, in South Africa. In North America, the African-American population has a somewhat reduced risk from that of the Caucasian population, but the risk is clearly greater for African Americans with their diverse genetic background than for native Africans.

A so-called north-south gradient has been confirmed in several studies. Living in more temperate areas, such as the northern United States, involves a somewhat greater risk than that seen in populations living in the South. This has been a subject of great interest and controversy but has not as yet been fully explained. According to one theory, there is an environmental factor, perhaps a virus infection, which is more prevalent in one region than another. Or, perhaps sunlight related to vitamin D metabolism is at work. Another believable argument is that the genetic background of patients differs from one region to another, and the relative prevalence of MS is due to the increased number of northern Europeans living in more temperate areas. The highest known occurrence of MS is in Scandinavia and the islands of northern Scotland, and MS is also more common in descendents of immigrants from these areas. Without doubt, MS can be considered primarily a disease related to Northern European ancestry; it is observed 20 times more often in Northern Europe than in the Far East, and occurs even less often in Africa.

These observations clearly pose the question: Is MS an inherited (genetic) disease? This question has been the source of intense worldwide investigation over the past eight to ten decades and, while highly useful information has emerged, the final answer is not yet in. Without doubt, MS occurs more often in some families and racial groups. But is this due to environmental exposure or inborn genetic risk? One way of approaching this question is to study the occurrence of MS in twins, assuming that both twins had common or similar childhood experience (i.e., infections, etc.). Most, but not all, of these studies have shown that monozygotic (identical) twins, who have the same genetic make-up, have approximately a 25% chance of both developing MS. In contrast, dizygotic (fraternal) twins only have a 5% chance of developing the disease. Close relatives, siblings, or parents also have a 4% to 5% chance of developing MS, which is still much higher than the general population of similar ethnic background.

There has also been a concentrated search for specific genes that may increase the risk of the disease. This has led to the conclusion that MS requires multiple genes that may determine not only the risk, but perhaps also the severity of the final disease state. Conclusions from multiple independent studies show that the primary genes contributing to MS are on what is termed the major histocompatibility complex (HLA) region of a chromosome 6, with additional contributing genes on chromosomes 19 and 17. These findings have implications for the "gene therapy" efforts now of considerable interest, suggesting that this therapeutic approach may be complex and difficult.

The Cost of Multiple Sclerosis

When considering the impact of MS or any chronic neurologic illness, one of course first focuses on the issue of increasing disability or the patient's ability to function in society. This applies to performing what are termed *activities of daily living* (ADLs), from walking and climbing stairs to gainful employment to caring for family and, finally, to participating in and enjoying social and recreational activities. During the 25, 30, or more years of adult life during which patients must deal with the increasing challenges of MS disability, the quality of life declines. This in turn generates enormous personal psychological consequences, first for the patient but also, spreading like a wave, to involve the family, close friends, and even society. An additional, and always present, negative impact of chronic MS is the direct financial cost that the illness inflicts on the patient and usually the family.

These include obvious direct medical costs—drugs, physicians, and hospitalizations—which may or may not be underwritten by insurance or various government programs. It also includes the indirect costs imposed when a patient loses or reduces employment and, finally, both paid and unpaid caregiver time and cost. It comes as no surprise that the cost of dealing with MS increases with progressive increases in disability. It is possible to relate the cost of MS care directly to increasing disability as measured by the EDSS. Figures published in 2007 showed that the annual cost of MS—including medical costs, employment losses, paid and unpaid medical care, and patient leisure-time losses—amounted to $10,064 per year when the patient had an EDSS score of 1, which implied only slight disability. When the patient reached EDSS 6 with disability levels demanding (among other challenges) the use of constant walking aids, the yearly cost reaches $51,697. When viewed over a lifetime lasting two-and-a-half to three decades from onset, this figure shows how MS negatively impacts the patient, his or her family, and society at large.

The disease that shatters dreams also shatters family budgets and savings, while thrusting major new burdens on government and society. Untreated, MS creates enormous costs for the patient, the family, and society. No doubt this has led to the unending pressure to find a safe, proven treatment.

As the years roll on, each patient must live with the daily anxiety and fear of a new relapse, or the grim struggle to function as increasing disability robs life of its nobility and pleasure. When will there be relief?

2

Multiple Sclerosis Heroes:
Two Participants in Clinical Trials

Every medication that requires a physician's prescription, the so-called "innovative" as contrasted with "over-the-counter" drugs, must be approved before coming to market by appropriate national regulatory authorities. In the United States, this is the Food and Drug Administration (FDA). Federal law demands that any new medication be shown to be both safe and effective for its primary treatment purpose. This requires that each potential medication goes through a complex process that is usually quite long and expensive. It involves a human trial—a population of similar patients, usually numbered in the several hundreds or more. These participants are divided into two groups, one of which receives the experimental therapy and the other a placebo (a preparation that has no medical or biological activity). This is the so-called *placebo-controlled, double-blind* trial, in which neither the patients nor the physicians and coordinators conducting the trial are aware of to which group each patient is assigned. Only after the trial has been completed is the assignment of each patient revealed; in the case of multiple sclerosis (MS) drugs, this often requires over 2 years of observation. This process is an attempt to reduce or remove biases and clearly demonstrate a significant therapeutic benefit of the experimental therapy, or lack thereof. Only after such a human trial is completed and analyzed can the company, usually called the sponsor, approach the FDA with the request that the compound or medication of interest be allowed to be marketed as a prescription-controlled drug. The details of this process will be considered later in Chapter 9.

This legally required process means that some patients might be exposed for long periods to experimental substances which may be dangerous and, in some cases, even life-threatening, while others might be exposed to a placebo without therapeutic value for long periods, during which their disease may progress. In fact, the placebo group must show increased disease progression to identify the usefulness or benefit of the treatment. For example, one of the beta-interferon trials for MS, for a drug that was ultimately approved by the FDA, was continued for over 4 years. This meant that some patients injected themselves with a useless placebo every other day for this entire period, and did indeed worsen to a greater extent than those receiving interferon.

Many individuals contribute to the process of discovering and bringing new and improved therapies to the marketplace for the benefit of patients who suffer from the entire spectrum of serious and often life-threatening diseases. Among those involved are basic science researchers, often members of a university faculty; scientists working in the pharmaceutical industry; company executives, who must make decisions requiring the expenditure of millions of dollars; and many others, all of whom contribute to the discovery of therapies that improve human health. Another critical and essential group, often overlooked, that contributes fundamentally to the development of new and better therapies includes the many patients who volunteer to participate in controlled clinical trials. They willingly take part in inconvenient and possibly dangerous procedures that may include the risk of taking the experimental medication on one hand, or taking a placebo that will mean the lack of useful therapy for their ongoing disease on the other. Although often forgotten, these patients should be considered the true heroes in the complex process of discovering new therapies for human diseases.

Two MS heroes are described here. Their stories are told to illustrate real-life examples of the course of early MS, and to acknowledge their unique and essential contributions to the improved control of MS relapses. For each patient, we will return to their lives and disease course as we consider how they managed during the conduct of the Cop 1 (copolymer one) trial.

Case 1

V.J. was a 20-year-old college student when, in March 1990, he noticed decreased sensation and numbness in his left leg that ascended to his waist over a matter of 3 days. A magnetic resonance imaging (MRI) scan showed a lesion at the thoracic (T12) level of his spinal cord, as well as other lesions in the periventricular area of his brain (further defined in Chapter 3). His cerebral spinal fluid was normal. He was given anti-inflammatory high-dose steroid therapy intravenously, and his symptoms soon disappeared.

A few months later, in September 1990, he suddenly became aware of visual trouble in his left eye (what appeared to be a blind spot in the center of his vision) and pain in the left orbit when he moved the eye from side to side. The eye doctor said he had acute optic neuritis. Once again, the symptoms resolved with steroid therapy.

Eleven months later, in August 1991, he developed weakness of the left leg, with poor balance and difficulty with his gait. Examination showed an increase in the deep tendon reflexes in the left leg and a pathologic reflex (a Babinski response) in the left foot. A third course of intravenous steroids partially reversed the symptoms.

He reported that a maternal cousin had clinically definite MS; however, his two siblings were well.

On a screening visit in October 1991, prior to enrolling in an MS treatment trial, he had improved but still had difficulty with tandem walking—that is, walking heel to toe—and had decreased sense of vibration in his left foot. His Expanded Disability Status Scale (EDSS) level (described earlier) was 1.5. After he read about the details of the

Cop 1 trial, including the fact that he had a 50% chance of receiving a placebo for 2 years and had to inject himself every day, he consented to enroll.

Case 2

In September 1987, D.D. first experienced numbness of the entire right side of her body, as well as incoordination of her right hand, which interfered with writing and other fine movements. These symptoms developed over 3 days. After an extensive medical evaluation, a diagnosis of MS was considered; she was given high-dose intravenous steroids and quickly improved.

For 3 years she was well; however, in March 1990, she developed numbness and mild weakness of the entire left side, which affected walking and again included some left-sided numbness. A diagnosis of clinically definite MS was made, and she was again treated with high-dose intravenous steroids. Once again she improved.

Eighteen months later, in October 1991, the left-sided numbness returned, along with disturbed walking due to weakness of the left leg. Once again, she improved partially with steroid therapy.

At the time of screening for the Cop 1 clinical trial in January 1992, she still displayed mild weakness of the left leg, increased deep tendon reflexes of the left arm and leg, and a mild left arm tremor whenever she attempted to reach for or grasp objects.

D.D. had two children, ages 2 years and 6 months, and she was frightened by the prospect of further MS relapses and increasing neurologic impairment at a time when she had the responsibility of her enlarging family. She reported that an aunt had MS.

3

The Central Nervous System

This book describes the unique historical partnership of two Israeli organizations, the Weizmann Institute of Science and TEVA Pharmaceuticals, which joined together to develop the first treatment proven to benefit the course of multiple sclerosis (MS) relapses. To understand the enormous contribution made by this partnership to MS patients everywhere, it is first necessary to have some understanding of MS and how the disease affects patients and shatters their dreams (Chapters 1 and 2). It also will help to appreciate some fascinating features of the central nervous system (CNS), the single organ targeted and damaged by MS. Finally, some idea of how damage to the CNS occurs during MS will help to explain the symptoms and disability that patients endure.

Without doubt, the human nervous system is the most complex and intricate object on earth, and probably in the solar system. It is capable of immediately attending to multiple functions, ranging from perceiving the external environment, stimulating movement, learning and thinking, developing, storing and recalling memories, and experiencing the entire scope of human emotions. Both in its structure and in its function, the nervous system is divided into two related parts: the peripheral nervous system (PNS) and the CNS. Multiple sclerosis affects only the CNS. The CNS is composed of the brain, a small object weighing only 3 pounds and housed within the skull; the spinal cord, a structure about as thick as a woman's little finger, which runs down through the vertebral canal in the back; and the optic nerves, which grow out from the base of the brain and pass through a bony canal into the retina at the back of the eyeball. All of the organs of the body, including the heart, lungs, liver, and kidneys, exist primarily to maintain and promote the health and function of the brain. Even reproductive organs can be thought of as means of advancing the activities of the brain to the next generation.

Nature has accommodated to the primary status of the brain by protecting it in numerous ways. The brain is the only organ encased in a protective bony structure, the skull. Likewise, the spinal cord descends down the back enclosed in a tube or canal that is composed of multiple vertebrae that provide protection while allowing movement. Two membranes surround the brain and spinal cord: the thick fibrous *dura* and the thin *pia* membrane that covers the surface of the brain and spinal cord. Between these membranes is a space filled with spinal fluid, which serves as a shock absorber to further protect the CNS. The CNS is also protected internally. The blood—brain barrier is a series of cells and membranes that separate the blood from the CNS tissue. This barrier helps to exclude toxins, viruses, bacteria, and other substances that may circulate in the blood but must not be allowed to enter and damage the CNS. This barrier has important implications when describing how MS therapies may work

The PNS is composed of nerves that branch out from the CNS and course through the limbs, conducting sensation (touch, pain, etc.) to the CNS or carrying commands from the CNS to the muscles to initiate movement. Multiple other PNS activities relate to transporting impulses or messages to control the blood vessels that maintain blood flow and pressure, and control the functions of the large and small bowels, respiratory activity, heart rhythm, etc.

Imagine the complexity of how the CNS forms and retains memories, perceives and reacts to music, internalizes emotions both good and bad, or visualizes religious images. For example, consider such a simple act as touching a hot stove and withdrawing your hand before suffering serious injury. The nervous system is made up of millions of specialized cell types, each of which serves specialized functions. There are neurons or nerve cells, oligodendrocytes (often called oligos, astrocytes, or microglia), and various supporting cells and structures, such as blood vessels and the cells covering the CNS. In the center of the brain are two comma-shaped cavities, the *ventricles* where cerebrospinal fluid is formed, circulated, and stored. The *ependyma*, another specialized cell membrane, lines the ventricles.

Neurons, which may be considered royalty—the essential premiere cell of the CNS—have developed in an enormous number of highly specialized subtypes, all of which share several essential features. Each has a cell body that consists of fluid-like cytoplasm surrounding the nucleus, which, among other things, contains the chromosomes, which in turn contain the genes. Several *dendrites*, like branches on a tree, allow many contacts to be made to each neuron, so that numerous messages from other cells can reach it. Every neuron also has a single extension, called an *axon* or *nerve fiber*, which may be as short as a millimeter or very long, in some cases extending from the top of the brain to below the waist. The axon is uniquely designed to rapidly conduct an *impulse* or message in a combined chemical-electrical fashion. Most neurons have novel roles; for instance, some can perceive light in the eye and conduct a message or impulse from the retina in the back of the eyeball to other neurons that relay the impulse through other neurons to the back of the brain, where conscious vision occurs.

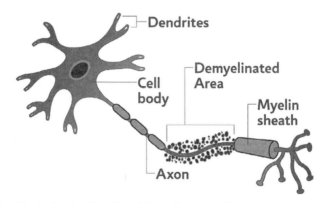

Neuron and cell body, showing the effect of demyelination on the axon

In the example of withdrawing a hand from a hot stove, neurons conduct a sensory impulse from the skin to the brain, first via the peripheral nerve, then the spinal cord. The brain senses the impulse as pain and reacts, sending a message that travels back through the spinal cord and peripheral nerves and initiates motor commands to the muscles, which then contract and immediately withdraw the hand from the hot object. All of this occurs in milliseconds, while at the same time visualizing the stove surface results in sending images from the eye to another area of the brain, which instantly remembers a previous unpleasant experience with a hot object.

The rapidity with which the axon can conduct a message is accomplished by the presence of a distinctive insulating substance called *myelin*, which allows the impulse to jump from point to point along the axon rather than flowing continuously along its surface like water flowing along a river bed. We will return to myelin later, when we consider how it plays a major role in understanding the development of Cop 1, the subject of this book.

The insulating myelin is formed and maintained by the *oligodendrocyte* or oligo, a cell that is capable of wrapping the axon with a myelin membrane composed of lipid (fat) and protein molecules. Myelin can be envisioned as a sheet or plate of lipid layers into which several different proteins are inserted in precise locations. The proteins, very long strings of amino acids, are folded into compact bundles. The myelin membrane or sheet is then wrapped around the axon several times, giving it the appearance of the cross-section of a jelly roll obtained at the bakery. Axons, with their surrounding myelin, end at a structure called the *synapse*, where the electrical impulse stimulates the release of a chemical into a microscopic space, which initiates the beginning of a new impulse or message in another neuron or, in the case of movement, at the surface of a muscle cell, stimulating contraction or shortening of the muscle.

Cells called *astrocytes* form a matrix—a network or skeleton—that holds neurons and oligos in place. Among their many functions is the ability to form scar-like tissue that is not too different from the scars that may form in damaged skin. In fact, the term "multiple sclerosis" comes from the early recognition that the astrocytic scars felt hard or *sclerotic* when a finger was run across the surface of the cut brain at autopsy. Cells called *microglia* act to remove debris from damaged CNS tissue, but also have immunologic capacities that will be considered later.

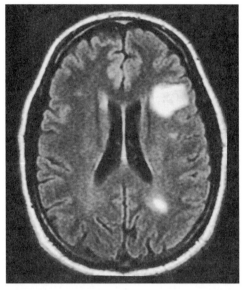

Cross-section of the human brain, showing lesions (white) representative of multiple sclerosis.

The CNS is, somewhat simplistically, composed of two major types of tissue; the *gray matter*, made up primarily of billions of neurons, all with specialized functions, and *white matter*, which is composed of the axons with their myelin covering. The axons form into large bundles or tracks that carry impulses that relate to specific functions such as vision, sensation, motor or movement activities, etc. The gray matter or *cortex* is found on the surface of the brain, and is approximately ½-inch in thickness, whereas the spinal cord has the gray matter in a butterfly shape in the middle with the white matter tracks of axons surrounding it.

Changes in the Brain with Multiple Sclerosis

By the mid-19th century, many physicians, scientists, and pathologists, including Jean-Marie Charcot, recognized that the brains of patients with the disease that would come to be known as MS had local areas or spots in the white matter. These had a tan rather than cream color, and seemed firm to the touch, rather than having the soft gelatinous feel of the rest of the brain. Similar spots also were noted in the white matter of the spinal cord. These spots came to be known as *plaques* or—by the more general term—*lesions*. They were of various sizes, some being hardly visible and others larger than a man's thumb nail. The plaques were scattered quite randomly throughout the white matter, although there was a general tendency for more to develop adjacent to the ventricles, when they were referred to as *periventricular plaques*.

Microscopically, these spots often had a blood vessel at their center, suggesting some relationship between the plaque and the blood circulation. This is where the blood–brain barrier is located. Microscopic examination showed that the plaques had an inflammatory component: there were large numbers of white blood cells in the plaques, mainly lymphocytes; increased space or fluid between cells, known as edema; and plasma cells, a specialized type of white blood cell called a B-lymphocyte, that later was recognized as the cell that produced immunoglobulin or antibodies. Also present in the plaque were microglia, the cells often associated with cleaning up debris after tissue injury.

It was also apparent that the myelin wrapping on axons was frequently damaged or destroyed, giving rise to the term *demyelination*, which has ever since been recognized as a fundamental aspect of the MS pathologic process. While damage to the myelin was most obvious, it was also recognized, even in the 1860s, that some of the axons in the plaque were damaged or even cut or destroyed. In what appeared to be the more mature or older plaques there appeared to be more evidence of axonal destruction than in what appeared to be fresh plaques, where the inflammatory and demyelinating features were most prominent. Also, the "older" plaques contained more astrocytes, forming hardening, sclerosis, or scarring.

While the three pathologic features of inflammation, demyelination, and axonal loss were all described in the mid-19th century, this triad was often lost sight of throughout much of the 20th century. The MS plaque was described as inflammatory-demyelinating. Only in the 1980s and onward was the component of axonal damage again reemphasized.

As the concept of clinical-pathologic correlation emerged in the 19th century, these pathologic brain changes came to be associated with the clinical patterns or symptoms that most people with MS experience. At the onset, during the relapsing-remitting phase described in Chapter 1, it is commonly thought that the symptoms are due to the rapid localized inflammation that defines the early features of an MS plaque in the CNS white matter. Later on, as the plaque matures and more and more axonal damage and loss is incurred, the brain's ability to transmit or send messages between neurons is at first delayed, then lost. The more disabling secondary-progressive stage of MS then evolves, characterized by an increase in neurologic impairment that is generally irreversible. Walking becomes difficult, and a cane or wheelchair is needed; bowel and bladder complications appear; and cognitive decline may disturb quality of life. All of these relate to the spreading loss of axons or their inability to conduct impulses.

The scattered distribution of MS plaques throughout the CNS white matter also helps to explain the unique clinical pattern that each patient experiences. Thus, for instance, if a new plaque develops in the optic nerve, the patient will have difficulty with vision and may also experience pain because the optic nerve is stretched during movement as it travels through the bony canal at the base of the skull. Alternatively, if a new plaque develops in the spinal cord, the axons carrying sensory messages or movement commands will be affected. As a result, the patient will most likely notice numbness, loss of sensation, and perhaps weakness in the limb served by sensory and motor neurons in the area of the CNS that controls that function.

Throughout much of the last century, MS was considered a "white matter" disease, involving an attack on myelin and axons. Over the last decade, we increasingly appreciated the significance of attacks and the formation of lesions or plaques in the gray matter, where the neuron cell bodies are located. Previously, because these lesions cannot be seen on routine magnetic resonance imaging (MRI), they were not understood to be part of the MS process. Recently, they have been recognized to develop early in the MS disease process, and are probably of major importance in the permanent disability, the brain atrophy, and even the cognitive decline characteristic of most MS.

Abnormal changes typical of MS also are noted in the spinal fluid, which surrounds and generally protects the brain. The spinal fluid appears clear like water, but contains small numbers of white blood cells. These cells are increased in MS, and there is also an elevated concentration of proteins, the most important of which are the *immunoglobulins*, a complex mixture of antibodies. Immunoglobulins can be measured in two ways in the laboratory; one shows an abnormal amount, the IgG or immunoglobulin index, and the other, the presence of abnormal populations of immunoglobulins measured by placing the spinal fluid in a gel, which is then subjected to an electric field to separate the proteins by their electric charge. In the spinal fluid of patients with MS, the immunoglobulins separate as collections, called *bands*, not seen in normal spinal fluid. Despite enormous effort in many laboratories, these spinal fluid abnormalities have not led to the hoped for clues to the cause of MS. However, the spinal fluid changes do indicate that an immunologic abnormality is developing, which is now known to be a central part of the MS disease process. The measurement of MS spinal fluid changes has become an important diagnostic tool, especially early in the disease process.

The pathologic changes observed in every MS brain or spinal cord at autopsy, as well as the spinal fluid changes observed in over 90% of cases of MS during life, strongly suggest that MS is one of a number of human autoimmune diseases in which the immune system, usually thought of as protective and beneficial, instead turns back to attack and produce CNS tissue damage, neurologic symptoms, and permanent disability, the central features of MS.

4

The Search for a Multiple Sclerosis Model

No naturally occurring disease similar to multiple sclerosis (MS) has ever been discovered in wild, domestic, or laboratory animals. This has hindered attempts to study and understand the disease, and may have delayed the search for a treatment or cure. One giant advance over the past 70 years has been the discovery and extensive development of a useful animal model, *experimental allergic encephalomyelitis* or EAE which, while not identical to MS, has many similar features. The interesting, still-evolving, story of EAE could start in many ways and locations, but perhaps returning to France in the late 19th century is the most plausible beginning.

In July 1885, a 9-year-old French peasant boy, Joseph Meister, was mauled and bitten by a rabid dog. Rabies was common, and it was well known that once the rabies virus was injected via a bite, universally fatal rabies (hydrophobia) was sure to follow, even though there might be an incubation period of several weeks or even months. Luckily, the boy was quickly taken to the famous French scientist, Louis Pasteur, who, in addition to his major contributions to the understanding of microorganisms and inventing ways to preserve both wine and milk (pasteurization), had been experimenting with microorganisms—including viruses—that could be made into protective vaccines by passing them repeatedly through a series of animals. Even though Pasteur had suffered a brain hemorrhage in 1868 that affected the left side of his body, he continued his exploration of vaccines. Fortunately for little Joseph, he had been working with rabies virus, hoping to develop a vaccine by injecting central nervous system (CNS) tissue of infected rabbits repeatedly from one animal to another until he observed and developed what is known as a "fixed strain" that no longer appeared to produce disease in the animal. Meister was

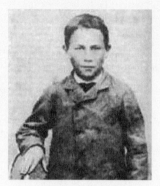

Joseph Meister, 1876–1940

brought to Pasteur (who was not a medical doctor and had never treated a human), and he agreed to try his vaccine on the boy. Meister was given 13 injections over 11 days of the "fixed" rabies virus contained in rabbit spinal cord. The child survived and was thus the first of many thousands of victims exposed to rabies virus to be saved by the Pasteur vaccine. Within 3 years, in 1888, the Pasteur Institute was formed to treat patients exposed to rabies virus. This institute has grown to become a major international medical and scientific organization in the decades since.

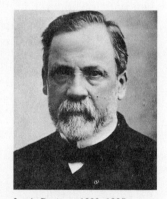

Of interest, a second child, a shepherd named Jean Jupille, was bitten by a rabid wolf and also treated by Pasteur, in October 1885. He survived as well. As adults, both

Louis Pasteur, 1822–1895

Meister and Jupille worked at the Pasteur Institute in Paris. (Meister is known to have committed suicide in 1940 at the age of 65, said to have become despondent over the German invasion of Paris in World War II.)

The Pasteur vaccination process, used to protect thousands of people exposed to rabies virus, required 14 to 21 injections of the fixed rabies virus contained in rabbit brain or spinal cord tissue. Over time, it was recognized that approximately one of every 4,000 vaccinated persons would develop an acute neurologic reaction. This was usually characterized by fever, paralysis, and occasional seizures, and was not uncommonly fatal. Pathologically, abnormalities were confined to the CNS and consisted of patches of inflammation and demyelination in the white matter.

A similar disease or reaction was also occasionally observed after use of vaccinia virus as a vaccine for smallpox, as well as after acute measles and other virus infections. This condition became known as *acute post-vaccination* or *post-infectious encephalomyelitis*, and was recognized as a significant medical problem. It still appears at times in modern neurologic and pediatric clinics, usually after some acute viral infection.

EAE

Several investigators carried out experiments trying to explain the vaccine reaction, with limited success. However, in the early 1930s, Thomas M. Rivers and colleagues at the Rockefeller Institute in New York began a series of experiments asking the question "Was the post-vaccinial encephalomyelitis due to some component of the vaccinia virus or to repeated injections of CNS tissue?" In a number of fairly complex experiments, two of eight monkeys that were exposed both to vaccinia virus and the CNS tissue developed inflammation and demyelination that was fairly typical of post-vaccination encephalomyelitis. In a second critical series of experiments, eight monkeys were given repeated intramuscular injections of emulsions and extracts of rabbit brain. No virus was involved.

After between 46 and 85 injections given three times per week, seven of the eight monkeys developed a paralytic neurologic disease; at autopsy, all showed typical lesions or plaques of demyelination and inflammation similar to the human rabies vaccine reaction. This appeared almost certainly to be a disease produced by an immunologic or allergic reaction to the injected brain tissue and not to an infectious agent. It was the beginning of a vast and still ongoing scientific effort to unravel what became known as the study of experimental allergic encephalomyelitis, or EAE. This research field has occupied the activities of hundreds, if not thousands, of laboratories worldwide and has been supported undoubtedly by several billion dollars of research grant money in the past 60+ years. A recent search of the scientific literature uncovered over 6,000 publications devoted to EAE, which is probably a modest count.

The study of EAE was greatly advanced when it was found that, by combining the injected CNS tissue (called the *antigen*) with *complete Freund's adjuvant*, an immunologic booster composed of mineral oil and inactivated and dried microbacteria (usually the bacteria causing tuberculosis), EAE could be produced with a single injection, rather than requiring the 60 plus injections used by Rivers. The experimental disease, which appeared to only affect the brain and spinal cord, developed routinely within 10 to 20 days after the injection.

Experimental allergic encephalomyelitis provided scientists with a reliable laboratory disease, a tool that could be used to study immunologic diseases that affect the human CNS, such as acute post-vaccination encephalomyelitis or possibly even MS. It was soon discovered that EAE could be induced in virtually every experimental animal species, even though there were disease variations, being more severe in monkeys than in rats for instance. It was also found that brain tissue from most, if not all, mammalian species could be mixed with Freund's adjuvant and injected to produce EAE in a variety of species and tissue types, from rabbits to guinea pigs, from cows (bovine) to human tissue.

This was a stunning discovery. Here was an attractive, quick, and relatively inexpensive research tool; an experimental animal disease that could be uniformly produced in one of several laboratory species, of which mice, rats, rabbits, and guinea pigs have most often been used. Only one organ system in the injected animal, the CNS, shows disease. The pathology is very reproducible; it includes inflammation and, to a lesser extent, demyelination in focal patches in the white matter. The experimental disease appeared predictably, usually within 15 to 20 days of the injection.

After the decades-long fruitless search for a natural animal disease that displays the characteristics of human MS, there has been great interest in any experimental disease that could support useful research to increase our understanding of the cause and treatment of MS. Two fundamental themes of investigation have dominated the field: first, the possibility that MS is an unusual infectious process probably due to some virus, and, second, that it is an immunologic process probably appearing in individuals who have a genetic predisposition to develop the disease. These two themes are not mutually exclusive, and there is evidence that MS may be related in some way to a viral infection. However, the search for an "MS virus," which has now lasted for decades, while generating numerous unconfirmed claims, has not led to the discovery of a virus that causes MS. Despite many widely heralded claims, there has been no convincing evidence of an MS virus that could be reproduced in other independent laboratories. Thus, the immunologic theme, based primarily on knowledge and scientific sophistication gained from thousands of EAE experiments, has been a primary field of interest, pursued with enormous scientific vigor.

Following Rivers' publications in 1935, it soon became possible to induce EAE in virtually any experimental mammal, especially after the discovery that combining CNS tissue with Freund's adjuvant accelerated the process. In fact, a similar field of investigation has developed using peripheral nervous system (PNS) tissue to produce a disease called *experimental allergic neuritis*, which has likewise contributed greatly to the understanding of immunologic diseases of the PNS.

It is said that every scientific discovery prompts more questions than answers, and that is certainly true with EAE. The obvious question was: What substance or even molecule was contained in the brain of every mammal, including humans, which, under the right conditions, had the potential to stimulate a serious and at times fatal disease in the brain of an injected mammal? Scientists soon began to segment or separate the brain into its chemical components. There were clues. EAE developed in the white matter, where the axons, oligos, and their product myelin were located. It was not long before myelin became the suspected tissue where the *antigen* or material that triggered the immune attack of EAE could be found.

Seventy percent of the dry weight of brain is made up of myelin. This can be seen in the figure in Chapter 3, and it is clear that white matter is the most abundant brain tissue by volume. Myelin is made up of two substances, lipids (fatty material) and proteins. The protein that soon attracted most interest was *myelin basic protein* (MBP), which makes up about 30% of the myelin proteins. Two other minor proteins, *myelin-associated glycoprotein* (MAG) and *myelin oligodendroglial glycoprotein* (MOG), also have been shown to be efficient triggers in stimulating EAE.

Further cementing the immunologic basis for EAE was the demonstration that *lymphocytes* (white blood cells) removed from lymph nodes of animals with acute EAE symptoms could be injected into well animals not previously injected, and that EAE would appear in them in 10 to 15 days (transfer EAE). These lymphocytes contained the "immunologic knowledge" to recognize and attack myelin in the recipient animal.

Myelin basic protein is composed of 170 *amino acids*, the fundamental building blocks of every protein. These amino acids are strung together like beads on a necklace. In nature, MBP, like all proteins, is folded in a complex way and inserted into the myelin membrane which, in turn, is wrapped around the axon, as shown in Chapter 3. However, in trying to understand EAE, it is easier to envision the amino acids in a long string. There are in nature only 20 amino acid molecules (such as alanine, lysine, tyrosine, or glutamic acid), which must be strung together in a precise sequence to make up each and every protein. Some amino acids may appear several times at precise locations on the long chain making up the MBP protein. It was soon found that purified MBP, obtained from the brain of virtually any species of mammal and injected with Freund's adjuvant, could produce EAE, demonstrating that this was a widespread if not universal reaction.

Using many innovative experiments employing various species of laboratory animals, especially inbred strains of mice, it was in time possible to reproduce many of the pathologic changes and characteristics of MS. The CNS pathology could be shifted to show more inflammation or more demyelination and, in some experiments, even induce a repeating or recurrent disease pattern, in which an injected animal would show acute neurologic symptoms, recover, and then weeks later become ill again. This was much like the relapsing-remitting stage of MS.

Using modern protein chemistry, scientists soon began to break the long MBP molecule into small segments of 8, 12, or 20 amino acids called *peptides*, which then could be mixed with Freund's adjuvant and injected into experimental animals. These peptides maintained the same sequence of amino acids found in the parent MBP and, depending on how the experiment was designed, could predictably cause EAE. An extremely important discovery was that some of these small purified peptides induced EAE, whereas other peptides from MBP could protect the animal from developing the disease. Such protected animals were immune to subsequent exposure to MBP or its peptides. Could this be the answer to treating MS? Could some peptides act as a vaccine to protect against animal EAE or even protect humans from MS?

Unfortunately, it's not that simple. It soon became apparent that an MBP peptide that protected one species, such as guinea pigs, would produce EAE in another species, such as rats. The short string of amino acids, the peptide which caused EAE in the guinea pigs, was found to be sequence 114–122 of the 170-amino acid MBP molecules or string, whereas sequence 44–89 produced disease in rabbits and rats. In monkeys, a 14-amino acid peptide at the end of the MBP molecule was the active site. Other peptides from MBP were protective, inhibiting the production of EAE in each of these species. In considering these discoveries, in hoping to develop a treatment for MS, there was the real danger that an MBP fragment or peptide that protected monkeys, for instance, might result in serious or even fatal EAE if injected into humans. This disappointing discovery suggested that MBP, other myelin proteins, or their peptides might not be the long-sought answer to treating MS.

Despite the intense ongoing creative investigation of EAE—even now, the research focus of laboratories worldwide—a vigorous debate continues about its status as a model for MS and its value in understanding the disease. Even with its hundreds of reproducible variations, EAE is not a true model for the human disease. Multiple sclerosis is much more complex, evolving over time in the heterogeneous genetic environment of outbred humans, rather than in the inbred strains of laboratory animals. The immunologic intricacy in humans and the attack, not only on myelin in the CNS white matter but also on the neuron-rich gray matter of the cortex, has never been adequately replicated in any EAE model.

Has the enormous effort and expense of studying EAE been worth it in trying to unmask the mysteries of MS? Without doubt it has, by contributing enormous insight into many aspects of MS. Also, EAE has been the platform from which the search for many potential therapies for MS has been launched. Virtually every therapeutic idea that has been or is being tested in MS has first been tested in EAE. Animal experiments are faster, less expensive, and critical in uncovering unsuspected dangers rather than proceeding directly to human trials of new therapeutic ideas.

Unfortunately, a large number of experimental MS drug treatments, even if they showed great promise in several EAE systems, have still failed when tested in MS clinical trials. Some were ineffective, some were toxic and produced serious side effects, and some even made MS worse.

PART II

The Weizmann
Institute of Science

5

The Weizmann Institute of Science, Rehovot, Israel

The first treatment to positively change the course of multiple sclerosis (MS), copolymer 1, also known simply as Cop 1, was developed at the Weizmann Institute of Science in Rehovot, Israel. When one thinks of the development of modern effective drugs for serious human diseases, the first places that come to mind are the major national or multinational pharmaceutical concerns based in New Jersey or suburban Philadelphia, the research triangle of North Carolina, or perhaps the large pharmaceutical concerns located along the Rhine River in Basel, Switzerland. Not only was Cop 1 unusual in the location of its development but also, rather than being the product of numerous—even hundreds—of chemists, pharmacists, and other applied scientists working collectively in industry, it was developed by only three individuals: Michael Sela, Ruth Arnon, and Dvora Teitelbaum, working alone on the project for over a decade. They will play a large role later on in this story.

Rehovot, also called Rehovoth, is located on a relatively fertile plain along the Mediterranean Sea. Tel Aviv lies approximately 12 miles and 30 minutes by train to the north, and Jerusalem is approximately 30 miles up through the Judean Hills to the east. The border with Gaza is about 44 miles to the south. Rehovot was founded in 1890, by a group of Jewish immigrants from Warsaw, Poland. Later on, a large population of Yemenite Jews also settled there, in part because of the agricultural opportunities available. The Hebrew University Faculty of Agriculture is located adjacent to the Weizmann Institute of Science in Rehovot. From the beginning, Rehovot was noted for its productive citrus groves, and it is now a center for fruit packing and the manufacture of citrus concentrates. The government-run Volcani Institute of Agricultural Research is also in Rehovot.

In many ways, Rehovot serves as the geographic intersection for the many interests of Chaim Weizmann, a true giant in the history of modern Israel. He was a notable scientist, leading Zionist, effective political leader, and international visionary. Born in 1874, in Motol, Russia, the son of a timber merchant, Weizmann showed an early interest in science. Following high school in Pinsk, he studied at the Polytechnic Institute in Darmstadt and later at the Royal Technical College in Berlin, before going to the University of Fribourg in Switzerland, where he was awarded a degree in chemistry in 1899, at the age of 25. By 1901, he had become an assistant lecturer at the University of Geneva.

Making what would become a fateful lifetime decision, in 1904, Weizmann decided to relocate to Manchester, England, although apparently he knew little English, had few contacts, and possessed neither a job nor any money. Within a year, he was working as a chemistry demonstrator at the University of Manchester and had begun a research program at the local Clayton Analine Chemical Factory. A gifted chemist, he soon developed a fermentation process to produce acetone, which was expensive and in short supply. Among its many uses, acetone was essential for the manufacture of cordite, a military propellant or explosive that was the major component for artillery shells, both on land and for the British navy. It was employed in both World Wars I and II.

Because of these and many other scientific discoveries related to bacterial activity, Weizmann was recognized as the father of industrial fermentation. Among other scientific interests was his participation in the development of synthetic rubber. This was of enormous importance, especially during World War II, when the availability of natural rubber was cut off by Japanese control of rubber plantations in Southeast Asia. During his life, Weizmann was awarded over 100 patents for his creative scientific work. These scientific and industrial activities, essential for the war effort, brought him in contact with leading British government officials, contacts that he used to great effect for his second lifelong passion, Zionism, a movement devoted to setting up a Jewish

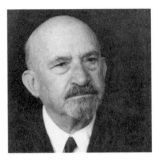

Chaim Weizmann

national or religious community in Palestine. (Incidentally, Weizmann became a British subject in 1910.)

Zionism had become a movement of immense interest to the Jewish communities throughout Europe, but especially in Great Britain, at the end of the 19th and beginning of the 20th century. The effort was apparently rather fragmented in London, but was quite focused in Manchester, and Weizmann joined and soon became a leader in Zionist activities there. In 1903, he had attended the Sixth Zionist Congress in Basel, and in 1920, he became president of the World Zionist Organization, a position that he held until 1931, and again from 1935 to 1946.

The early decades of the 20th century were formative for the worldwide Zionist movement. This was especially true in England. Palestine had been ruled by the weak Ottoman Empire, from Istanbul, Turkey, since 1517. With the final crumbling of this Empire, Palestine came under British control, and was occupied by the British military under a League of Nations program known as the British Mandate, which was activated in 1920. An important, hotly debated issue at that time was the vision of a homeland for Jews in Palestine. This concept had received a major advance in November 1917, with the Balfour Declaration, which recommended the separation of Palestine into Arab and Jewish states. Arthur Balfour, the British Foreign Secretary, was an enthusiastic proponent of Zionism.

Weizmann, apparently because of his substantial links to the British Cabinet established through his scientific efforts in aiding the war effort, was able to influence this declaration. In 1918, he led the

Zionist Commission, arranged by the British, to begin to determine the future of Palestine. Not limiting his interests only to political and scientific activities, however, Weizmann during this period began to lay the foundation for the creation of the Hebrew University of Jerusalem as an essential center for learning, an effort that also attracted the interest and support of Albert Einstein and other international Jewish leaders. In 1925, Weizmann, now 51 years of age, was pleased to be at the official opening of the Hebrew University on Mount Scopus overlooking Jerusalem.

After 30 years as a British subject, Weizmann and his pediatrician wife Vera decided to leave England and move to Rehovot. In 1936, they commissioned the acclaimed architect, Erich Mendelsohn, to design a unique house on a Rehovot hill facing on one side the distant Mediterranean Sea and on the other the Judean hills. This large, distinctive, modern white house still stands, having been donated by the Weitzmans to the State of Israel. It is now open as a public museum. It is built in a unique U-shaped design surrounding a swimming pool, and still holds the Weizmann's furnishings and art. Weizmann and his wife are buried near the house.

The turmoil and war clouds beginning to form over Europe with the rise of the Nazis during the 1930s again formed an intersection for Weizmann with the town of Rehovot. Returning to his friends and close Zionist contacts from his early years in Manchester, Weizmann appealed for help from his close friend, Israel Sieff. Another Russian Jewish immigrant, Michael Marks, had come to England in 1884. In 1894, he and Thomas Spencer established a department store named Marks and Spencer, which has over time expanded to become a substantial retail company, operating numerous department stores throughout Great Britain and Ireland. Michael Marks' daughter, Rebecca, married Israel Sieff in 1910, and in time Sieff rose to become the first Lord Sieff, Chairman and President of Marks and Spencer. He was throughout his life a strong supporter of the Zionist cause.

Weizmann had conceived of a new research institute as a professional home for German and other European Jewish scientists who were forced to leave Europe to escape from the Nazis. Plans were made for them to immigrate to Rehovot, where they could live in safety and continue their scientific studies. This led to the establishment, in 1934, of the Daniel Sieff Research Institute, named in memory of Israel's and Rebecca's son, Daniel. At its onset, the Institute had only ten scientists and ten technicians. It grew and prospered, and in November 1949, with the agreement of the Sieff family, was renamed and formally dedicated as the Weizmann Institute of Science in Rehovot.

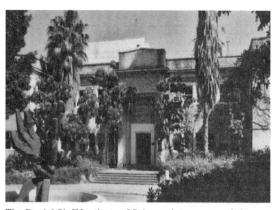

The Daniel Sieff Institute of Science, later renamed the Weizmann Institute of Science

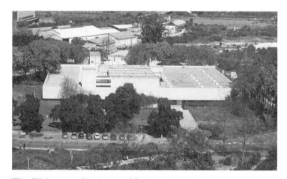

The Weizmann Institute of Science today

The Weizmann Institute of Science has prospered; in 2005, its staff numbered over 2,500 scientists, technicians, and research students. It now comprises 18 departments organized into five faculties—Biology, Biochemistry, Chemistry, Physics, and Mathematics and Computer Science. It is recognized as one of the top-ranking multidisciplinary research institutions in the world. In 2005, *The Scientist* magazine rated the Weizmann Institute of Science as the best university in the world for life scientists to conduct research.

The singular career of Weizmann had yet one final chapter to play out. The period from 1947 to 1948 were evolving as critical years in the extended history of Zionism and the potential for the long-held dream of an independent Jewish nation in Palestine: the State of Israel. The

British Mandate was ending, the British declared that they would leave in May 1948, and active warfare had broken out between Jews and Palestine Arabs, especially around Jerusalem. The vision of the establishment of a Jewish State of Israel was at stake.

It became apparent that, with the end of the British occupation, the United States would have to become a primary political player and potential supporter if there was going to be a State of Israel. Once again, Chaim Weizmann, now 73 years of age, chronically ill, and partially blind, was called upon to assume a leading role in the Zionist cause. He alone, it was thought, could make a final desperate appeal to American President Harry S. Truman, who had been unwilling to support the concept of a separation of Palestine into two states, Jewish and Arab. Besides, Truman, sitting in the Oval Office in the White House, had other issues with which to deal. He was leading the drive to rebuild war-torn Europe through the Marshall Plan, and had recognized the rising threat of the Soviet Union and the beginning of the Cold War.

Weizmann traveled to New York, but all attempts to arrange a meeting with Truman were refused. Finally, one last unusual and long-shot appeal to Truman was conceived. Eddie Jacobson was the owner of a modest menswear shop in Kansas City. He was Jewish but not an ardent Zionist; however, he was at one time Harry Truman's business partner. Truman had never closed his Oval Office door to Jacobson, who now came to Washington to make a personal request that Truman meet with Chaim Weizmann. Truman at first refused but finally, after a long argument, he agreed to a meeting. Truman is quoted as saying to Jacobson,

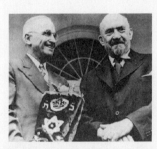

"You win, you bald-headed son-of-a-bitch, I will see him." The secret conversation occurred at the White House on March 18, 1948. At the end of the 45-minute meeting, Truman agreed to support continued Jewish immigration into Palestine, lift the arms embargo, and advocate the partition of the country into Arab and Jewish states.

President Harry S. Truman and Chaim Weizmann, 1948

With the withdrawal of British troops at the end of the Mandate, even though a desperate war broke out, the State of Israel was declared on May 14, 1948. It was recognized by the United States the next day.

Weizmann returned to his beloved home in Rehovot and, on February 16, 1949, was inaugurated as the first President of the State of Israel. He died on November 9, 1952.

The trip to Rehovot is always a memorable experience. Leaving the busy, dusty, noisy, frenetic hubbub of downtown Tel Aviv, the green agricultural origin of Rehovot is still evident. As seems to be the case throughout Israel, there is building everywhere, yet there are still citrus groves between the highways and railroads, where every acre is used. Approaching the Weizmann Institute, numerous modern glass and steel buildings that house the booming high-tech industry of contemporary Israel indicate the importance of Weizmann science to Israel, just as similar juxtapositions in Bethesda and Rockville, Maryland, point to the importance of the National Institutes of Health (NIH) to the biological and pharmacologic industry in the United States.

The Weizmann Institute of Science campus is of surpassing beauty, where numerous four- to eight-story laboratories housing the five divisions of the Institute are set among lawns, landscaping, and mature trees, and where gardens give color to the peaceful environment. In the spring, the yellow, orange, pink, and lavender masses of bougainvillea are magnificent.

The original Chaim Weizmann residence, now a state-owned museum, is set on a small knoll surrounded by lawns and carefully planned and pruned trees and shrubbery, which enhances the strikingly modern architecture of the white building. All of the Weizmann couple's original furnishings and art remain, including Vera Weizmann's custom-built grand piano. Adjacent to the circular driveway is a glass garage containing the black Royal Ford Lincoln Cosmopolitan limousine that was a gift from Henry Ford II to Chaim Weizmann when he was President of Israel. Only 18 of these cars were produced, according to specifications drawn up for the President of the United States.

The physical setting and the unique scientific environment of the Weizmann Institute at which the remarkable development of Copaxone would occur was slowly evolving.

6

Understanding Protein Structure and Function

Applying the scientific method into the cause and treatment of human illness over the past 250 years has totally transformed what we now know as modern medicine and has clearly extended the duration of human life and improved the quality of daily living.

Every successful experiment—as well as most failures—raises new questions and the need for further experiments, and often points to unexpected new directions of investigation. The never-ending expansion of scientific medicine is uneven, however. Each discovery or failure may raise many issues that must be recognized in order to direct future research into new, unexplored, creative, and perhaps surprising avenues.

Our previous description of experimental allergic encephalomyelitis (EAE) illustrates how this exciting but unpredictable journey may unfold. The observation that occasional patients who received the Pasteur rabies vaccine later came down with a severe neurologic complication led Rivers and his colleagues several decades later to ask whether it was the repeated injections of mammalian nervous tissue that led to the serious vaccine complication. This in turn led to the discovery of EAE, which—as described in Chapter 4—has stimulated thousands of subsequent experiments that have in turn helped to solve many of the mysteries of autoimmunity (the immunologic attack on one's own tissues).

The emergence of Copaxone® as the first successful treatment of multiple sclerosis (MS) occurred in the fertile intellectual environment of the Weizmann Institute of Science. This important therapeutic advance rests on the original observations of three creative scientists— Michael Sela, Ruth Arnon, and Dvora Teitelbaum, who were able to recognize that their early observations could be directed into new pathways, in a series of linked experiments lasting over 15 years. It was the genius of recognizing the potential implications of the unexpected outcomes of their initial experiments that led them to Copaxone.

Few, if any, medical discoveries emerge as unique events, like a bolt of lightning; rather, they are most often related to earlier or contemporary efforts, often involving one or many investigators working in the same field, frequently at independent sites throughout the world. In reconstructing the direct history of Copaxone, one might begin the story in 1946, when a young scientist arrived in Rehovot. He had been invited by Chaim Weizmann to work at the Daniel Sieff Institute, soon to be renamed the Weizmann Institute of Science. One could say that the stage was being set for the future work leading to Copaxone.

Ephraim Katchalski (Katzir), who one future day would become the fourth President of Israel (1973–1978), was born in Kiev, Ukraine, in 1916. In 1922, when he was 6 years old, his family, which included his older brother Aharon, age 9, immigrated to Palestine. They settled first in Tel Aviv, then a small coastal city, and a year later moved to Jerusalem.

At that time, the entire population of Palestine was only 752,000, and only 83,000—11%—were Jewish. Jerusalem, revered by Jews, Christians, and Muslims alike, was over 2,500 years old. It was then a small city built on several hills, Mount Zion, Mount of Olives, Mount Scopus, and others, often separated by rather deep valleys. Then, as now, most of the buildings were constructed of honey-colored stone, giving the city hillsides a warm attractive glow. The ancient center of Jerusalem, called the Old City, was surrounded by a high, thick stone wall. It was divided into Muslim, Jewish, Christian, and Armenian quarters. Most streets in the Old City are narrow, allowing only hand-cart passage. Many are lined with small shops, but there are also churches, synagogues, monasteries, convents, and centers of religious study. The most distinctive feature of the Old City was and still is the large stone-paved plaza of the Temple Mount, on which were built the huge Al Aqsa Mosque and the Dome of the Rock, with its universally recognized gold-colored dome, one of the most sacred sites of the Muslim world. One side of the Temple Mount is supported by the Western Wall, of major religious importance to devout Jews.

In 1922, most people in Jerusalem walked or used donkey carts. Katchalski states that, in 1932, when he enrolled in the new Hebrew University, "The ascent to Mount Scopus each day on my motor bike, one of the few motorized vehicles in Jerusalem in those days, was always an exhilarating experience, with the Old City in front of me flanked by the mighty Judean desert to the West and the stone-colored new city shining in the East."

Both Katchalski brothers were attracted to science, especially chemistry and biology. Ephraim followed his brother Aharon, who had 2 years earlier entered the new Hebrew University of Jerusalem's first class of biology students. Of interest, Moshe Weizmann, Chaim Weizmann's younger brother, taught organic chemistry to the Katchalski brothers. Ephraim was an energetic and creative student, participating early on in the publication of two volumes on organic chemistry that were used as high school textbooks for many years.

Following his undergraduate studies, Ephraim continued at the University and was awarded both master's and Ph.D. degrees in the Department of Theoretical and Macromolecular Chemistry. From the onset, his interest was focused on amino acids and peptides, especially basic amino acids and their electrochemical properties. In Jerusalem at that time, these amino acids were not commercially available, and he had to obtain blood from the local slaughterhouse in order to isolate the basic amino acids—lysine, arginine, and histidine—for his research. The ultimate goal of his early studies was to understand the nature—the structure and function—of proteins, the ultimate building blocks of all biological structures. All proteins are composed of chains of the 20 amino acids. Later, remembering his early studies at the Hebrew University, he stated that "Most intriguing was the revelation that proteins not only constitute the basic building blocks of elaborate cellular structures but also act as molecular machines that carry out a multitude of complex reactions within cells and tissues."

Life was not always comfortable or easy for the Katchalski brothers during the formative years of their scientific careers, or for the growing population of Jewish inhabitants of Jerusalem. As he stated, "In the 1930s and '40s, the local Arab population, angered by the increasing Jewish presence, often attacked the Jews. We had to protect ourselves, and this we did by joining the illegal Jewish defense organization, the Haganah, which later became the Israel Defense Forces." The Jewish population of Palestine had grown from 83,000 (11%) in 1922 to 553,000 (31%) in 1945 and, not surprisingly, tensions were rising.

As the immigrant Jewish population grew, and as the final days of the British Mandate were playing out in 1945–1948, strains and growing numbers of terrorist attacks by both sides were increasing, concentrated mainly in Jerusalem. By 1945, over 100,000 Jews resided in Jerusalem, and both the Zionist leaders led by David Ben-Gurion and the Arab leader Abul Khader Husseini realized the importance and vulnerability of this population. Husseini announced a siege and vowed, "We will strangle Jerusalem."

A siege and open warfare did indeed take place, and the Jewish community, which had to depend on food and supplies carried up over a single mountainous road from the Mediterranean coast and susceptible to ambush, had at times only 2 or 3 days of food rations available. In this environment, it must have been exceedingly difficult to study, carry on creative research, and establish what would become highly productive scientific careers by both Katchalski brothers.

With the declaration of the State of Israel in May 1948, Ephraim and his brother Aharon, then in Rehovot, along with three others, laid the foundations for the Israeli Army's scientific defense unit, Hemed, which developed new weapons and explosives and would grow in time to become Israel's future defense industry. A secret munitions factory was built in the basement of the local laundry in Rehovot, supplying guns and ammunition to the Jewish forces. Life was complicated and dangerous.

Still, despite the noise and turmoil of war, the love of science continued to call. For his graduate studies and early professional work at the Hebrew University of Jerusalem, Katchalski chose to investigate what had emerged as one of the great biology questions of the 20th century: understanding the genetic code and how proteins are derived. The fundamental pathway of DNA to RNA to protein is now well-known. It is the basis for the hugely important field of molecular biology, which has transformed medicine, agriculture, and in fact every

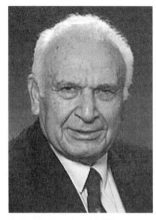

Ephraim Katchalski (Katzir), 1916–2009

sphere of biology. Katchalski's work predated and also contributed to that glorious avenue of discovery in the second half of the 20th century.

Proteins, the building blocks of all biologic structures, are composed of long chains or polymers of the 20 amino acids, linked in a precise sequence and then folded in an intricate manner. Proteins are the necessary structural components of skin, heart muscle, brain, and all other body tissues. They also act as critical functional machines, such as hemoglobin to carry oxygen, antibodies to protect against infectious disease, and as the agents of other critical processes. One of the most important functions of proteins is to act as enzymes to speed up chemical reactions. But how were proteins formed from precise chains of amino acid? Katchalski decided to start with the simplest structure or polymer, linking one amino acid, L-lysine to a second L-lysine molecule, which might serve as a model to begin to understand the construction of a basic protein. In time, this effort was successful and led to constructing many other synthetic amino acid chains or polymers. Traveling to the United States, to Columbia University, the Polymer Institute at Polytechnic Institute in Brooklyn, and shortly after to Harvard as a Visiting Scientist in 1948–1950, allowed Katchalski to share his ideas on the usefulness of simple poly-alpha-amino acids as models for proteins and receive a positive response from other international leaders in the field.

Work on synthetic polymers of amino acids as models for proteins rapidly spread to numerous laboratories throughout the scientific world. But new administrative duties also demanded his attention in the early years of his career. Following his brother Aharon, he relocated to Rehovot. During the turmoil and the War of Independence surrounding the establishment of the State of Israel, Katchalski was appointed acting head of the Department of Biophysics, and his brother Aharon became temporary head of the Department of Polymers at the Weizmann Institute of Science, appointments that were soon made permanent.

Not only the structure but also the function of proteins was receiving worldwide attention, including at the Weizmann Institute. In 1960, Drs. Michael Sela and Ruth Arnon, whose work led to the discovery of copolymer 1 (Copaxone), were both working in Katchalski's department. They will assume a leading role in this history in the next chapter. Arnon had joined Sela in 1957, as his Ph.D. student. They had begun to study why some proteins stimulated a response from the immune system while others did not. Together, they developed the first fully synthetic immunologic antigen, using amino acid polymer techniques already developed by Katchalski, to show that such molecules stimulated some of the same biologic responses as natural proteins.

As Katchalski's work was continuing in Rehovot, momentous earth-shaking discoveries were occurring in the field of biology. In 1953, Watson and Crick, working in England, reported their discovery of the double helix of DNA, which led the way to the explosive advance of molecular biology and genetics in the second half of the 20th century. A daunting question remained, however: What was the code that translated the nucleic acids of RNA to link amino acids, the building blocks of proteins? Marshall Nirenberg and his co-workers at the National Institue of Health (NIH) found that the three-molecule combination, or triplet, of uracil (codon) was the code of the amino acid phenylalanine. In their experiments in Bethesda, Maryland, a polymer of multiple linked molecules of L-phenylalanine produced in an RNA model proved to be identical to the poly L-phenylalanine produced synthetically at the Weizmann Institute. Sela, then a visiting scientist at the NIH, worked with Nirenberg on further deciphering the genetic code, using amino acid polymer techniques devised at the Weizmann Institute to verify the synthesis of proteins by RNA. Nirenberg was awarded a Nobel Prize in Medicine in 1968, for his pioneering discoveries on defining the genetic code.

As an increasingly successful biochemist of international reputation, Katchalski, in 1966, accepted the responsibility of heading a committee to advise the Israeli government on organizing future scientific and technological activity. This included promoting collaboration between governmental institutions, institutes of higher learning, and industry. In 1967, he served as Chief Scientist of the Defense Ministry during the crucial Six-Day War. These and other governmental responsibilities led Prime Minister Golda Meir to recommend him to stand for President of Israel, a position to which he was elected by the Knesset, Israel's parliament, in 1973. At that time, he changed his name to the Hebrew name, Katzir.

As Katchalski-Katzir has written,

The President is elected by the Knesset, Israel's parliament, for a 5-year term. Israelis look to their President for moral rather than political leadership and choose an individual noted for intellectual activities rather than political experience. Running the country is the responsibility not of the President but of the prime minister and his/her cabinet. He therefore serves, both at home and abroad, as a symbol of the State of Israel. Symbolizing the state means not only supporting it in its successes but also defending it in its failures. It means being a source of moral strength and inspiration, acting sometimes as a father figure and always as an example. It means raising the national morale in time of trouble. Two of the most momentous events in Israel's modern history occurred when I was President. I refer to the Yom Kippur War and the visit of President Anwar Sadat of Egypt to Jerusalem. It was not until Anwar El-Sadat came to Jerusalem in November 1977 that the way was opened to peace with one of our erstwhile enemies. The visit came at a very short notice and took us all by surprise. Its direct outcome was the peace treaty between Egypt and Israel, signed by President Sadat, Prime Minister Menahem Begin, and American President Jimmy Carter at Camp David in Washington on March 26, 1979.

I remember with mixed pleasure and sadness the close personal relationship that I developed with President Sadat during his brief but momentous visit to Israel and until his untimely death. This was a valued friendship, and one that I had hoped would help establish closer ties between our two countries. It was a bitter disappointment to find that zealots from both sides seemed to have ruined every chance for lasting peace. Sadat was murdered in Egypt by Moslem extremists, and Rabin, whom I greatly respected and admired, was assassinated by a Jewish extremist in Israel.

Violence and personal tragedy also touched Katchalski-Katzir during his term as President. "My beloved elder brother, Aharon, was murdered in May 1972, at Ben-Gurion Airport, by Japanese terrorists supported by local Palestinian groups. Of all those who touched my life, the one who had the greatest personal influence on me was my brother. Aharon was my closest friend and colleague, my guide and leader into the world of polymer research."

After leaving the Presidency of Israel, Katchalski-Katzir remained active in science and administration well into the first decade of the 21st century. He led the development of the Department of Molecular Microbiology and Biotechnology at Tel Aviv University, which expanded the expertise of biotechnology in Israel. He and his group also maintained an active scientific program at the Weizmann Institute of Science. He died in 2009 at the age of 93.

Katchalski-Katzir established the laboratory and department but—perhaps more importantly—set the scientific stage for biologic polymers so that Sela, Arnon, and their young colleague Dvora Teitelbaum could begin their pioneering work leading to copolymer 1 (Copaxone).

7

Scientific Serendipity I

The high adventure of science is the unexpected discovery—never knowing for sure where the next experiment may lead. One would not predict that the first drug ever to improve the course of multiple sclerosis (MS) and become a major commercial success would be the outgrowth of a basic research effort that was conceived with the goal of an opposite purpose. Neither would one expect that the drug would be the result of work by three dedicated scientists, toiling for over 29 years from first concept to a successful and emotional conclusion before a U.S. Food and Drug Administration (FDA) advisory panel. This story must be considered legendary in modern pharmacologic drug development.

This improbable but true tale begins in the small city of Tomaszow, Poland, where Michael Sela was born in 1924. His grandfather and father were successful industrialists who specialized in weaving high-quality worsted fabrics. His parents were well educated, his father attending a university in Vienna and his mother studying philosophy in Warsaw and Rostow. When he was 11, the family moved from Poland to Bucharest, Romania, where his father was invited to create a modern woolen textile plant. This move was fortunate, for not too long after, the Nazis invaded Poland, where eventually 23 members of Sela's family were killed.

Proficient in languages, 15-year-old Sela was in the provincial city of Craiova, Romania, in 1939, when the senior Polish government fled the Nazis, staying there for a short period before moving on to France.

While in Craiova, Sela served the Polish officials as an interpreter, employing his knowledge of both Polish and Romanian. With the increasingly deadly turmoil in Europe, the family wisely decided to immigrate to Palestine in 1941, and in October of that year Sela began his studies of chemistry and physics in Jerusalem, at the Hebrew University on Mount Scopus.

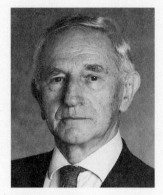

Michael Sela

Unfortunately, turmoil, danger, and conflict followed Sela to Palestine. He tells the story of preparing for his final examination in physics in 1946 at age 22. The day before the examination, he faced the conflicting decision for a student his age—studying physics or attending a dance at the Hadassah Medical Center adjacent to the University. He chose to attend the dance, where he and his partner were awarded first prize in dancing. The next day, his oral examination was interrupted by a thunderous explosion that rocked Jerusalem, the result of a terrorist attack by the Stern gang on the King David Hotel, in which 90 Arabs, Jews, and British were killed. This was one of the more notorious of many terrorist attacks carried out by both Jews and Arabs, leading up to the Israeli War of Independence in 1948. In spite of war and science, the dancing prize did stimulate Sela's interest in both modern and classic dance; he has maintained a lifelong interest, serving as an active supporter and leader for over 30 years of the Batsheva Society for Modern Dance, well-known throughout Israel. Successfully completing his studies, he was awarded a master's degree in chemistry from the Hebrew University in 1946.

Eager to continue his scientific education, Sela enrolled in the Ecole de Chimie at the University of Geneva. However, after 6 months, the events in Palestine overtook him, and he moved from Switzerland to Italy, where he became involved in immigration efforts helping Jews to reach Palestine. He then moved on to Prague, where he was named Secretary of the Commercial Section in the Legation of the new State of Israel to Czechoslovakia.

Science continued to beckon young Sela however, and in 1950, he returned to Israel and became a graduate student in the recently established Department of Biophysics at the Weizmann Institute in Rehovot, thus beginning his life-long association with his mentor and colleague, Ephraim Katchalski. In 1954, he received a Ph.D. degree from the Hebrew University for research carried out at the Weizmann Institute.

Over time, as his highly productive career unfolded, he became Head of the Section of Chemical Immunology at the Weizmann Institute, which in 1968 became the Department of Chemical Immunology. In 1975, he was elected to the first of two 5-year terms as President of the Institute, which continued to grow and prosper under his leadership.

From the beginning of his research at the Weizmann Institute, Sela was involved in the synthesis and use of poly amino acids as protein models, a field that had been successfully explored for several years by his supervisor, Ephraim Katchalski. Sela's Ph.D. thesis concerned the synthesis—or creation—of polymers of the amino acids tyrosine and tryptophan, using innovative methods already worked out in conjunction with Katchalski. This early work, and his becoming an expert in amino acid polymers and synthetic proteins, was critical in Sela's later work on copolymer 1, described later on. By 1955, his own work had advanced sufficiently for him to return to Europe to present papers on multi-chain poly amino acids at the International Congress of Chemistry in Zurich and the International Congress of Biochemistry in Brussels. His extraordinary career as a protein chemist had been launched.

After 5 years of working on protein models at Rehovot, Sela felt ready to go abroad for post-doctoral work, and chose to travel to the National Institutes of Health (NIH) in Bethesda, Maryland, in 1956, to work in the laboratory of Christian B. Anfinsen, Jr. This was clearly another providential choice for Sela; he has alluded to two principal mentors in protein chemistry with whom he had the good fortune to study and learn from: Ephraim Katchalski and Chris Anfinsen. Sela would, over time, arrange for prolonged stays with Anfinsen in Bethesda, in 1956 and 1957, 1960 and 1961, and later in 1973 and 1974. Anfinsen, in return, came to Rehovot for extended sabbaticals on several occasions, and later served as a valuable member of the Board of Governors of the Weizmann Institute of Science, including a number of years as Chairman of its Scientific Advisory Committee.

Anfinsen was an interesting person. Born in Monessen, Pennsylvania, to well-educated Norwegian immigrants, he studied chemistry at Swarthmore College and then entered graduate school at the University of Pennsylvania. In 1939, he received a fellowship to study new methods of analyzing the chemical structure of complex proteins—namely enzymes—at the Carlsberg Laboratory in Copenhagen, Denmark. However, the deteriorating and dangerous environment in Europe at the beginning of World War II forced him to return to the United States. He was offered a sought-after university fellowship in the Department of Biological Chemistry at Harvard Medical School, where in 1943, he was awarded his Ph.D. He taught Biological Chemistry at Harvard until 1950, when he was recruited to head the Laboratory of Cellular Physiology at the NIH. A Guggenheim Foundation fellowship allowed him to study at the Weizmann Institute in 1958 and 1959.

In 1962, he returned to Cambridge to assume the Chair of the Department of Biological Chemistry at Harvard; however, NIH soon wooed him back to Bethesda, where he was appointed Chief of the new Laboratory of Chemical Biology at the National Institute of Arthritis and Metabolic Diseases. In 1972, while at NIH, Anfinsen was awarded the Nobel Prize in Chemistry for his ground-breaking work on protein structure and function, specifically concerning the connection between the amino acid sequence and the biologically active conformation of the enzyme ribonuclease. Anfinsen followed Marshall Nirenberg as the second NIH scientist to become a Nobel laureate. With his protein chemistry knowledge, Sela had the opportunity to interact with both of them while at NIH. After an extended period in Israel, during which he converted to Orthodox Judaism, Anfinsen returned to the United States and joined the faculty of the Johns Hopkins University in Baltimore, as Professor of Biology, where he spent the final 12 years of his life. He died of a heart attack in May of 1995, a year short of his 80th birthday.

Even though Sela made significant contributions to the knowledge of protein chemistry alone and in conjunction with Katchalski and Anfinsen, his greatest contributions were yet to come in the realm of chemical immunology. He states that while he had great teachers in chemistry, he had no similar teacher in immunology, and he had to learn the field essentially by himself. He did, however, have a creative and productive colleague and career-long scientific partner in this effort, Ruth Arnon.

Arnon is a *Sabra*, a native-born Israeli. Her maternal grandparents and her father came from Russia and settled in Petach Tikva, northeast of Tel Aviv, now the location

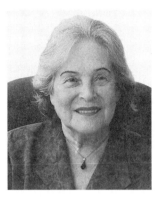

Ruth Arnon

of the Executive Offices of Teva. She received her undergraduate education at the Hebrew University in Jerusalem and served in the military from 1954 to 1956. After arranging a meeting with Ephraim Katchalski, she asked for a position as a graduate student and he agreed, stating that he required her to start work the following morning. Even though she had full-time employment, she was able to reschedule things to begin the next day. This was the beginning of what would become an impressive life-long career at the Weizmann Institute of Science.

Katchalski, with his students Sela and Arnon—who would soon become his research colleagues—was focused from the beginning not only on the structure but also the function of mammalian proteins. Their ability to create synthetic proteins or their simpler fragments, called *peptides* and *polymers*, led to highly complex and sophisticated science. A major question at that time, and one which continues to the present day, was how and why only some proteins are capable of eliciting a response from the immune system of an animal or human. The immune system is a fundamental protective barrier, capable of differentiating "self"—molecules and cells that belong in the body—from "non-self"—those that don't, such as the protein components of a virus or a bacteria—and then attacking and destroying non-self. This ability to detect a non-self protein not only is protective in nature but was also the basis for the development of vaccines, going back to the earliest work by Pasteur on rabies virus, which we discussed in Chapter 4. At times, this self/non-self division breaks down, and components of the immune system become capable of recognizing and attacking self proteins. This produces the family of *autoimmune diseases*, of which MS and rheumatoid arthritis are well-known examples.

Sela and Arnon, with their finely honed skills in producing synthetic proteins and peptides, soon began focusing their research on the structural and amino acid requirements of peptides that were capable of stimulating an immune response in a mammal. Using rabbits as their experimental animal, they explored what was required of a peptide in terms of amino acid content in order to elicit an immune response. The protein or portion of the protein that stimulates an immune response or reaction is called an *antigen*. They began to experiment with the necessary amino acid requirements that would produce an effective antigen, looking primarily for an antibody response in the serum of rabbits injected with the manufactured antigen.

Gelatin is a highly important structural component of collagen that is present in bones, tendons, or other fibrous connective tissue. Earlier studies had determined that, although it is a protein, gelatin generally is incapable of eliciting an immune response. Would it be possible to construct and attach small peptides, or even individual amino acids, to gelatin to turn it into an effective antigen? As part of her Ph.D. thesis, Arnon found that attaching tyrosine or tyrosine-containing peptides to gelatin turned it into a potent *immunogen*—a substance capable of eliciting an immune response.

Throughout the late 1950s and 1960s, Sela and Arnon made numerous notable discoveries that resulted in a number of significant publications. They were influencing, in fact leading, the entire field to define the link between protein chemistry and immunology. This junction of chemistry and immunology signified the biological connection between them and underlined the importance of this field. Five years later, in 1968, the Section had been elevated to the Department of Chemical Immunology. By 1963, Sela had been promoted to professor and appointed Head of the Section of Chemical Immunology at the Weizmann Institute. Arnon was appointed to this position when he assumed new administrative duties as President of Weizmann.

As their studies continued in increasing sophistication and complexity, they began to explore the difficult and interesting area in which lipids or fatty materials or even sugars would potentially function as antigens, especially if attached to synthetic copolymers or peptides. They chose to work with a tumor-associated lipid called *cytolipin* or *sphingolmyelin*, a nervous system lipid.

The publications resulting from the tremendous scientific productivity of Sela and Arnon did not go unnoticed. In 1959, Sela was awarded the Israel Prize in Natural Sciences for research on synthetic poly-peptides as protein models. In 1967, he became a foreign member of the Max Planck Society, and the next year was made an honorary member of The American Society of Biological Chemists. In 1968, he was also awarded the Otto Warburg Medal of the German Society of Biological Chemistry, and the Rothschild Prize in Chemistry for contributions toward the elucidation of the chemical basis of antigenicity. Both he and Arnon have continued to receive numerous international awards and recognition for their work in immunology.

8

The 180-Degree Turn

In May 1967, Israel was emerging from its adolescence and celebrating its 19th birthday as an independent nation. A question arose as to whether competitive, world-class biologic research could be carried out in the stressful and dangerous environment then surrounding Israel and Rehovot. Israel had a strong, reliable supporter in the United States and its President, Lyndon Johnson. However, to the north was Syria and to the south Egypt, and they were attempting a political union, the United Arab Republic (UAR), with the ongoing political support and supply of weapons from the Soviet Union. Tensions were continuously increasing, pointing to armed conflict in the region, with serious international undercurrents of the Cold War.

At the time, President Gamal Nasser of Egypt was quoted as saying, "If war comes it will be total and the objective will be Israel's destruction." In Syria, Prime Minister Zu'ayyin proclaimed, "We shall set the area afire and any Israeli movement will result in a final grave for Israel." During the spring of 1967, the Egyptian army crossed the Suez Canal and was soon within 75 to 100 miles of Rehovot, causing great concern and considerable stress to the Israeli population.

War broke out in June 5, 1967. Within 6 days, Israel had defeated both Egypt and Syria and had occupied the entire West Bank to the Jordan River and most of the Golan Heights above the Sea of Galilee, altering the geopolitical situation of the entire Middle East. This conflict, the Six-Day War, created an exclamation mark in Middle Eastern history which remains to this day. Now, over 40 years after the Six-Day War, tension, periodic terror attacks, and political uncertainty still prevail in the region.

The answer to the question of the ability of committed researchers to carry out productive and competitive science in this stressful environment was an emphatic *yes*. The research team of Sela and Arnon was now joined by a graduate student, Dvora Teitelbaum, who would be a vital contributing member of the team until her death from metastatic cancer in 2008, and they set out to plan a new, highly creative project, to unravel the immunologic mystery of experimental allergic encephalomyelitis (EAE).

They had, over time, gained considerable experience in creating combined protein or peptide-plus-lipid antigens. Sela reasoned that, because myelin was composed of a membrane containing both lipid and protein wrapped around the nerve fiber, it might be possible to make a synthetic peptide or polymer of just a few amino acids that would serve as a tool to investigate the immune steps leading to demyelination, a hallmark of both EAE and multiple sclerosis (MS). Sela contacted his friend, Otto Westphal of the Max Planck Institute, who was enthusiastic about the idea and even helped the Weizmann group to obtain a small research grant from the Freudenberg Foundation to support it.

They made three polymers or copolymers, consisting of four, seven, or 12 amino acids, all containing a large amount of lysine to give them a basic nature similar to that of myelin basic protein (MBP). The plan was to administer the agents, which they chose to call copolymers 1, 2, and 3, to guinea pigs by various routes and doses, along with complete Freund's adjuvant, to see if they would induce EAE. With these copolymers as tools, they might then peel back the immunologic secrets of EAE.

After a full year of concentrated effort, no guinea pig showed any evidence of EAE after injection of any of the three copolymers. Was their hypothesis wrong? Did they not understand the protein immunologic reactions that had been the foundation of their research for over a decade? Describing her feelings, Arnon used the emotion-laden single word—disappointment. They considered giving up on the project.

While they were carrying out the initial copolymer synthesis and animal testing, the group had also developed a simplified process for purifying bovine MBP and had shown that, when combined with complete Freund's adjuvant, it was a potent inducer of EAE in guinea pigs. From their knowledge of EAE, the broader immunologic literature, and their own experience, the creative idea of immunologic inhibition began to dawn. An awakening, an epiphany! If the copolymers had no encephalitogenic activity—that is, no ability to cause EAE—could they do just the opposite, that is, suppress EAE? This was a process which had been used to determine the specificity of other immunologic interactions. Could they turn their immunologic battleships in the opposite direction, a 180-degree turn?

They quickly began a new series of experiments to determine if the copolymers would suppress EAE that would otherwise develop in guinea pigs injected with MBP. As Arnon has written, "The results of the inhibition experiments were overwhelming." Of the three copolymers, the simplest, copolymer 1, seemed to be the most effective, and most subsequent experiments employed it in attempting to suppress or treat EAE even after its induction in the animal.

A number of closely coordinated experiments were carried out in guinea pigs to test their observations and gain confidence that suppression or prevention of EAE was in fact taking place. In each series of experiments, some animals were injected only with MBP and adjuvant to serve as active controls. All animals were observed daily for signs of weight loss and paralysis of the hind legs, which are the recognized symptoms of early EAE in the guinea pig. At the end of 4 weeks, all animals in each experiment were humanely sacrificed. The brain was removed for microscopic examination, searching for the typical pathologic signs of EAE, mainly signs of inflammation (an immunologic reaction) surrounding blood vessels. These studies were always coded, that is, the changes in brain tissue from the control versus the Cop 1 (copolymer one), 2 or 3 injected animals were not revealed until all microscopic observations were complete.

The experiments were divided into two groups, testing for prevention or suppression of EAE. For prevention, the guinea pigs were injected with the copolymer twice a week for 4 weeks and then challenged with MBP and adjuvant to see if EAE developed. For suppression or treatment, the animals were injected with MBP and adjuvant, and then the copolymer was injected twice a week, beginning 2 days after the MBP challenge. Injections under the skin and by an intravenous route were both tried. In every experiment, the appearance of EAE either by paralysis or pathologically in the tissue was markedly reduced if the animals had received copolymer injections. Following these and a number of other experiments to convincingly show that EAE could be prevented or suppressed by the three copolymers, a detailed scientific report was published in 1971, in the *European Journal of Immunology*, with Dvora Teitelbaum as the first author. The first steps on the long trail leading to an MS treatment had been taken.

Sela, Arnon, and Teitelbaum were pleased, relieved, and excited by the discovery that their copolymers were capable of suppressing EAE in guinea pigs but, as with science in general and certainly with EAE, every successful experiment raised new questions. The first question was the

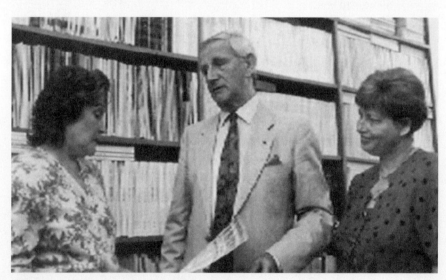

Ruth Arnon, Michael Sela, and Dvora Teitelbaum

source of the MBP that was employed, for it was known that MBP from some sources was more active. A series of experiments employing both bovine and human MBP were conducted and, regardless of the source of MBP, the suppression of EAE was still very effective.

Next they created a series of copolymers in which the amino acids were individually replaced with similar amino acids; in one copolymer aspartic acid replaced glutamic acid, while another was devoid of tyrosine. Although similar, these altered copolymers were less effective in suppressing EAE.

By 1970, the voluminous and growing EAE literature had reported quite clearly that the species of animal used in an experiment was critical in the type of immunologic reaction that resulted. As noted in Chapter 4, when whole MBP was split up into smaller peptides or fragments containing peptides of 10 to 15 amino acids in length, a peptide that produced EAE in one species of experimental animal could be suppressive, or could protect against EAE in another species. To explore this question, the Rehovot group conducted a series of experiments using rabbits as the experimental animal rather than guinea pigs; again, suppression especially by Cop 1 was successful. The result was similar with mice.

Was the route of administration important? It turned out that intravenous treatment with Cop 1 was most effective, and that multiple doses were much more effective than a single dose. A dose of 5 mg seemed to be optimal for both guinea pigs and rabbits.

As the group investigated multiple questions one after another, such as source of the MBP, dose of the copolymer, route of administration, and species (guinea pigs, rabbits, or mice), in each instance the effectiveness especially of Cop 1 as an EAE suppressant was confirmed. The exposure of the animals to the copolymers seemed to cause essentially no side effects or pathologic damage in other organs. It was also important to determine if Cop 1 had some specificity for suppressing EAE or was instead a general immunosuppressant. In a series of experiments using different antigens rather than MBP, with or without Cop 1, it made no difference. They all showed that Cop 1 was not a general, nonspecific immunosuppressant.

The type of pathologic damage in the brain induced by bovine MBP was then compared with that induced by human MBP. Human MBP produced a more pathologic change that showed some demyelination, whereas the bovine MBP only caused inflammation surrounding blood vessels. However, both types of pathology were inhibited or suppressed by Cop 1, indicating that both inflammation and demyelination could be inhibited. This immediately increased their interest, for they knew that pathology seen in MS shows both pathologic changes.

This long, sequential, and complex series of experiments carried out over many months vastly extended the knowledge of EAE suppression produced by Cop 1.

This impressive series of successes continued to encourage Sela, Arnon, and Teitelbaum, along with several other Weizmann colleagues who were participating in the laboratory studies. Now it was time to move into new realms of complexity, testing whether Cop 1 would suppress EAE in primates. Experimental allergic encephalomyelitis in monkeys is known to be a devastating disease, almost uniformly causing fatal disease approximately 3 weeks after the animal is challenged. Rhesus monkeys were the experimental primate chosen for the next series of experiments. Ultimately, ten animals were included. All were injected with 5 mg of bovine MBP in complete Freund's adjuvant on day 0. Five were controls, and all five developed severe EAE 16 to 24 days after the MBP inoculation that resulted in death. When examined pathologically, the brains of all five animals showed lesions, some of which could be identified on the cut surface of the brain even before microscopic examination. Inflammation was widespread and, in addition, local areas of hemorrhage were found, which are characteristic of fatal EAE in the rhesus monkey.

The team decided to observe whether Cop 1 could reverse EAE already appearing in monkeys injected with MBP. Therefore, the next five animals were given Cop 1 injections only after they had shown the first stages of paralysis from EAE. Relatively high doses of Cop 1 were used, beginning with 100 mg per day for the first seven injections, followed by a step-wise decrease thereafter. Each monkey began to show neurologic improvement approximately 4 days after onset of the Cop 1 injections.

The brains of four of the monkeys treated with Cop 1 and then sacrificed several months after the EAE challenge showed no evidence of any inflammation or other pathologic change typical of EAE. They had survived and apparently were free of EAE or its effects.

The fifth monkey in the group treated with Cop 1 was interesting and unique. It recovered completely during the first series of Cop 1 injections. However, 35 days after the last injection, it began to show neurologic symptoms. Cop 1 injections were reinstated at a dose of 50 mg, and within 3 days it once again seemed to recover. Ten days after the last Cop 1 injections, the monkey suffered an acute relapse and, despite the reinitiation of Cop 1 treatment, this animal died 5 days later, 3 months after the initial challenge with MBP and adjuvant.

The final series of nonhuman primate experiments were conducted using baboons, large animals that weigh approximately 30 kilograms. The experiments were done in three stages, each consisting of five animals. All of the animals were injected with bovine MBP and complete Freund's adjuvant, and two of the animals in each stage were thereafter not treated with Cop 1, serving as active controls. All six control animals, two in each of the three stages, developed severe EAE and died 4 to 11 days after showing the first neurologic symptoms of EAE.

Three baboons in each stage were started on Cop 1 therapy at the first evidence of neurologic symptoms and, even though they continued to deteriorate, most of them reaching a stage of almost complete paralysis, they then began to recuperate; seven of the nine showed full recovery. In addition to the daily clinical observations and microscopic review when the animal was sacrificed, one of the baboons was repeatedly filmed, recording the pretreatment phase, the serious paralysis of acute EAE, and the gratifying recovery with Cop 1 treatment. The remarkable results of these primate experiments were published in the *Israeli Journal of Medical Science* in 1977.

Beginning in 1967, with the stated goal of creating a laboratory tool to investigate the mechanisms operative in EAE, the Weizmann group over a period of approximately 8 years had produced three copolymers that, rather than inducing EAE to serve as a research tool, instead created something much more exciting and much more valuable. They were able to show that the small copolymers they had fabricated were able to suppress and even treat EAE in a variety of laboratory animals: guinea pigs, rabbits, mice, rhesus monkeys, and baboons. They had shown that both the clinical disease and the pathology in the animals was inhibited or treated with the copolymers, and that the process was not as a nonspecific immunosuppressant, but rather seemed to be quite specific for EAE. By themselves, this series of experiments must be considered exceptional and unique, yet they were only the beginning of what the group was hoping to accomplish in the immediate future. History-making in scope, these revolutionary studies are remarkable, carried out in Rehovot during a time when Israel was under great stress and challenge to its very existence. Regrettably, as this prodigious scientific program was underway, Michael Sela's son-in-law was killed on the front in the Yom Kippur War in October 1973, just a year after Ephraim Katchalski-Katzir's brother Aharon had died in a terrorist attack outside Tel Aviv.

9

Is It Effective, and Is It Safe?

The U.S. Food and Drug Administration (FDA) in the United States, and similar agencies that control or regulate prescription drugs in countries throughout the world, operates under several laws and numerous regulations concerning the sale and use of any prescription drug or treatment to be used therapeutically in humans. This is understandably an area of great complexity, but ultimately the two questions which must be answered by any company (often called a sponsor) seeking to receive permission to sell any drug are, "Is it effective therapy for a specific human condition?," and "Is it safe?" Safety is not absolute, and most effective modern drugs have some side effects and even serious risks. However, it is important to determine what the side effects and risks are and how they can be recognized, managed, and perhaps avoided. Safety is also relative; a treatment that may be approved for metastatic cancer that is expected to be fatal in a short time may not be acceptable for a disease such as multiple sclerosis (MS) that is variable and unpredictable, but does not generally shorten life significantly. People with MS may live for many years or several decades after diagnosis, so proof of long-term drug safety is a critical issue with medications to treat this disease.

In the early 1970s, after working diligently and persistently on Cop 1 (copolymer one) for several years, Sela, Arnon, and Teitelbaum came face to face with an enormous challenge: How could they bridge the wide gorge from their extensive animal experimentation to the risk of exposing humans to Cop 1? The first daunting question was whether it was safe, but there were also the related questions of dose and route of administration. Of critical concern was how and where they would choose the first human patients to be exposed to what could be real danger.

It is important to recall from Chapter 4 some of the important discoveries that had emerged from the long-term investigation of the MS animal model, experimental allergic encephalomyelitis (EAE). This serious, sometimes fatal, animal disease is produced by the injection of a myelin protein, usually in combination with a nonspecific immunologic stimulant, complete Freund's adjuvant. Thomas Rivers (Chapter 4) had shown in 1936 that multiple injections of central nervous system (CNS) tissue alone could produce EAE. It had also been discovered that it was not necessary to use the entire 170-amino acid sequence of myelin basic protein (MBP), but that EAE could be triggered by smaller fragments called peptides or polymers, composed of strings of only 10 to 15 amino acids. To add to the complexity of the situation, the MBP fragment that produced EAE in one animal species might turn out to be protective or to suppress the disease in a different species. It might also be recalled that Sela and Arnon, working with various synthetic amino acid polymers or peptides in Katchalski's laboratory (Chapter 6), had found that some of their synthetic polymers could be antigenic, that is, they could produce a serious immunologic reaction when injected repeatedly into an experimental animal. In anticipating the important and obviously very exciting possibility that Cop 1 might be the first unique and useful treatment for MS, the question of risk and safety had to be confronted head on.

By the 1970s, the same question of safety was also being considered in other laboratories investigating the role of amino acid polymers or peptides in neuroimmunologic diseases, including MS. Barry Arnason, a well-known and productive neuroimmunologist working at Harvard in Boston, was using poly-L-lysine, a string of linked molecules of the amino acid lysine, as an experimental tool to investigate EAE in guinea pigs. One might remember that this was one of the first synthetic amino acid polymers created by Katchalski at the Hebrew University in Jerusalem in the 1930s and 1940s. In a paper published in 1975, Arnason wrote "It will be recalled that encephalogenic determinants (peptides or fragments) on myelin basic protein are not the same in different species." This, of course, echoes the earlier discoveries made throughout the long history of EAE. He goes on, "These results point out the inherent risk in anticipating that synthetic agents, because they suppress a given auto-allergic disease (EAE) in one species can be expected to do so in others, a point of some importance when assessing treatments for EAE as potential therapies for multiple sclerosis in man." Here was the vexing dilemma: What was the risk of injecting Cop 1 into humans? Would it act to benefit MS, or would it induce the serious damage of EAE?

The Weizmann investigators decided to enlist the advice and help of Oded Abramsky of the Hadassah University Hospital in Jerusalem to cautiously approach this fundamental, all-important question. Abramsky was a neurologist and, importantly, a well-trained neuroimmunologist who had received both his medical and Ph.D. degrees from the Hebrew University of Jerusalem, followed by neurologic training at the Hadassah University Hospital. He had also worked as a visiting scientist at the well-known neuroimmunologic laboratories at the University of Pennsylvania in Philadelphia.

At that time, Abramsky was engaged in research on the immunology of diseases of the peripheral nervous system (PNS) at the Weizmann Institute, under the direction of Arnon, and was actively collaborating with Dvora Teitelbaum and others working on the Cop 1 project. This was during the time that monkeys were being exposed to Cop 1. After extensive discussions with the Cop 1 research team about the potential benefit or danger of injecting humans with Cop 1, a proposal was submitted to and approved by the Israeli Ministry of Health to proceed. Abramsky was well aware

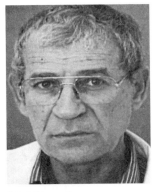

Oded Abramsky

of the potential dangers to humans and considered injecting himself. However, he had recently had a laboratory mishap and had accidentally injected his hand with an antigen mixed with complete Freund's adjuvant. This resulted in massive but temporary swelling of his arm. Because of this incident, he was advised not to inject himself with Cop 1. Two of his scientific colleagues who were healthy volunteered, and received injections of Cop 1 with no reaction or side effects. This was probably the first human exposure to injections of Cop 1 and could be considered a small but important Phase I trial by the FDA definition of human drug development (see below).

Abramsky recommended that the first patients would be those with acute disseminated encephalomyelitis (ADEM), which was considered to be a close human counterpart to EAE. Recall from Chapter 4 that this disease had been identified in humans exposed to various vaccinations (rabies and vaccinia for smallpox) but also following one of several acute viral diseases (acute post-infectious encephalomyelitis). A second group of patients he suggested to be considered were patients in the more advanced stages of MS. The wards and clinics of Hadassah Hospital in Jerusalem were searched to identify such patients.

Two of the selected ADEM patients at the Hadassah, aged 14 and 12 years, had developed convulsions with paralysis or coma 1 or 2 weeks after recovering from measles infection. (Before the widespread use of measles vaccination, ADEM was a relatively common complication of measles.) A third ADEM patient, recovering from mumps, had developed optic neuritis or acute visual impairment, along with mild signs of encephalitis. In this patient, the electroencephalogram was diffusely abnormal and the spinal fluid contained an abnormally large number of lymphocytes, which would be expected in ADEM.

Four patients with longstanding and severe MS were also recruited. These included:

- a 40-year-old man who had had MS for 8 years and was bedridden;
- a 23-year-old man who, although only 3 years into the course of his disease, was paralyzed in both arms and legs and had severe

incoordination; he was unable to eat or talk and had to be fed with a stomach tube;

- a 30-year-old woman with a short MS history of 2 years, who had weakness in her legs and serious incoordination; and
- a 40-year-old woman with MS for 10 years, who had paralysis of her legs and was confined to a wheelchair.

These seven Hadassah patients, three with ADEM and four with advanced MS, must be considered pioneers or, perhaps more importantly, patient heroes. They were willing to volunteer and accept the risk of being the first humans exposed to a potentially dangerous but also possibly beneficial MS therapy.

The three ADEM patients all received daily injections of Cop 1 for 2 weeks at a relatively low dose of 2 mg. All three recovered completely. Of two other untreated ADEM patients, who could be considered a small control group, one recovered while another had long-term persistent neurologic symptoms.

The four MS patients received injections of 2 or 3 mg of Cop 1 every 2 or 3 days for 3 weeks, then a weekly injection for 2 to 5 months. Overall, the patients were treated for 3 to 6 months. Two showed some improvement in speech and visual function, one was unchanged, and one, treated for 3 months, suffered an MS relapse at that time and the injections were stopped.

There were no observed side effects or abnormalities in any laboratory test in any of these original seven patients, the first ever exposed to Cop 1. Here, then, was the first hint that Cop 1 might fulfill one of the essential requirements: It might be safe to use as a human MS treatment.

A report of this study was published in the *Journal of Neurological Sciences* in early 1977, authored by Abramsky, Teitelbaum, and Arnon. It retains its place as one of the important guideposts on the long journey to a successful treatment for MS.

The journey from the first human exposure to Cop 1 to the time when it could be registered by the FDA and made available as an MS prescription drug turned out, as is often the case, to be long, expensive, and full of unanticipated delays. A similar path is often followed by many modern therapies for significant human diseases. The history of the regulatory framework that governs the development of prescription drugs is quite fascinating, and each new chapter in this story is frequently stimulated by some unexpected disaster resulting from adulterated or otherwise toxic side effects of a food or drug. As early as 1202, King John of England proclaimed the first English food law, which prohibited the adulteration of bread. In the United States, in 1848, Congress passed the Drug Importation Act, which required that the U.S. Customs Service inspect incoming shipments for adulterated drugs. Of interest, President Lincoln, in 1862, appointed a chemist, Charles M. Wetherill, to serve as a safety officer in the newly formed Department of Agriculture. This might be considered the direct predecessor to the modern FDA.

The original Food and Drug Act was passed by Congress in 1906, and signed into law by President Theodore Roosevelt. It prohibited commerce in misbranded and adulterated foods, drinks, and drugs. Numerous new laws and regulations were passed in the ensuing decades, often brought on by some widely publicized public health event, such as the finding in 1937 that elixir of sulfanilamide contained a poisonous solvent that resulted in the death of 107 people, many of them children. By 1938, it was necessary for Congress to pass a new, much more comprehensive law, the Federal Food, Drug, and Cosmetic Act, stating that new drugs had to be shown to be safe for human use before being marketed to the public. Following up on this increasing concern about drug safety in 1940, the FDA was transferred from the Department of Agriculture to the Federal Security Agency; in 1953, this agency became the Department of Health, Education, and Welfare. Two years later, it was discovered that widely distributed polio vaccine, thought to have been inactivated, in fact contained live polio virus that was associated with 260 cases of paralytic polio. A new Division of Biologics Control was established; it was initially located within the National Institutes of Health (NIH).

Following on the recurring theme that public health disasters are the stimulus for new regulations, in 1962, a unique sleeping pill, thalidomide, was found to have caused birth defects, mainly limb deformities, in thousands of babies born in Western Europe. This tragedy led to the Kefauver-Harris Drug Amendment, which stated that drug manufacturers are required to prove to the FDA not only the safety but also the effectiveness of their products. This was a revolutionary change, because it required, among many other things, that sponsors or manufacturers also had to establish that drugs were an effective treatment for a specific disease through adequate well-controlled clinical trials.

This usually demanded that candidate treatments had to be more effective than a placebo by being tested in a *randomized, double-blind, placebo-controlled trial*, meaning that participants are assigned to either the treatment or to the placebo category, but neither they nor the investigators, usually physicians and nurse coordinators, are aware of which group they are assigned to. This requirement added substantially to the cost and size of each trial, the duration of observations, and a much greater emphasis on the biologic mechanisms by which a drug functioned to improve, control, and treat a specific human disease. By 1972, the regulation of biologics such as serums, vaccines, and blood products which—as noted above—had been within the purview of the NIH was transferred to the FDA.

Recognizing that relatively rare diseases were less likely to gain attention by commercial drug companies, in 1983, Congress enacted the Orphan Drug Act. This Act enabled the FDA to promote research and marketing of drugs needed for the treatment of rare diseases. This law has direct application to the treatment of MS and the development of Cop 1.

In 1981, the FDA and the Department of Health and Human Services expanded and strengthened a number of regulations for the protection of human subjects in any type of medical research. Basic to these new regulations were two fundamental principles. First, all research participants must be carefully educated about the purpose and risks of a trial, and then give their own personal informed consent prior to participation. Second, each institution conducting human research, such as a hospital or medical school, must establish an institutional review board or internal review board (IRB) to ensure that all human volunteers recruited to research studies are appropriately enrolled, and that the conduct of each trial is ethical and conforms to all applicable federal regulations. This is of some importance because each IRB, composed of locally chosen, interested persons, including not only medical researchers but also clergymen or lawyers and perhaps common citizens, is involved in making sure that research subjects are informed and protected. All clinical trials then must receive permission not only from the FDA at the federal level but also from the IRB at a local level before and during the conduct of any drug trial.

The first plateau that must be reached in the long journey from an idea to FDA approval for any new drug is the requirement for preclinical studies. There must be some rough concept of how a drug might work, something of its structure or biologic composition, and—of course—why it might be useful for a specific human disease. Most potential drugs start with *in vitro* studies, laboratory studies showing chemical composition and activity. Animal studies are usually required in which different doses of an experimental drug are tested, ultimately determining the lethal dose for that species. These *in vivo* studies are generally conducted in at least two species of animals and often are carried out for several weeks to several months, depending on the potential drug use in a specific human disease. In most cases, studies must also be conducted in pregnant animals to get some sense of the risk to the pregnancy or fetus. Other studies, often lasting several months, are done to determine *oncogenesis*, the chance that a potential drug could produce cancer in animals and thus carry some risks to humans exposed to the experimental treatment.

Once extensive preclinical studies have been completed, the sponsor, usually a pharmaceutical company, must apply to the FDA for an Investigational New Drug Application or IND. This permits the sponsor to conduct human trials. The IND process is most commonly divided into three phases.

Phase I trials involve the initial exposure of humans, usually healthy human volunteers, to the experimental drug, in order to gain some perspective on side effects or dangers, often after increasing doses are given. Hopefully, some information about the metabolic and pharmacologic actions of the drug in humans will be gained. During Phase I studies, the human volunteers remain under close observation for a number of hours in the clinic or—in some cases—are admitted to an inpatient facility so that unexpected side effects can be adequately managed and treated. Commonly, between 20 and 80 patients are recruited to Phase I trials, depending on the treatment in question.

Moving to Phase II trials, and relying on the results from Phase I, an effort is made to begin to determine the potential effectiveness of a drug on the disease or condition in question. Patients with the disease are kept in some type of controlled setting for ongoing observations, or they may return to the clinic for frequent evaluations, especially for side effects. Laboratory evaluations are essential. Hopefully, some relatively clear evidence of the pharmacology of the drug and some sense of its possible effectiveness will emerge during Phase II.

Phase III trials, often referred to as *pivotal trials*, are complex, long, and costly studies that hopefully will lead to the success of the drug or, much more commonly, to its failure. Phase III trials are almost always randomized, double-blind, placebo-controlled studies which, in the case of MS experimental treatments, rarely last for less than 2 years. The patients are recruited if they not only have clinically definite MS, but also have specific characteristics such as the number of recent clinical relapses, defined levels of disability or—in rare cases—specific magnetic resonance imaging (MRI) characteristics. *Placebo-controlled* indicates that the study is set up to compare the clinical results or the drug effects of the group receiving the experimental drug with the other group receiving placebo. Neither the patients nor the investigators can choose to which group they are assigned, and neither knows the group assignment until the end of the trial.

Both treated and placebo patients are cared for identically and are evaluated at regular clinic visits, often at monthly intervals, when they will be checked for side effects, as well as undergo blood tests and other laboratory tests such as an electrocardiogram (EKG) or MRI. If patients experience increasing disease activity or have new side effects, they are required to immediately contact the investigating center so that their condition will be recorded and they will be treated if necessary.

Phase III trials are commonly carried out at a number of independent clinics or centers, usually associated with medical schools and large hospitals. They may also be conducted simultaneously in several countries at well-qualified clinical centers. If unexpected or severe side effects occur, including even deaths, the trial of course can be terminated or put on hold. Looking over the sponsor and the investigative centers are independent safety data monitoring committees that receive periodic secret access to laboratory studies, safety issues, and even beneficial possible effects of the therapy. This committee can stop the study if there are unacceptable safety issues or, in some cases, can even recommend an end to the study if the beneficial effects are so great that it would be unethical to continue to expose the placebo group to a useless compound when the effect of the experimental drug is significantly better.

The FDA requires strict record-keeping, usually on detailed forms that must be kept not only during the trial but maintained for many years after it has been completed. Also, the FDA may evaluate the records unannounced at any time, to ensure that the data are adequate and that the safety and welfare of all participants are being considered. If all goes well for the entire duration of the trial, the records from all of the participating centers are collected and the data covering the entire trial are analyzed by complex, sophisticated, statistical methods. Only when this has been completed are the sponsor, the investigative centers, and the patient groups given any indication of whether there was a beneficial treatment effect. Finally, a public hearing is held that almost always is exciting, emotional, or disheartening, depending on the results. In the case of Cop 1, that experience will be described in detail further on in this book.

In 1977, this long, complex process was just beginning for the Weizmann group, even though they had already dedicated over a decade to the search for a successful treatment for MS. Hope for the discovery of a treatment for the "disease that shatters dreams" carried them forward. Over 350,000 MS patients in the United States and many more elsewhere facing a depressing future of more debilitating MS relapses, also hoped desperately for a therapy to elevate their dreams.

10

Expanding Human Exposure

With promising results—or at least gain in comfort—about safety from the small human exposure to Cop 1 (copolymer one) at the Hadassah Hospital in Jerusalem, a new light shone on the dark horizon, and a ray of hope had been created for the million plus sufferers of multiple sclerosis (MS), although none of them was aware of it at the time. Immediately, a new challenge confronted the Cop 1 team at the Weizmann Institute. Where would an appropriate location be to begin to test the potential efficacy and safety of Cop 1 as an MS treatment? A decision was made to look toward Germany, but also to the United States for expanded human testing, even though the compound itself would continue to be produced at the Weizmann Institute.

In Germany, a small preliminary trial was conducted under the leadership of Helmut J. Bauer in Göttingen. Bauer had a large MS clinic and was recognized as an international MS leader during the last third of the 20th century. The German trial recruited 21 patients, ten of whom had early MS and were injected with a daily dose of 2 mg of Cop 1. The other 11, who had fairly advanced MS, received a daily dose of 20 mg. The study duration for all patients was 1 month. Some improvement may have occurred in the patients with early disease; however, with its short duration and without a control population, it was impossible to establish any clear clinical effect. Still, the trial was very important in demonstrating that Cop 1 seemed safe, even with relatively large doses of 20 mg.

In September 1973, in the attractive port city of Barcelona, Spain, where the outrageous, unique, and beautiful cathedral created by the architect Antoni Gaudi is located, elite neurologists from around the globe gathered for the World Congress of Neurology, an event held every 4 years. A satellite scientific session on MS attracted an audience of between 150 and 200, small in comparison to the huge groups numbering well over 2,000 that would gather once new treatments for the disease became available in the mid-1990s. Nevertheless, many scientific notables were there, including Jonas Salk, Albert Sabin, and Hillary Koprowski, all of whom had played important roles in the development of polio vaccines. Also in the audience were several lay persons with a personal commitment to the MS effort, including the one-time child movie star, Shirley Temple Black.

Among those invited to present lectures on new developments of MS interest was the young Israeli immunochemist, Ruth Arnon, who described interesting animal experiments using a new agent, copolymer 1, which suppressed experimental allergic encephalomyelitis (EAE) in laboratory animals. Her mentor and colleague, Michael Sela, was in the audience. The scientific basis for this approach was unfamiliar to the audience, and it was thought to be an unusual concept at a time when most attention was focused on viruses as a cause of MS. The information excited moderate interest but was probably filed away as one more agent that affected laboratory animals with EAE but was unlikely to have an impact on MS treatment. One person in the audience, however, Dr. Murray Bornstein from New York, was quite interested and approached Arnon after the session to ask if he could obtain some Cop 1 for investigation in his laboratory and perhaps even for clinical studies.

Bornstein was to become one of the pivotal figures in the development of Cop 1 as a successful MS drug. Born in 1918, in Patterson, New Jersey, he graduated from Dartmouth College in New Hampshire in 1939. Attracted to science, he enrolled at McGill University in Montreal, where he received a master's degree in physiology. He then moved to the University of Geneva in Switzerland, where he continued his basic science studies, receiving a second master's degree in physiology before entering medical school in Geneva, where he was awarded his M.D. in 1952. Of interest, he may have been a student in Geneva at the same time that Michael Sela was studying there, although Sela does not remember meeting him.

Following training as a resident in clinical neurology at Mount Sinai Hospital after his return to the United States, Bornstein became a research fellow at Columbia University in New York in 1956, and began his highly productive studies on the immunology of MS. In 1958, he became a lab director at Mount Sinai Hospital in Manhattan, where he remained until 1966, before joining the Albert Einstein School of Medicine faculty in the Bronx. There, he continued his scientific work for 22 years until his official retirement in 1988, although he remained active at Einstein until 1994.

Although Bornstein's career and legacy will perhaps always be identified with his singular, pioneering work on the development of Cop 1 as an MS treatment, his scientific career is much more expansive and illustrates his single-minded interest in understanding MS using complex laboratory tools. Beginning in 1956, while he was still a research fellow at Columbia University, he began the study of cultures of mammalian nervous system tissue, showing that it was possible to grow organized components of the nervous system—that is neurons, axons, oligodendrocytes, and myelin—and that these organized cultures could be used to investigate important questions of nervous system structure, pathology, and immunology. The cultures were grown in what was called a Maximow slide assembly, which allowed fragments of brain or spinal cord tissue to mature and differentiate over 21 days. They could then be exposed to an experimental agent (serum, spinal fluid, virus, etc.) and allowed to grow for another 2–3 weeks before being analyzed to see what changes developed in the cells and tissue.

An example of the unique pioneering and widely cited studies conducted with his Mount Sinai colleague, Stanley Appel and Stanley Crain of Columbia University, Bornstein added serum from rabbits with EAE or serum from MS patients to myelinated cultures that had been grown from rat cerebellum. The mature myelinated nerve fibers in the cultures were completely demyelinated by the serum from animals with EAE or humans with MS, but not after exposure from control serum from normal animals or individuals. Follow-up studies showed that the antibody or immunoglobulin component of the sera was responsible for the damage to myelin, and that sera from normal rabbits or healthy humans produced no similar effect. These studies attracted widespread interest and were published in the renowned jour-

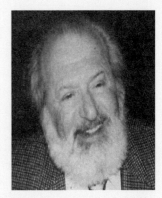

Murray B. Bornstein, 1917–1995

nals *Science* and the *Journal of Experimental Medicine* and were described in an article in *TIME* magazine on June 11, 1965.

From 1958 until 1995, he and his colleagues authored over 120 papers explaining how these organized central nervous system cultures might show the way to answering many neuroscience and immunologic questions. They employed the most up to date neuroscience techniques as they became available; from biochemistry to immunology to physiology, and finally ultrastructure using the electron microscope. Seldom has a scientific career been so focused and productive over a 30-year span. During this time, he became recognized internationally as a creative, important leader in neuroimmunology, especially in the area of MS and its laboratory model EAE.

Bornstein was always interested in what one might call soluble or humeral immune factors. These may well be a critical part of the MS story; they are the factors in solution in serum and spinal fluid (as opposed to cells such as lymphocytes) that might play a role in damaging the MS brain. It was possible to ask these questions using Bornstein's cultures because he and his staff could add serum or spinal fluid from patients with MS or animals with EAE to the organized cultures and observe changes in them. These culture systems also lent themselves to asking important questions about how various viruses may affect the nervous system. This has been a scientific area of continuing interest to MS researchers over the last 100 years, especially when it became possible to isolate specific viruses suspected or known to cause chronic neurologic infectious diseases which might be linked to the cause of MS.

It is of some current interest that, after several decades of research focused primarily on lymphocytes and other immunologically active cells (which are undoubtedly important in MS), new information in the 21st century is emerging about how the cerebral cortex is damaged by the MS process. Recently published studies are again bringing humeral factors, especially factors circulating in the spinal fluid, back to the attention of MS researchers.

Colleagues remembered Bornstein as an energetic, robust person. Other descriptions were that he was enthusiastic, optimistic, and outgoing. He was always notable when entering a room sporting his well-developed, well-trimmed, gray, bushy beard. One colleague commented that Murray always reminded him of a Jewish Santa Claus. Senior lab director, Vincent Spada, a key figure in the program at Albert Einstein, remembered Bornstein as an ideal boss, always concerned about the 20 or so technicians and others in the laboratory. Spada recalled that when grant funds declined from time to time, as they always do in a program dependent on competitive grants from the National Institutes of Health (NIH) or elsewhere, Bornstein would even decrease his own salary temporarily to help pay valuable members of the laboratory staff.

Following their return from Barcelona, Arnon to Rehovot and Bornstein to New York, they soon began to correspond and plan how laboratory and clinical studies might be conducted at Einstein Medical School in the Bronx. Discussing the future of the Cop 1 project, three potential opportunities were becoming clear to the Weizmann team. They were, after all, superb immunochemists and the mysteries of Cop 1 were important and exciting to them. How did Cop 1 work to suppress EAE in so many species of animals, and what was its mechanism of action? This question alone could probably occupy all of the resources of the laboratory for years to come. While they were not physicians, they had always been scientifically linked to medical and health problems in their work with proteins and peptides, and suddenly the idea that they may have a treatment for an important disease like MS was highly energizing. There were no known MS therapies: Could this be the first? If Cop

1 was a therapeutic success, could it have commercial value? To this end, the group prepared patent applications in Israel and elsewhere, and patents for Cop 1 were granted in the early 1970s.

But serious new challenges also confronted the Cop 1 investigators. If Bornstein or others were able to initiate clinical trials in humans with MS, an enormous new responsibility would be laid on the shoulders of the Rehovot investigators. It was assumed that the injections would be done daily and might need to be continued for not only months, but perhaps even for years, in relatively large numbers of trial patients. This was not like animal experimentation in the laboratory, where the duration of observations was short and the entire program could be mapped out and resources allocated in advance. The Cop 1 had to be available for patients month after month, and perhaps year after year. Also, it had to be *standardized*; that is, it had to be safe, free of bacterial contamination; and it had to be *active*, meaning that it had to effectively suppress EAE. What were they getting themselves into?

Work began long before daylight in Rehovot. The initial synthesis of each batch of Cop 1 was the responsibility of Israel Jacobson, whose work and dedication would become essential to the success of the project. Jacobson trained as a pharmacist in Europe, but was forced to leave when the Nazis came to power, arriving at the Sieff Institute in 1938, shortly after its establishment (it became the Weizmann Institute in 1949). He worked with Katchalski on the preparation of amino acids, peptides, and proteins, then came to work with Sela and Arnon in the early stages of the Cop 1 program. Each batch of Cop 1 took over 2 weeks to synthesize and, as time passed, well over 120 batches were prepared in what Arnon calls a continuous production line stretching out over 10 years. Once prepared, each batch had to be tested for its chemical characteristics and also for its ability to suppress EAE in guinea pigs. Dvora Teitelbaum was responsible for this essential work of standardization.

As this activity was going on a few miles from the eastern shore of the Mediterranean Sea, complementary work was under way a few miles from the shores of the Atlantic Ocean in the Bronx. There, Vince Spada shouldered equally serious and responsible duties. Each batch of Cop 1 was received in a frozen and powdered form, which had to be dissolved in sterile water containing sodium chloride and then dispensed into individual vials, each containing a final injectable dose. Each batch was retested for sterility in New York and, over the course of the three major clinical trials conducted by Bornstein, only one failed the sterility test.

In early 1978, Bornstein had the great good fortune to be joined by a serious, enthusiastic, well-trained young neurologist, Aaron Miller, who had recently completed research training in neurovirology, first at Johns Hopkins in Baltimore and then at Einstein.

After extensive planning by Bornstein, Miller, statisticians, and others, a preliminary trial of Cop 1 was initiated in April 1978. The Einstein team had very little on which to base their decisions, and they had to be aware of the potential safety risk to which they were exposing their patients. The early Bronx trial finally recruited 16 patients, 12 with what was described as chronic progressive disease (some patients were confined to bed or in a wheelchair) and four with early relapsing-remitting MS, who were fully active. They all came from Bornstein's practice and were well known to him. The U.S. Food and Drug Administration (FDA) granted permission to start this preliminary trial, and all patients agreed and gave written consent. To ensure adequate observation if any safety complication arose, the patients were hospitalized at the General Clinical Research Center at the Albert Einstein College of Medicine. Blood and cerebrospinal fluid were collected for laboratory analysis. All patients were examined frequently by Miller. The initial hospitalization was for 3 weeks.

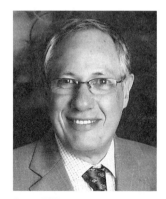

Since the only experience of treating MS patients with Cop 1 had come from Abramsky and Bauer, the investigators in the Bronx were certainly probing in the dark. They had no information about dose, frequency of injections, or route of administration. All had to be determined while watching carefully for any safety issues.

Aaron Miller

As confidence of the safety of the product increased, hospitalization was eliminated. Initially, the patients were given a dose of 5 mg of Cop 1 intramuscularly five times a week for the first 3 weeks, three times a week for the next 3 weeks, twice a week for the next 3 weeks, and finally once a week for the planned 6 months of the trial. The team had the impression that the patients showed improvement early on, but then returned to their pre-study condition as the dose was lowered. One patient was only injected for 3 weeks, but several received Cop 1 for many months. Eight continued to receive injections for several years. Once the initial 6-month program was completed, the dose was slowly increased up to 20 mg given daily by subcutaneous injection. No serious clinical or laboratory abnormalities were observed during the study. By 18 months, the dose had been increased to 20 mg 7 days a week, and 12 patients were maintained on this dose for over 2 years.

Reviewing the results after approximately 2 years, it was concluded that two of the four patients with early relapsing-remitting disease and three of those with chronic progressive disease had, in fact, shown objective improvement; that is, five of the 16 originally recruited seemed to be better. Safety and patient acceptance of the dose appeared to be excellent. All patients had been seen at regular intervals and were carefully examined by Miller. Systematic records were charted and maintained for potential FDA review.

Looking back on these early studies, enormous strides had been made even though the Cop 1 MS project was only in its first stages. Patients with MS had been exposed to the drug in three different clinics: in Jerusalem, in Göttingen, Germany, and in the Bronx. Various doses had been employed, and some glimmer of hope that there was a therapeutic effect had been recognized.

Perhaps just as important, progress in synthesizing and testing the material for chemical standardization and the ability to suppress EAE in guinea pigs had been accomplished in Rehovot. In the Bronx, there was early reassurance that researchers were on the right track and that new clinical research steps should be taken enthusiastically. Could the thick impervious armor of the disease that shatters dreams, that had resisted all treatment efforts for over a century, finally be dented or even pierced?

11

The Bornstein Trials

The stage had been set. Even though the preliminary trials in Jerusalem, Göttingen, Germany, and the Bronx had given an early sense of safety, and had even pointed toward a dose of 20 mg given subcutaneously every day, fewer than 50 multiple sclerosis (MS) patients had been treated with Cop 1 overall. Perhaps there had been some therapeutic effect, but this was only a personal impression by the various investigators. The time had come to put Cop 1 (copolymer one) to the test, to challenge it in a rigorous, scientifically valid placebo-controlled trial.

Most, if not all, U.S. Food and Drug Administration (FDA)-approved drugs must be tested in one or more placebo-controlled trials, the "gold standard" for proving drug safety and efficacy. The complete description for such human studies is "a randomized, double-blind, placebo-controlled trial" carried out with appropriate monitoring for a scientifically reasonable length of time, which in the case of MS, generally means an investigation lasting at least 2 years. As described in Chapter 1, MS is a highly variable and unpredictable disease, and any treatment observations of less than 2 years might give results that were due purely to chance. Chapter 9 describes the various FDA Phases employed to finally determine the safety and value of any drug.

Briefly, the word "randomized" means that patients entering a trial are placed either in the group receiving active drug or the group receiving placebo. A secret selection process is used to guarantee that neither the patient nor the investigator has any choice in or knowledge of the selection. Both the patient and the investigative team must be "blinded," or unaware throughout the trial of the group in which each patient is placed. All patients are observed at regular intervals and will be seen promptly if there is any evidence of new MS activity or of some safety concern. Only after the trial has run its full course is the "code broken" and the group—placebo or active treatment—to which each patient had been assigned revealed. Then, statistical analysis determines if there had been a "significant" result; that is, whether there is at least a 95% likelihood that the final result was not due to chance. Of course, if unexpected safety concerns occur, there may be a need to halt the trial for a time or even terminate it to ensure that patients are not at risk of disease or injury. An independent safety monitoring committee with no direct communication with the investigative team or the patients periodically reviews the accumulating data to ensure that no unforeseen safety issue or injury is occurring.

Bornstein, Miller, statisticians, neuropsychologists, and numerous others met to design what is called "the protocol," that is, the rules or road map for conducting the trial. How many patients would be recruited? How often would injections be given, and at what dose? How often would patients be evaluated neurologically? How often would blood be drawn for safety analysis? Where would the patients come from, and how would they be recruited? All of these and many other questions had to be considered in designing the protocol. Once these questions were resolved, discussions had to be carried out with the Rehovot group to determine if a continuous supply of Cop 1 could be assured.

The final protocol, which Bornstein, Miller, and their team designed, has been recognized as a superb example of how to carry out a clinical trial in MS. As a result, their Cop 1 protocol has served as a model for many subsequent clinical trials of potential MS treatments. The trial would be called "a pilot trial of Cop 1 in early relapsing-remitting MS patients" and would include 50 patients equally randomized to receive active treatment (Cop 1) or placebo, which in this trial would be a weak sterile salt solution. The dose would be 20 mg of Cop 1 injected under the skin (subcutaneously) every day. The trial would be carried out in the Department of Neurology at the Albert Einstein College of Medicine in the Bronx, and the patients would remain ambulatory, without the need for hospitalization. The Committee on Clinical Investigation of the College of Medicine and the FDA reviewed every detail and then gave approval to go forward. Because trials to test new drugs are always very expensive, and there were no resources at the Weizmann Institute and no commercial sponsor had been identified, Bornstein successfully applied to the National Institutes of Health (NIH) in Bethesda, Maryland, for a grant to underwrite the costs of the trial.

Since this trial would be conducted only in the Bronx, all patients had to be recruited from the New York metropolitan area. To identify potential participants, Bornstein chose to advertise the trial both on television and in newspapers in the New York area. While this method has been criticized, it was a very effective way to find suitable and willing patients. At that time, there was certainly a huge unmet medical need for an MS drug of any kind, and it is not surprising that 932 potential volunteers completed a questionnaire describing their individual MS experience. The Einstein group reviewed all the questionnaires and chose 140 candidates, who were evaluated at the College of Medicine using both neurologic and psychosocial examinations. Fifty patients were finally accepted into the trial, 25 randomized to receive active Cop 1 and 25 randomized to the placebo group. The selected patients had very active MS with a history of between two and eight MS relapses in the 2 years prior to entry into the trial. They were spread across the various levels of disability as measured by the Expanded Disability Status Scale (EDSS) previously described in Chapter 1. For example, six in the placebo group and four in the active drug group were at EDSS 6 level and required some kind of daily walking aid to compensate for their gait impairment.

At the beginning, all patients were instructed about the purpose of the study and the method of self-injection, and were then asked to sign a consent form before receiving their study materials. They visited the clinic 1 month later and then every 3 months for the balance of the 2 years of the trial. At each visit, they were examined by a neurologist who was unaware of their randomization group. Only the clinical assistant lab chief, Vincent Spada, was aware of the patient group assignment, and only he was allowed to gather information on side effects from the patients. In speaking to several members of the research team, it is obvious that the blinding mechanism was well maintained throughout the course of the 2-year investigation. Both blood and urine analysis were undertaken every 3 months to help assure patient safety during this critical trial.

When any completed clinical trial is reported in a medical journal, the bare facts are clearly laid out. They include the type of drug or agent and the details of the protocol followed; these details include the length of the trial and the final results, comparing the treated and placebo groups to establish whether the study was significant or not. While these reports are the scientific backbone of clinical medicine and are of considerable interest to physicians and other investigators, they are usually not recommended for relaxed bedtime reading!

None of the actual day-to-day activity involved in a trial or the work that consumes the clinic or—more importantly—the personal feelings of the participants, are described or make it to the final scientific publication. In fact, clinical trials are hard, everyday work. For instance, for the 2-year Cop 1 pilot trial there were approximately 400 patient visits to the Bronx MS Clinic, all of which had to be scheduled, usually by a study coordinator. On the day of the visit, in addition to questions about safety, the patient was examined by a neurologist and specimens were collected for the laboratory. Personal concerns and patient anxieties had to be addressed. Clinical trials are serious scientific experiments, and the FDA demands meticulous record-keeping on specially designed forms that must be completed and available for unannounced audits or examination by the FDA at any time. In addition, all records are carefully preserved for 7 or more years after the trial is completed. If presumptive MS relapses occur—and they always do in MS trials—the patient must be evaluated within a short period of time, usually within 7 days, when a decision is made as to whether this is a side effect of the drug, an MS attack, or some other safety issue that must be immediately attended to. In the Cop 1 pilot trial, approximately three out of every four patients who experienced an MS relapse were prescribed steroids by the investigative team—the standard form of therapy to reduce the severity of MS relapses.

For each patient volunteering for this or any MS trial, life changes, taking on a new meaning and rhythm. First, the patients commit to visiting the clinic every 3 months and, of course, must faithfully inject their study medication (Cop 1 or placebo) every day. At the time of the Cop 1 pilot trial, there was still a serious question of safety and the risk of a dangerous reaction to the drug. The patients all realized that they had a 50% chance of being randomized to the placebo group. However, they were also personally aware that it would never be possible to prove that Cop 1 was a useful MS drug if they were unwilling to agree to that chance. In fact, every patient, both those receiving active drug and those receiving placebo, provided equally valuable information to the final outcome of the trial.

Most patients participating in this or any other MS trials will, in time, find the experience to be a positive one. They have the sense that they may be helping themselves to find a treatment for their life-long, life-defining disease. They also recognize that they may be contributing to the well-being of the entire MS population that would benefit from Cop 1 or any therapy that improved the course of the disease. Over time, patients accommodate to the rhythm of the trial and even look forward to meeting with the study coordinator and the neurologist involved. Unlike their life before they received the diagnosis of MS, they must now live every day carrying the image of that distant black cloud on their personal horizon, of the risk of a new serious relapse. The chance to avoid or at least reduce that risk urges them on.

In spite of meticulous screening and careful decision-making in the patient selection process at the Bronx MS clinic, it turned out that two of the 50 patients were psychologically unable to participate; thus, the final study population was 48 patients. Five patients dropped out over the 2-year trial duration, but four of these participated well into the second year and provided useful information.

The *principal endpoint* is a fundamental concept in understanding how clinical research trials work. Prior to the start of any trial, the investigative team must identify and state a principal endpoint that they plan to achieve. That is, they must declare that the study drug will be more effective than the placebo in one well-defined aspect. This must be stated in the protocol and agreed upon with the FDA prior to onset of the trial. There is a good reason for this. Many endpoints may be considered and analyzed in an MS trial; these might be, for example, the number of relapses experienced by each group, the duration of time between relapses, the number of patients who experienced no relapses during the course of the trial, or even some measurable difference in the increase in disability between the two groups (those taking the active drug and those receiving the placebo). One endpoint must be chosen as the principal one to avoid the possibility that, at the trial's conclusion, only one endpoint of many would be positive and the investigators would argue that the drug should be approved by the FDA even if all of the other endpoints failed to achieve significance. The choice of the principal endpoint can never be selected in hindsight.

The Bornstein group chose as their principal endpoint "the proportion of relapse-free patients," that is, the number of Cop 1-treated patients who completed the trial without suffering a relapse would be significantly more than the group of patients who had received placebo and had no relapses. This was a formidable endpoint to choose. In addition, the research group would analyze the number of attacks in each group (called the *relapse rate*) and also—critically important for both investigators and patients—the average amount of increased disability that was experienced by each group.

The trial continued—some would say plodded on—over the 2 years as the patients came and went, yet each visit, each relapse, and each safety check added to the accumulating mass of facts, the database which would spell success or failure for Cop 1 as an MS therapy.

A sense of excitement began to grow both in the Cop 1 discovery group at the Weizmann Institute and the clinical trial group in the Bronx, but there was also a sense of anxiety as the investigators began to anticipate receiving information about the final outcome of this pilot trial, which had been so long in coming. The last patient came for a final visit by May 1985, the last report form was placed in that patient's binder, and the final report had been received from the clinical laboratory. A preplanned statistical analysis program had been developed, and the statisticians had the tens of thousands of bits of information to condense into the outcome or final picture of the results. It was time for the "code to be broken." Who had injected Cop 1 and who had received placebo? And how did each fare?

The results were stunning. At least in this small placebo-controlled trial, there seemed little doubt that Cop 1 had a very significant beneficial effect on early relapsing MS. Six of 23 patients in the placebo group (26%) and 14 of 25 patients in the Cop 1 group (56%) had no exacerbations or relapses during the 2 years of study. For this principal endpoint, there was a clear, significant difference favoring Cop 1. Sixty-two relapses were experienced by patients in the placebo group and only 16 in the Cop 1 group, meaning, on average, that each patient injecting placebo had 2.7 relapses whereas the patients injecting Cop 1 had only 0.6 relapses over the 2 years of careful observation. The effect on relapses seemed to be more obvious in those patients who had less evidence of neurologic disability when they entered the trial. Cop 1 also had a significant beneficial effect on avoiding the accumulation of disability during the 2 years of observations. While receiving Cop 1, on average, the treated group only declined by half an EDSS unit, whereas those who had received placebo had worsened by 1.2 EDSS units.

There was also clear evidence of safety, defined as a low risk of side effects. More brief injection site reactions or evidence of skin irritation at the injection site were noted for patients who received Cop 1 (copolymer one), and a rare systemic reaction consisting of facial flushing, chest tightness or pain, rapid heartbeat, and anxiety was experienced by a few patients immediately after making the Cop 1 injection; fortunately, this reaction was self-limited, lasting only a few minutes, and it appeared to be benign.

Once the results were announced, Vincent Spada, the study coordinator in the Bronx, described how Bornstein kept asking the statisticians to recheck the numbers to be sure they were right. On seeing the results for the first time, Miller confessed that he was dumbfounded. The investigators in Rehovot and those in the Bronx were finally convinced. They stared at each other and asked, "Have we done it, have we finally found a treatment that can, for the first time, benefit MS patients, and that might also be safe to use on a long-term basis?" Time would tell.

Charcot had made his dismal assessment of MS treatment prospects an incredible 119 years earlier. In well over a century following his remarks, virtually hundreds of potential MS treatments had been considered, tried, and failed. Now there was tentative evidence of a long-term, safe treatment that would benefit the course of MS.

Barely able to control their excitement and relief, the collaborators in the United States and Israel plowed into the task of writing an account of the Cop 1 trial in early MS and submitting it for publication. After carefully considering every word and constructing a number of figures and tables that clearly explained the results, a manuscript was submitted to the *New England Journal of Medicine* by the 15 authors who had contributed to the success of the study. It was accepted and published on August 13, 1987, a date that will remain throughout MS history as a landmark turning point.

The response to the article was interesting but mixed. Patients cheered and of course wanted access to Cop 1 immediately, but it was not available and—as events unfolded—would not be on the market for almost another decade. The reaction in the medical community was more reserved. While potentially important, the trial was, after all, quite small—only 48 patients in what was correctly termed a pilot trial. How did Cop 1 work? What was its mechanism of action? Could it be even called a drug when it was described as a mixture of polymers quite unlike the single-molecule drugs doctors had been used to ever since their pharmacology classes in medical school? Even Dr. Bornstein's rather extroverted personality and his use of public media to attract patients to the trial were discussed. More evidence was needed.

The Chronic Progressive Multiple Sclerosis Trial

As noted in Chapter 1, MS is a highly variable and unpredictable disease; however, observations over long periods show that patients almost always start with a relapsing-remitting phase which, after an average of 10 to 15 years, changes to what has been called the chronic progressive stage. These two stages are not easy to identify as the change is occurring, but looking back, a doctor can clearly see how the disease pattern had changed. In the chronic progressive stage, patients are likely to have many fewer relapses but instead begin to show progression; that is, their level of neurologic disability increases. While at one time patients might have had relapses that almost completely resolved, over time they begin to notice difficulty with walking or some other neurologic dysfunction. They begin noticing difficulty with climbing stairs, often with some sensory changes; then, several months or a few years later, they notice that they can no longer walk very far unaided and must depend on a cane, a crutch, or another ambulatory aid to get around at all. This was called the *chronic progressive* stage. Recently, the terminology has changed, so that now neurologists talk about the relapsing-remitting stage followed by the secondary progressive stage. This implies that the patient at one time experienced relapses but now notes either unrelenting increases in disability or disability interspersed with periods of stability before the progression once again surfaces, robbing the patient of independence and often reducing the ability to function at home and in society. In time, this impairs patient homemaking, parenting, employment, and even the ability to fully participate in social activities.

This was all well known to Bornstein and his colleagues when they first began to plan their placebo-controlled trials, and it seemed logical to run two trials; one for relapsing-remitting patients and a second one to test Cop 1 in chronic progressive patients. In fact, there was some overlap in the two trials, even though the relapsing-remitting one was carried out and completed prior to the conclusion of the second one, which was entitled "A Placebo-Controlled, Double Blind, Randomized Two-Center Pilot Trial of Cop 1 in Chronic Progressive Multiple Sclerosis."

Whereas the first trial was conducted only in Einstein, in New York, Bornstein decided that the progressive trial would be more rapidly enrolled if two centers cooperated. He reached out to his old colleague from his early laboratory days, Stanley Appel, who had become Chairman of the Department of Neurology at the Baylor School of Medicine in Houston, Texas.

The protocol, or design, of the chronic progressive trial is quite sophisticated and rather complicated, requiring that recruited patients demonstrate that they had entered the progressive stage. They had to be between the ages of 20 to 60 years, with clear neurologic disability up to the point at which that they might require some kind of an external walking aid. Using their previously successful method to get the word out, the trial was widely advertised in both New York and Houston, and a total of 2,270 interested patients were screened either by phone or questionnaire. Of these, 370 were selected for neurologic and psychological evaluations. From these, 169 patients were actually selected and entered into an innovative pretrial study period that lasted for between 6 and 15 months, when objective evidence of increased neurologic worsening or progression based on repeated neurologic examinations was observed.

Due to the demand for evidence of progression before the patients were even randomized, only 106 patients ultimately qualified for entry into what was planned as a 2-year trial. Of these, 55 were at Einstein in New York and 51 were at Baylor in Houston. The dose of Cop 1 was still in question, and it was decided to require two injections under the skin each day. For those patients randomized for active Cop 1, a dose of 15 mg per injection (a total of 30 mg per day) was chosen. The placebo patients also were required to make two injections a day to maintain the blinded nature of the trial. The Cop 1 continued to be made either at the Weizmann Institute or at a commercial laboratory attached to the Weizmann, the Bio-Yeda Company, also located in Rehovot. The patients were examined by the blinded neurologist every 3 months, and side effects were only revealed to the clinic coordinators at the two institutions to maintain blinding.

For a time in the mid-1980s, the two pilot trials overlapped, and the demand for Cop 1 was greatly increased. In fact, for 1 month, no Cop 1 was available to supply the chronic progressive trial, and the patients who had been randomized to active drug had to be switched to placebo for 30 days. Neither the patients nor the investigators were informed of this temporary switch until later, and neither patients nor neurologists noticed any change in the patients' status or side effects during this brief period.

Multiple sclerosis is never a simple disease to follow and analyze, even in the course of a treatment trial. Recognizing change in neurologic disability is considered to be more difficult than simply counting relapses. In order to improve the understanding of what was going on, a concept of confirmed or sustained progression has evolved as a well-established component of most MS trials. Using this concept, the investigators not only had to determine that the patient had worsened in some defined way using the EDSS scale, but also that the worsening was maintained or even increased at a subsequent visit 3 months later. This required that the examining neurologist not only be an expert in how to measure the EDSS but also that, if at all possible, the same examiner be available to evaluate each patient at each 3-month interval throughout the course of the trial.

The principal endpoint was time to reach a confirmed progression; that is, each randomized patient injecting either Cop 1 or placebo would either worsen and maintain that worsening for at least 3 months or be neurologically stable or perhaps even improved. A minimum of eight neurologic examinations were required, and all were entered into the accumulating database.

The patients chosen at the two centers were very similar, with an average age of 42 years; 54% were women. They were quite disabled, with an average EDSS score of 5.7, meaning that almost all had considerable difficulty with walking, and about 65% required some kind of aid in walking, such as a cane or a crutch. In spite of their advanced level of neurologic disability, 81% of patients were able to complete all of the requirements of the study; that is, they continued the twice-daily injections until they either worsened for at least 3 months or completed the 2 years of observations in a stable or improved condition.

When all of the data from both centers had been collected and analyzed at the end of 2 years, it turned out that nine patients who had received Cop 1 and 14 patients who had received placebo had shown confirmed progression. Although this was a positive trend in favor of Cop 1, it did not reach a statistical level of significance. Subsequent analysis on the patients at each center showed a surprising and disappointing difference, which made for further confusion in understanding the final results. For those patients studied at Einstein, significantly more placebo patients progressed, whereas at Baylor the two populations, Cop 1 and placebo, experienced almost the same chance of progressing or worsening.

The safety profile was similar to that observed in the relapsing-remitting pilot trial, with no serious safety issues. More patients receiving Cop 1 displayed brief injection site reactions in the skin, and 12 patients who received Cop 1 displayed short periods of flushing, chest tightness, fast heartbeat, and anxiety, which developed right after the injection. This lasted 3 to 10 minutes and produced no serious after effects.

In discussing the somewhat disappointing results of this chronic progressive trial, the investigators noted the peculiar discrepancy between the fact that all of the patients before entering the trial had shown evidence of progression, whereas only 23 continued to progress during the 2 years when they received injections, either Cop 1 or placebo. Also of note was the fact that there was evidence of MS progression in the placebo group at Einstein, but no evidence of progression in Baylor, a finding that is still unexplained. Nevertheless, the opportunity to demonstrate that few safety issues surfaced in a larger population of MS patients injected with a larger dose (30 mg per day) was encouraging in considering further development of Cop 1 as an MS drug.

Later, another approved MS drug, beta-interferon, was shown in repeated trials to be efficacious in relapsing-remitting patients, yet failed when tested in chronic progressive patients. Continuing observations show how difficult it is to influence MS in its more advanced stages.

12

Could Cop 1 Be a Successful Drug?

By the middle of the 1980s, Sela, Arnon, and their young colleague, Teitelbaum, could already look back on fruitful and highly productive scientific careers. After helping to pry open the black box of protein structure and learning much about the manufacture of synthetic amino acid polymers and peptides in the laboratory of their mentor, Ephraim Katchalski, they had journeyed on independently. The area they chose to explore was of critical importance in biology: What were the features of a protein that allowed it to act as an antigen? That is, why did some proteins stimulate a response from the mammalian immune system, whereas others did not? This, of course, was critical to understanding how the interaction between proteins and the immune system could work both in a protective way, for instance as a vaccine, or as a destructive force, as in an autoimmune disease.

All of this meant that they were pioneers in uniting protein chemistry with immunology. Their success in this field was not long in coming, and had far-reaching consequences. They received recognition and honors not only in Israel but also in Europe, the United States, and in several Asian countries. Their program in immunologic chemistry was elevated to a department at the Weizmann Institute. Sela became the first chairman of this department but later, as his administrative skills became increasingly apparent and he assumed the responsibilities as president of the entire Weizmann Institute of Science, Arnon became the acting chairman of the department.

Sela's influence and impact on science were not restricted to his activities at the Weizmann Institute in Rehovot. During his tenure as a visiting scientist at the National Institutes of Health (NIH) in Bethesda, Maryland, he contributed directly to those scientific discoveries that led to the award of two Nobel Prizes, first for helping to decipher the genetic code with Marshall Nirenberg, and later for proving the understanding of the structure of enzymes with Chris Anfinsen.

What is surprising, remarkable, and impressive is that this world-class scientific activity was not being performed in the safe, ivy-covered walls of academia in Western Europe, the United Kingdom, or the United States. It was being conducted in the regionally unsettled environment of Israel, where wars were close at hand, and danger and turmoil were never far away.

It was in this unique juxtaposition of highly creative scientific progress and achievement and regional turmoil and danger that the Weizmann team confronted their next challenge and a perplexing dilemma. They had been pursuing their dream of a treatment for multiple sclerosis (MS) for almost 20 years. They had studied Cop 1, an unusual four-amino acid copolymer, in the laboratory and in innumerable animal experiments in several species. And, with their medical partners in Jerusalem, Germany, and New York, they had tested its action in MS patients. Where to turn next? How could Cop 1 be taken to the next critical and most important level—a commercially available MS treatment that could benefit tens of thousands, perhaps even hundreds of thousands of people with MS?

The answer was clear. They had to find a partner in the commercial pharmaceutical industry, one that had interest and financial resources, could review the vast amount of animal and increasingly impressive human data, and would agree to sponsor the large human trials required. That partner would have to take on the daunting task of maneuvering through the complex international regulatory environment and initiate an expensive marketing campaign that would finally bring

Cop 1 to the bedside, into the daily lives of MS patients, and begin to improve the outlook of victims of the disease that shattered dreams.

The Search for a Commercial Partner

Arnon immediately began the quest for a reliable partner. Refining the data from the human trials in Israel, Germany, and especially the United States under the leadership of Bornstein, she created an impressive therapeutic history of Cop 1. To this, she added collected animal data, including the movies of the baboon that recovered from acute experimental allergic encephalomyelitis (EAE). Then she set out for the United States.

Her first visit was to Johnson & Johnson in New Jersey, followed by a trip to Upjohn in Kalamazoo, Michigan. At each company, she met with leaders in the clinical research departments and in each case the final result was the same. They marveled at the persistence of the Weizmann group, they were amazed by the immunologic and chemical activity of this strange therapeutic approach that could not be defined as a single-chemical molecule. Finally, they decided that because the drug had not evolved from their own laboratory efforts, or perhaps because it was targeted for a relatively rare disease, they were unwilling to recommend Cop 1 to company management. Arnon later recounted that perhaps if she had sought out company leaders in marketing, rather than in research, she would have received a more positive answer.

Sela was always uneasy with the approach to foreign pharmaceutical companies, the so-called "big pharma." As a scientist, not a business person experienced in the development of commercial drugs, he was uneasy about forming a partnership—in fact a bond—with people in corporations that were far removed from his world of scientific openness and transparency. Where else could they turn?

The Israeli company, Teva Pharmaceutical Industries Ltd., had consolidated with other small Israeli pharmaceutical and chemical firms. It was renowned in Israel but was certainly very modest by international standards. In fact, when the Weizmann laboratories were having difficulty manufacturing and supplying Cop 1 for the Bornstein clinical trials in the United States, the Weizmann team had approached Teva about aiding with its manufacture. A young scientist who had recently come to Teva, Dr. David Ladkani, went to Rehovot and worked with Israel Jacobson on the benchtop Cop 1 manufacturing process. Could Teva be the

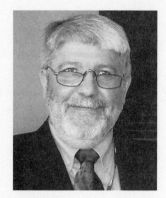

David Ladkani

long-sought partner in its further development? Did this modest Israeli company have the knowledge and resources to develop Cop 1 into a viable international commercial product, which the Weizmann scientists envisioned?

As Sela sat at his desk at the Weizmann Institute considering further options for the development of Cop 1 as an MS treatment, he reached behind his desk and took a box off the bookshelf. He carefully took out and opened a leather-bound book in which, for many years, he had collected autographs of visitors to the Weizmann. It was an intimate record of important leaders in many fields of enterprise who had visited him in Rehovot. There were signatures from stars of the entertainment world—Kirk Douglas and Grace Kelly, Princess of Monaco; from productive world leaders in science, especially biologic science, among them Byron Waxman, formerly of Harvard and Yale, and then head of the research program at the National Multiple Sclerosis Society; from political leaders, such as Henry Kissinger; and from luminaries from the world of the arts, including his close friend, Zubin Meyta, conductor of the Israel symphony.

As his fingers traced down the incredible list of talented individuals who had contributed so much to society, it stopped at the name of Eli Hurvitz, the President and CEO of Teva Pharmaceutical Industries for many years, and a friend of Sela and of the Weizmann. Could Teva, well-known in Israel but miniscule among the pharmaceutical giants of the world, be the partner that could take Cop 1 to commercial success and bring the first successful drug to the hundreds of thousands of people with MS?

Sometime in 1985, Sela and his wife, Sara, invited Hurvitz and his wife, Dalia, to dinner. Sela asked Hurvitz to arrange for a slide projector and screen, and the four of them looked carefully at the animal and human data that had been accumulated over the past 17 years. Hurvitz was intrigued and, as Sela says, he had the vision and courage to consider negotiating a contract with the Weizmann to develop Cop 1 as an innovative drug for MS. As Sela has said, "The rest is history." A partnership had been struck between two giants on the Israeli scene (albeit very small players on the world stage)—Teva and the Weizmann Institute. This led, over the next decade, to a huge medical and commercial success.

PART III

Teva Pharmaceuticals

13

Teva

Teva Pharmaceuticals of Israel has, over the last three decades, enjoyed outstanding—almost unbelievable—success and growth, with the first decade of the 21st century probably being the most remarkable period of all. The company is now ranked among the top 20 pharmaceutical concerns in the world, and among the ten largest companies on NASDAQ. For several years, it has been listed as number one in generic prescription drug sales in North America, Europe, and elsewhere. Truly global in scope, Teva now has manufacturing and/or marketing locations in the United States, Canada, France, Italy, Great Britain, Hungary, Holland, and a variety of other worldwide locations. But how and when did this remarkable success story begin?

The arc of history hovers over few areas of the globe as it does over the region adjacent to the eastern shores of the Mediterranean Sea. A narrow level plain only 10 to 15 miles in width runs along the eastern end of the Mediterranean. To the south is the arid Negev desert and to the north the mountains of Lebanon. This relatively narrow path has been used as a major human highway since prehistory, and could conceivably have even been the ground traveled by early humans when they first emerged from Africa. For thousands of years, camel caravans have transported goods from or to Africa and the Far East, north to Anatolia (now Turkey), and on to many western and northern lands, including Greece and Rome.

This corridor has trembled beneath chariot wheels and the cadence of hundreds of thousands of military sandals as the land was invaded and fought over. The Hittites came south out of what is now Turkey, the Egyptians marched north, the Assyrians and Babylonians came from the east, and Alexander and his Greek armies, and later the Romans, came from the west. From Europe, Crusaders marched into the area inflamed by their goal of capturing Jerusalem. Perhaps hundreds of other tribes, nations, and empires invaded this region. For the local inhabitants of each era, these centuries of incursions were at best unsettling and probably much worse. Then, for three or more centuries prior to the beginning of the 20th century, this area, which came to be called Palestine, was relatively calm. It was controlled by the government of the great Ottoman Empire, held in place under the Sultan, who lived in and ruled from the Topkapi Palace in Constantinople (now Istanbul).

Palestine stretches east from the Mediterranean beaches across the coastal plain and up over the Judean Hills, rising almost 3,000 feet to the ancient, historic, and religiously unmatched city of Jerusalem, which is spread over several mounts or hills. The land then drops precipitously into a deep valley, the site of the Sea of Galilee, which receives water from the mountains of Lebanon and Syria before flowing into the Jordan River, which empties into the mineral- and salt-laden Dead Sea several hundred feet below sea level. To the south are the deserts of Egypt and to the north mountainous Lebanon.

After centuries of comparative quiet, at the onset of the 20th century Palestine would again become roiled in strife, and periods of turmoil and war would again threaten the population. The Ottoman Empire was becoming weak and fragmented under pressures radiating from the conflict of World War I being waged in Europe. As the war was winding down, two powerful European imperial nations, France and Britain, focused their interest on the general region of the Middle East. They began between them to draw what sometimes were artificial boundaries to create new nations for which they selected new leadership groups. From this practice of nation building, fostered by the League of Nations, emerged the new states of Iraq, Syria, Lebanon, Trans Jordan, and Palestine.

On December 11, 1917, British General Allenby marched with his Army through the Jaffa Gate into Jerusalem, and in July 1920, a civil administration—the British Mandate for Palestine—took over under the authority of the League of Nations. For the first time since Crusader days, Jerusalem was again a capital city. Palestine, in fact, was rather advanced among the new Middle Eastern nations created by this practice of imperial fabrication and domination.

Somewhat earlier, in the spring of 1901, three entrepreneurs, Salomon, Levin, and Elstein, celebrated the establishment of a wholesale drug distribution company in a storefront-like building in Jerusalem. Their plan was to develop a regional business, even though many of their products were, by necessity for that time and place, carried by donkey carts and camels. Tel Aviv was only a tiny village; however, there was gateway port activity at Jaffa and at Haifa along the Mediterranean coast. Further afield were large, well-established, and ancient cities, such as Beirut and Damascus, although they were not then national capitals but rather outposts of the crumbling Ottoman Empire. The new company certainly supplied both Jewish and Palestinian Arab retail establishments, because the population of Palestine was only about 11% Jewish in 1901, out of a total population of about 600,000. (All population numbers from this era are questionable, for there was no distinct district of Palestine and for various reasons [taxes, etc.], the population avoided census procedures.) Women, children, and Bedouins (migratory Arabs living in the desert) were certainly undercounted.

In spite of the decline of the Ottoman Empire and the increasing turmoil in the Middle East, the small drug distribution company of Soloman, Levin, and Elstein, Ltd. continued to be successful. It is hard to imagine just how business was carried out in this region during the first three decades of the 20th century. Stimulated by the large immigration of European Jews, there were Arab riots, attacks, and even massacres of Jews in 1921, 1929, and especially between 1936 and 1939, when thousands of Jewish farms and orchards were destroyed and their owners forced to flee to safer areas.

In 1935, expanding on the past, Elsa Kuver and Dr. Gunter Friedlander established a new concern within the business regulations of the British Mandate. They chose the name *Teva*, which means "Nature" in Hebrew, as all their initial products were based on natural substances. They established, in Petah Tiqva, close to the rapidly expanding city of Tel Aviv, a pharmaceutical manufacturing facility, Assia. At around the same time, other pharmaceutical plants were established in Palestine; Zori in Tel Aviv, Ikapharm in Kfar Saba, and Abic. Eventually all merged to become part of Teva.

At least three forces were converging on the society of Palestine in the 1930s, which surely influenced the history and growth of Teva. First was the international Zionist movement that was promoting worldwide efforts to encourage the immigration of Jews into Palestine. Second was the British Mandate, which leaned toward separation of the country into two political entities, one of which would be a Jewish homeland. This had been established by the Balfour Declaration of 1917. The third was Nazi persecution of German and other European Jews, which forced many people to flee Germany and central Europe, a large number of whom made their way to Palestine. By 1948, over 600,000 Jews were living in Palestine. In 1940 alone, over 60,000 Jews relocated there, often confronting poor and even miserable living conditions.

Between the two 20th-century world wars, Germany had become an international pharmaceutical powerhouse. Schering and Merck were well-recognized pharmaceutical giants, for example. Large numbers of Jewish physicians, pharmacists, chemists, and other scientists with expertise in the pharmaceutical industry had been forced to flee Europe and had immigrated to Palestine. For example, by 1940, there were 40 physicians for every 10,000 Jews in Palestine, the highest concentration in the world. Next in physician numbers was Switzerland, with 17 per 10,000 inhabitants. Among Arabs in Palestine, there were only 2.9 physicians per 10,000, still the largest concentration among Middle Eastern countries. Thus, there was a large concentration of exceptionally well-trained individuals to help foster a new pharmaceutical industry in Palestine and the soon-to-emerge State of Israel.

During World War II, when military action raged throughout much of Europe and into the Middle East, transportation lines were severed and the only source for medications and other medical supplies was from local concerns such as Teva. The company grew rapidly. In 1951, only 3 years after the new State of Israel was declared, a new financial entity, the Tel Aviv Stock Exchange was established and Teva was one of the first to become a publicly traded company on that exchange, allowing it to raise new capital through stock offerings. Other embryonic pharmaceutical and chemical companies were being established in the early days of the State of Israel, driven by the large population of well-educated, talented, and entrepreneurial immigrants. Two other Israeli drug companies, Assia and Zori, had acquired a controlling interest in Teva and, in 1976, the three firms merged to create the modern Teva Pharmaceutical Industries. This was just the beginning of a program of acquisitions and mergers that led to the creation of the giant pharmaceutical company that Teva has become today.

The 1976 merger resulted in a highly valuable addition that may not have been fully recognized at that time. The new Teva acquired the talents of a person who would undoubtedly in time be recognized as one of the business executive geniuses of Israel, Eli Hurvitz. Hurvitz was born in Palestine and trained as an economist at the Hebrew University after serving in the Israeli Defense Forces in Israel's War of Independence in 1948. He started his career in 1953, at Assia, and rose in the levels of management of that company. With the consolidation in 1976, he became the general manager of the newly created merged entity Teva Pharmaceutical Industries.

From his appointment as head of Teva in 1976, until he ended his term as President and CEO to become Chairman of the Board in 2002, Hurvitz has "made his mark," not only on Teva but on the business climate of Israel and on Israel itself. He has served as Chairman of the Israel Export Institute and President of the Israel Industrialists Association. He has been Chairman of the Institute for the Development of Jerusalem, and Chairman of the Executive Council and Committee of the Weizmann Institute and the Ben Gurion Uni-

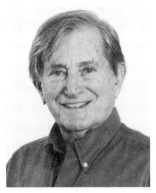

Eli Hurvitz

versity. He was awarded the Israel Prize-Lifetime Achievement Award and, more recently, a similar award from the Israel Ministry of Industry and Trade for the development of Israel's exports. Internationally, Hurvitz served as a member of the International Counsel of the Belfer Center for Science and International Affairs at Harvard University.

In 2004, the Eli Hurvitz Institute of Strategic Management was established at the Tel Aviv University to provide advanced professional and executive business training.

Even though successful, Teva was, in 1976, still a small regional company doing business primarily in Israel and Africa. It had no market influence in Europe or—more importantly—in the United States, the largest market for pharmaceutical products in the world. In 1980, Teva took over another Israeli company, Ikapharm which, with government assistance, had built a state-of-the-art pharmaceutical manufacturing plant in Kfar Saba, another suburb of Tel Aviv. This plant was capable of manufacturing drugs to U.S. Food and Drug Administration (FDA) standards, and in 1982, was approved by the FDA for manufacture of products that could be marketed in the U.S. This, of course, was a monumental step, allowing Teva to potentially view the United States as a market for its generic drugs.

Beneficial activities on the other side of the Atlantic were underway in the 1980s. In 1984, the U.S. Congress passed the Hatch-Waxman Act, which allowed for the sale of generic copies of prescription drugs that had lost patent protection. This Act opened the door for the huge generic prescription drug industry that we now take for granted. Concurrently, Teva went through a profound process of strategic thinking and reached the conclusion that the U.S. generic market was its number-one opportunity for growth.

By this time, Teva had gained the expertise to manufacture quality generic drugs that met FDA standards under license from a long list of major global pharmaceutical companies for consumption in Israel, and it had recently acquired the manufacturing plant to make this possible. What it lacked was capital and connections to get a foothold into the U.S. commercial market. With careful planning, in 1985, Teva entered a 50/50 joint venture with the W.R. Grace conglomerate of New

York to create TAG (Teva and Grace) Pharmaceutical, to which Grace contributed 93% of TAG's $23 million starting capital base while Teva contributed $1.5 million and its decades of experience and expertise. This allowed TAG to acquire Lemmon Pharmaceuticals from its German parent for $12.7 million. Lemmon, a Pennsylvania generic drug manufacturing and marketing company, had a somewhat rocky corporate history over its 15 years in business and, at the time of acquisition, had sales of about $20 million. Importantly, Lemmon opened the door to the U.S. generic market as the sales and distribution arm for generic drugs manufactured by Teva in Israel. This venture was immediately successful. At the time of the Lemmon acquisition, Teva sales were $17 million, whereas 2 years later sales had grown to $40 million. At the time, Teva was marketing seven generic versions of branded drugs in the U.S. Furthering its U.S. presence, in 1982, Teva was listed for the first time on NASDAQ, one of the major U.S. stock exchanges. By 1989, sales had increased to $268 million. Just as the consolidation in Israel had brought the unique executive talents of Eli Hurvitz to a leadership role, acquiring Lemmon allowed Teva to gain the knowledge and experience of another gifted leader, William Fletcher.

Born in Liverpool, England, Fletcher completed a degree in international marketing, and then moved to Paris and became involved in the European pharmaceutical industry. After 7 years, he was, as he says, "getting restless" and began looking for a position in the U.S. because "all marketers wanted to work in the U.S." He had joined Lemmon in 1980, and had experienced some of its corporate turmoil, including its purchase by a German company that had added several poorly aligned activities and products to its inventory. Buying into Teva's culture and vision in 1985 allowed Fletcher to blossom and add to the stirring success that Teva's U.S. thrust was building.

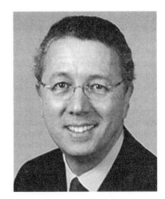

William Fletcher

In 2002, in reviewing his 26-year tenure as President and CEO of Teva, Hurvitz stated, "I would like to summarize the strategy we adopted in the '80s. We decided that in the first stage, we would become a global generic company; we aimed to enter the United States, and then, 'when we felt comfortable,' we would go into Europe. In the second stage, in addition to our regular activity, we would find niches for generic activity with added value. In the third stage, we would enter the field of innovative products. We estimated that each stage would take five to seven years. And indeed, in 1985, we entered the United States, and in the early '90s, we saw real profits from generics. In 1997, we put Copaxone, our first innovative product, on the market. Everything went more or less according to plan."

Like a plane taking off from an Israeli runway in the mid-1980s, Teva had been launched on a new journey. With 80 years of history behind it, the company had exceptional leadership at the controls. It had the ability to manufacture quality generic drugs that were accepted by regulatory agencies at the FDA and elsewhere. A foothold had been established in the dominant U.S. market. A vital regulatory law had been passed in 1985 that would probably reduce business turbulence as Teva flew forward. Modern Teva Pharmaceuticals was on its way, with the stated goal of joining the major international pharmaceutical companies of the world.

14

The U.S. Pivotal Trial

Approaching a bridge, especially on a journey to an unexplored land, both anticipation and apprehension rise: Is it safe? What about traffic competition? Are there tolls at the far end? Is there a clear path, or are there difficult obstacles beyond the span? In 1987, having concluded negotiations with the Weizmann Institute of Science to develop Cop 1 as an innovative drug for multiple sclerosis (MS), the Teva management team faced major, possibly project-defeating challenges, crossing the bridge from generics to its own innovative product. Rapid success had materialized in the strategic goals of creating a profitable global generic drug company and the penetration of the huge U.S. market. But the third goal that Eli Hurvitz had outlined in the 1980s—entering the innovative drug competition—involved an enormous increase in complexity, cost, and risk.

Teva had never sponsored a placebo-controlled pivotal trial for any drug or indication prior to Cop 1. The Bornstein relapsing MS trial, while significant, was much too small to convince regulatory agencies to grant permission to market Cop 1. In addition, Food and Drug Administration (FDA) regulations in the U.S. at least, required that there be two independent Phase III trials of adequate size and duration before a new drug application (NDA) could even be prepared and submitted for approval. Where should a Phase III "pivotal" trial be conducted: In the United States, in Europe, or both? Israel was too small and had an inadequate population of MS patients to consider doing a large trial there. Vigorous internal discussion was undertaken.

Multiple sclerosis was a mysterious disease to the leaders at Teva. Its clinical pattern was variable and unpredictable, divided into various phases: relapsing-remitting, chronic progressive, or primary progressive, any of which could be the therapeutic target of a trial of Cop 1. There must be advantages to choosing one phase versus another to test the benefit of Cop 1 on MS. Was MS even a suitable disease to consider when anticipating the development of Teva's first innovative drug product? Did the total number of cases comprise too small a population to invest in, in developing a commercial product? It certainly was an appropriate scientific subject for the investigators at the Weizmann Institute, who were interested in the immunology of the drug and the medical consequences of treatment. That did not necessarily mean that Cop 1 could be developed into a commercial success for Teva.

A daunting topic of discussion and analysis was the high cost to develop an innovative product. The more patients required to get an answer and the length of time they had to be observed would multiply the cost. A revolutionary but costly new scientific tool, magnetic resonance imaging (MRI), which was emerging during the 1980s and changing the field for diagnosis of MS, might convincingly magnify the validity of any findings from a clinical trial. But MRI was not fully understood even within the FDA, and including it was certainly a complicating and costly variable in planning a clinical trial.

Potential competition from other MS agents then being tested also had to be considered and weighed in the balance before committing to Teva's development of Cop 1. The decade of the 1980s was a period when the role of interferons as MS therapies was of increasing interest to both the international MS therapeutic community and to commercial companies. It was possible that Teva would be embroiled not only in a race to market, but also in a fierce competition over relative efficacy should both an interferon and Cop 1 pass FDA scrutiny and emerge as commercial drugs. Other as-yet-unrecognized competitors could also appear in the near future to challenge Cop 1 as a creditable and financially successful MS therapy.

The complexity of the situation Teva was facing was not limited only to sponsoring an expensive Phase III clinical trial in some distant part of the world. There were the internal challenges of producing Cop 1. The drug that the Weizmann Institute provided for the Bornstein trials had been manufactured "at the bench," in the laboratory, literally in glass beakers; it had been a long and difficult experience. It may be recalled (Chapter 10) that during Bornstein's chronic progressive MS trial, it had been impossible to produce enough Cop 1 for a short period, and the patients who had been randomized to receive the active agent had, in fact, been switched temporarily to placebo. Teva was faced with the need to produce considerably greater quantities of Cop 1 for new trials and, if they were successful, of producing even larger amounts to market in the U.S. and then the international MS community.

Quantity was not the only issue; there was also the question of the quality and reproducible immunologic activity of the manufactured product. At the Weizmann, the batch-by-batch level of therapeutic potency had been measured by the expensive, slow, and cumbersome process of inhibiting experimental allergic encephalomyelitis (EAE) in either mice or guinea pigs. This biological assay proved to be variable, capricious, and costly. It could never be relied upon as the sole measure of effectiveness for a commercial product or even for a large-scale clinical trial. Somehow, the chemists at Teva had to devise a method of measuring the biologic effectiveness of batch after batch of Cop 1, using a true and reliable measure of drug potency that would be convincing to the FDA. More importantly, the patients who were randomized to receive Cop 1 in a clinical trial, or ultimately the patients who were prescribed the drug in medical practice, had to perceive a measurable benefit to their MS. Could Teva produce vast amounts of Cop 1 that would be effective not only occasionally, but continuously and reliably, so that the FDA and the MS community would trust it?

The mountains to climb were high, the complex clinical trials and production problems were daunting, and a sense of worry began to invade the decision-makers at Teva. In fact, looking back, several participating discussion leaders at the company during that time said that they doubted that the project could be successful, and they actually recommended that it not be undertaken. It was the steadfast vision, confidence, and courage of Eli Hurvitz that led the group and the company forward.

Gathering in a conference room at Teva in Petah Tiqva in the spring of 1988, the Cop 1 development team began to plot the course for future trials. The location for the next clinical trial, the so-called "pivotal trial," was at the top of the agenda. In 1985, Bornstein had conceived of a large multinational trial that would include several MS clinics at American universities, but also centers in Canada, Belgium, France, The Netherlands, Switzerland, Denmark, and Finland. This program would have been costly, and it was never initiated because research grant funds could not be raised. Discussions at Teva led to the decision that the pivotal trial had to include the United States, for numerous reasons. The United States was the location of the rapidly expanding market for Teva's generic drugs. There were more than 350,000 MS patients and numerous well-established MS centers at important U.S. universities where the trial could be conducted. That the United States had a unified regulatory agency, the FDA, at which the rules for conducting clinical trials were well established and where the Bornstein trial had already been successfully recorded, made planning easier.

To advise it on how to proceed, Teva decided to hire as a consultant Dr. Bruce F. Mackler of Washington, D.C., a lawyer and earlier a successful academic immunologist with considerable experience in FDA regulations and practices.

In September 1988, the European Committee for Treatment and Research in Multiple Sclerosis (ECTRIMS) meeting was held in a conference center on the outskirts of Rome. Among the attendees was Ruth Arnon from the Weizmann, one of the creators of Cop 1, accompanied by a young Israeli immunologist, Irit Pinchasi, who had recently obtained her Ph.D. and had joined the staff of Teva as the Assistant Director for Innovative Research and Development. Much later, she would write, "People here were few and inexperienced, and we all had to learn on the job. But what we lacked in experience, we compensated for with enthusiasm and commitment. It was all very pioneering and entrepreneurial in spirit."

I also attended, and I gave a presentation on experiments currently under way in the United States and Canada on a topic of some interest: the use of beta-interferon as a potential MS therapy. The Israeli scientists approached me with the question of how I might design a clinical trial of Cop 1, in light of the recent publication of the Bornstein relapsing-remitting MS trial. The discussion was informal, and the use of MRI as a marker of MS activity that might be influenced by a therapy such as interferon or Cop 1 was mentioned.

A month later, at a small conference center on Jekyll Island off the coast of Georgia, the U.S. National MS Society sponsored an international meeting of MS investigators on the topic of how best to conduct clinical therapeutic trials in MS. This island had been a private sportsman's reserve for wealthy New Yorkers and had gone into decline, but was being reestablished as a vacation area and conference center. Among the conference attendees was Pinchasi from Teva, and during the meeting she approached me to ask if I would be interested in assembling a multiuniversity group to conduct a pivotal trial of Cop 1 in the United States. Several expert MS neurologists at the meeting from universities across the U.S. expressed interest and agreed to come to a preliminary investigators meeting in Baltimore if such a trial was likely to be initiated.

The University of Maryland

Three weeks later, close to Thanksgiving in 1988, Pinchasi and Mackler traveled to Baltimore to begin serious discussions about conducting a large multicenter pivotal U.S. trial, with the administrative center at the University of Maryland. Later, when asked why Teva had decided to consider the University of Maryland, several conditions previously discussed at Teva were cited. These included substantial experience with conducting MS clinical trials, a large and active MS clinical center, close proximity to Washington and the FDA, and the impression that our group had a good working relationship with the National MS Society, which might be the source of funds to help support the trial if a competitive grant request was successful. A major additional benefit was that the able administrator of the Department of Neurology, Bryan Soronson, and the Grants and Contracts office of the University campus, seemed willing to act as the central contacts that would receive funds from several sources and then disperse them to the participating U.S. universities, thus relieving distant Teva of handling this complex task from Israel.

During the short and dark days of January 1989, there was the sense that the Cop 1 project was accelerating, moving more quickly toward the ultimate goal of producing a treatment to control MS and benefit people with MS everywhere, even though they were not, of course, aware of any such activity on their behalf. Twenty-one years, after all, had passed since the research group at the Weizmann had performed their first Cop 1 experiments with the goal of finding a tool to unravel the mechanism of EAE and then, a year later, switched their scientific direction 180 degrees to investigate whether Cop 1 might suppress EAE and hopefully benefit MS. Hiring Bruce Mackler as a consultant to help demystify the path through the technicalities of the FDA was a major step, and selecting the University of Maryland MS Center had given Teva direct access to the clinical research expertise of a number of academic MS centers throughout the U.S.

A Cop 1 clinical trial planning meeting took place on Monday, February 6, 1989, in the Bressler Research Laboratories Conference Room on the 12th floor of the University of Maryland School of Medicine. Representatives from five clinical centers—the University of Maryland, the University of Pennsylvania, Wayne State University, the University of Southern California, and the University of Texas at Houston—attended, as did representatives from the National MS Society and the National Institutes of Health (NIH); very significantly, Dr. Paul Leber, Director of the Division of Neuropharmacological Drug Products at the FDA, also attended. Traveling from Israel were Ben-Zion Weiner, Ph.D., Director of Innovative Research and Development at Teva, and Irit Pinchasi, Assistant Director. Dr. Murray Bornstein was invited to review the previous human trial work on Cop 1. Mackler also represented Teva.

After long, at times intense, but always cordial discussions, the meeting adjourned with a general sense of enthusiasm and confidence that the trial could be rapidly rolled out and carried to an important conclusion. Expressing the desperation felt by MS sufferers everywhere, the investigators urged that a trial be started soon, and promised to search for suitable patients to enroll.

The Baltimore meeting marked the beginning of what might well be the final test of Cop 1 as a therapy for MS: Up or down, success or failure, this trial would be of critical importance to Teva but, much more importantly, would help determine the possible direction for future treatment of MS throughout the world.

One issue actively discussed in Baltimore was the role that MRI might serve in the Cop 1 or any MS trial. Magnetic resonance imaging was in daily use as an MS diagnostic tool by then, and everyone was aware that it was being used in the ongoing interferon beta-1b trial then under way in the United States and Canada. Teva's leaders, to their later regret, decided not to include an MRI component in the Cop 1 trial, but to rely solely on a clinical outcome: the difference in the number of MS relapses between the two groups. The decision to forego MRI was probably financial. Teva was just getting started as a global generic drug company and, as Hurvitz has said, "we could commit $1 million, we could commit $5 million, but we could not commit the whole company to the Cop 1 program."

Clinical trials of new treatments for any disease are extraordinarily complicated and costly, among the most expensive of all medical experiments. It must be emphasized that these are in fact human experiments, in that patients are, in most studies, separated or randomized into those receiving active drug or placebo. Patients receiving placebo are expected from the onset to worsen; that is, their disease is expected to continue on its natural course, which often means that these patients will at the end of the trial be worse off or with more symptoms or even more disability than when they entered. Other potential outcomes, some bad, face the group selected or randomized for active treatment. They face the risk that the treatment may be useless, in which case they also might worsen; they may suffer from serious side effects caused by the test medication; the experimental medication might trigger the disease, resulting in more symptoms and disability; and they could even experience a fatal outcome. These unpleasant possibilities and risks are explained when patients are first considered as research subjects, and they must consent in writing that they understand the purpose of the experiment and are aware of its risks. Patient consent is especially important in an MS trial because of the length of observations required in this highly variable disease. Trial volunteers are the ultimate heroes who make therapeutic progress possible.

In reflecting on the complicated and expensive nature of human trials, perhaps it would help to enumerate the numerous groups, organizations, and committees that must smoothly interact if the study is to succeed. First is the sponsor or manufacturer of the drug, along with various consultants who advise on the construction and conduct of the trial. Second are the multiple MS centers, commonly in academic or university settings, which must identify, treat, and then carefully observe those patients who are chosen, recording every detail of the experiment. A safety monitoring committee composed of physicians, scientists, and statisticians, all knowledgeable about the disease and sworn to secrecy, evaluates the accumulating data and shoulders the responsibility of identifying potential emerging dangers of the treatment, which could require that the study be aborted or stopped to ensure safety of all participants.

Finally, an operational organization, commonly called a clinical research organization (CRO) tends to the "nuts and bolts" of the trial. The CRO usually distributes the treatment, placebo, or active agent and monitors the ongoing performance at each site by making regular visits to ensure that all rules of the trial are being closely observed. The CRO also is responsible for creating a patient binder, placed in a secure place at each investigative site, in which all the details of the trial are recorded: Was the medication distributed to the patient? Were the mandatory clinic visits accomplished? Were all the adverse events or side effects recorded? Were all laboratory results considered and maintained? Were all relapses or neurologic changes fully described?

Were there any changes in the personnel conducting the trial at each site noted?, and so forth. The accumulating records, recorded on detailed forms, must be available for unannounced audits by the FDA at any time, and all records must be securely maintained for a minimum of 7 years after the conclusion of the trial for later FDA audit. Each investigative site is staffed by neurologists and research coordinators, usually but not always nurses, who are in regular communication with the patients and available to respond to any patient change or problem.

Each patient assumes major responsibilities; he or she must come for the scheduled visits, and must submit to a careful examination, laboratory studies, or other diagnostic tests. Any changes or symptoms potentially related to the treatment or to new MS disease activity must be promptly reported. In most cases, participants begin to adjust to the rhythm of a trial. At the end of the experience, the majority find it to have been a positive one, in which they became comfortable with the coordinators and physicians, achieved a sense of security that their well-being was being considered, and accepted the risk knowing that, in the end, there could be improvements in MS treatment for themselves and for thousands of others.

All of this activity is expensive and must be paid for; many trials ultimately cost tens if not hundreds of millions of dollars. To help support the Cop 1 U.S. pivotal trial, Teva was able to obtain substantial grant support from two organizations, the FDA and the National MS Society. Cop 1 was considered an "orphan drug" because it potentially would affect hundreds of thousands but not millions of individuals. The U.S. government, through the FDA, provides a mechanism of trial support for such drugs, the explanation being that the treatment is necessary, even if only for a limited population, and that their serious need must be considered even though the financial rewards at the end might be modest or even nonexistent for the sponsor. Mackler used this FDA orphan drug process to apply for and successfully obtain a grant that aided Teva in supporting the trial.

The U.S. National MS Society accepted as its responsibility the welfare of MS patients and therefore was willing to provide partial support of the Cop 1 trial as a promising treatment with positive preliminary evidence obtained in the Bornstein trial. Both the FDA and the National MS Society grants were administered by the Grants and Contracts Office at the University of Maryland in Baltimore, along with substantial funding from Teva.

Planning across eight time zones was a daunting process as the clinical study protocol was painstakingly developed. In 1989, communication was a challenge for the sponsor in Israel, the administrative center in Baltimore, the FDA advisor in Washington, the CRO in Hartford, Connecticut, and the 11 clinical sites stretched across the United States. The Internet and e-mail were still years in the future. Frequent conference calls were scheduled, and fax machines were universally available, even though thermo-sensitive paper was still the norm and messages arrived on thin, tan, brittle paper.

When finally completed, the protocol carried the long but detailed title "Long-Term, Double-Blind, Placebo-Controlled, Multicenter Phase III Study to Evaluate the Efficacy and Safety of Copolymer 1 Given Subcutaneously in Patients with Relapsing Multiple Sclerosis." The protocol described and carefully detailed every aspect of the trial, including the type of patient to be recruited, the precise number of scheduled visits, the distribution of drug, and the number of items on each clinical form which would go into the patient's binder. The statistical methods that would be used to determine if the primary outcome was positive or negative, the manner in which side effects would be identified, and numerous other components added up to a document of 54 double-spaced pages. Attached were another 25 pages of appendices that defined the methods used to detect neurologic change, such as the Expanded Disability Status Scale (EDSS) described in Chapter 1. The responsible officials at Teva, Mackler in Washington, and myself in Baltimore, all supplied useful input to the final protocol. Teva chose the National Medical Research Corporation of Hartford, Connecticut, as the CRO, and work began on forms to record every detail of the study.

The protocol called for a comparison of the number of clinical MS relapses experienced by the Cop 1 and placebo enrollees treated for 24 months. The patients would contact their center at once if new symptoms arose and would be examined within 7 days. Each patient would be fully examined for their neurologic condition, static or changed, every 3 months, at which time laboratory studies would also be obtained. At the end of the study, these quarterly visits would permit the investigators to detect progression or decline of neurologic status. All information was charted on the forms in the patient binders and collected at regular intervals by monitors from the CRO. If Cop 1 was effective, it should be apparent on the completed forms. Of course, because the study was "blinded" and none of the investigators, coordinators, monitors, or patients were aware of what was being given to each patient, the final outcome was still unknown.

Once the time-consuming and laborious process of developing the protocol and getting buy-in from all of the collaborating organizations was finished, Teva began to prepare an extensive application to the FDA that itemized earlier drug development, previous animal and human studies, the description of how and where the drug would be manufactured and then tested, and the so-called good manufacturing procedures or GMP. Once this document was approved, Teva would receive a new drug application approval or an IND indicating that the human trial could proceed. The final mandatory step before the first patient could be recruited was approval by the local internal review board (IRB) at each treating site. The IRB is a committee of knowledgeable investigators, lawyers, clergymen, and regular citizens who must agree that each human subject's rights and safety are adequately protected and that an appropriate consent form described the purpose and risks of the trial.

Patient issues, clinical effects, drug safety and, of course, monetary concerns were not the only items on the discussion agendas at this time. A burning question that continues to bedevil the drug development universe even now was, "Who owns the data?" The academic community to which the 11 Cop 1 investigative sites belonged has always been committed to open discussion and the publication of complete scientific data, positive or negative, good or bad, whereas commercial companies developing new products or conducting studies comparing their drug with a competitor's might wish to suppress data that are not favorable to their product. This dilemma was purely theoretical, as Cop 1 was entering a new phase of development, yet the question and an agreed-upon solution was required. Rather heated legalistic discussions occurred between Mackler, representing Teva, and the University of Maryland lawyers representing the 11 investigative sites and academic orthodoxy in general.

In the end, a simple solution evolved and was written into the agreement between Teva and the University of Maryland Grants and Contracts office. The clinical trial data would be jointly owned by Teva for commercial endeavors and by the universities for academic purposes and for publication. Teva agreed that it would not attempt to suppress data regarding the trial, but did insist on the right to review manuscripts for proprietary manufacturing information prior to their being sent to a journal editor. This agreement satisfied both parties and has functioned very well throughout the history of Cop 1's rise to become the most prescribed of all MS treatments.

As this time-consuming process was going on, investigators at each university site were searching for suitable patients who were willing to participate. In 1989 and 1990, no drugs were available to improve the course of MS. The investigators at each site were prepared and anxious to proceed, willing patients called regularly to ask when the trial might begin, yet time dragged on with no message from Teva that everything was in place to begin.

The Gulf War

Just then, as had happened repeatedly in Israel's history, rumors of war and war itself again overran the Middle East. On August 2, 1990, Saddam Hussein invaded Kuwait, setting off the Gulf War. From the outset, Hussein threatened to destroy Israel, and the entire country went on high alert. It was well known that Hussein not only had missiles capable of reaching from Iraq to Israel, but also that he had

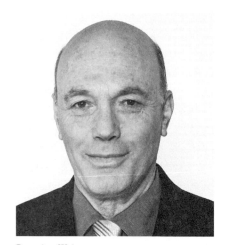
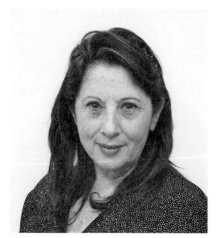

Ben-zion Weiner   Irit Pinchasi

poisonous gas weapons that he had already used on his own people, the Kurds, earlier in his regime. All Israeli citizens were issued gas masks, which were always available even when Tel Aviv citizens attended concerts at Mann Symphony Hall in the center of the city.

Conference calls continued as the plans for the U.S. pivotal Cop 1 trial were finalized. We later learned that Pinchasi took the calls from the basement of her suburban Tel Aviv home with a phone in her hand and her gas mask within reach on her desk. Weiner had been called back into the Army and was a Consultant for Special Activities in the Chief of Staff's command, serving in a secure bunker underground in Tel Aviv. In his uniform, in the bunker, he also participated in the Cop 1 pivotal trial conference calls. Hussein did launch 38 SCUD missiles that fell inside Israel, but none contained poisonous gas.

At the same time, Teva chemists were feverishly searching for a sophisticated chemical method to assay each batch of Cop 1 for immunologic activity, but they still had to test each batch with the original costly, slow, and cumbersome method of inhibiting EAE in mice. The special inbred strain of mice required for the EAE assays came from a laboratory in New Jersey and—due to the shipping difficulties of the Gulf War—the mice often failed to be shipped or to arrive on time.

Time continued to drag on and the U.S. participants were becoming impatient, in some cases even threatening to move their patients to other emerging MS clinical trials. The patients, too, became impatient.

On a steamy, hot August evening in Baltimore, my phone rang and I was surprised to hear Hurvitz's voice coming from suburban Tel Aviv with the very welcome news that the troubling issues concerning the standardization and manufacture of Cop 1 for the trial had finally been overcome. A pharmacology team from Teva would arrive in a few days for a conference at the FDA headquarters, with the hope that it would agree to the chemical standardization of the Cop 1 product and give the green light to the U.S. pivotal trial. The FDA team listened and was satisfied with the manufacturing process and immediately lifted the hold on the trial. The Teva group, relieved and excited, traveled to Baltimore where, with the University of Maryland investigators, a bottle of champagne was opened to toast the upcoming trial.

After informing the investigative sites of the good news, the CRO distributed the final data forms. The anxious patients were relieved. The first patient entered the U.S. pivotal trial on October 23, 1991.

During the delay in part due to the Gulf War, the landscape had changed and new MS treatment competitors had appeared. The traffic on the theoretical highway leading to a drug to help MS patients had become crowded. At least two companies with a beta-interferon product had started their own trials, and a sense of urgency invaded the headquarters of Teva in Israel. The first decision was to increase the number of investigative sites in the United States to speed up recruitment of new patients, and six additional university MS clinics were recruited, all of which were recognized for their excellence in MS studies. They included Yale University in New Haven, the University of Rochester in upstate New York, the University of Wisconsin in Madison, the University of Utah and the Veterans Administration Hospital in Salt Lake City, the University of New Mexico in Albuquerque, and a second site in Los Angeles at UCLA.

The investigative trial leaders included Hillel S. Panitch, University of Maryland, Baltimore; Benjamin R. Brooks, University of Wisconsin, Madison; Jeffrey A. Cohen, University of Pennsylvania,

Philadelphia; Corey C. Ford, University of New Mexico, Albuquerque; Robert P. Lisak, Wayne State University, Detroit; Lawrence W. Myers, UCLA; John W. Rose, University of Utah/VAMC, Salt Lake City; Randolph B. Schiffer, University of Rochester, Rochester, New York; Timothy Vollmer, Yale University, New Haven, Connecticut; Leslie P. Weiner, USC, Los Angeles; and Jerry S. Wolinsky, University of Texas, Houston. The university centers were distributed throughout the country to ensure that a broad population of MS patients with precise characteristics were chosen, as defined in the final protocol. Of course, no single investigator could carry out the duties called for, and several sub-investigators and clinic coordinators worked at each center. Also, some changes in personnel would occur during what would become a long-term Cop 1 investigation stretching over 15 or more years, but all 11 centers continue to participate, and the personnel were remarkably stable, ensuring that the collected data would be uniform and of high scientific quality.

All involved centers received site visits by CRO personnel and soon began recruiting patients. Rising to the challenge, all 11 sites recruited well-characterized patients and, by May 1992, the final group of 251 patients had been entered, 126 randomized to Cop 1 and 125 to placebo.

Recognizing that Teva needed a hands-on presence in the United States to help coordinate the trial, plans were completed for a young chemist, Dr. Yafit Stark, to relocate with her family to suburban Philadelphia, to help manage the day-to-day details and challenges of the trial. She met with the entire U.S. group, 11 investigative groups with their coordinators, as well as members from the CRO group, at a study meeting in Seattle, where she was introduced by Pinchasi. Looking back, her energy, commitment, and minute-to-minute attention to every detail were essential to the successful conduct of the trial.

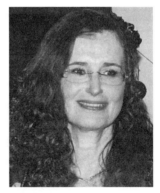

Yafit Stark

By and large, due primarily to the experience and commitment of the 11 site investigators, the trial went forward smoothly. When problems occurred, such as the difficulty at one site in maintaining records up to the expected standards, or at another site with the use of neurology residents rather than experienced investigators to evaluate the patients, the issues were recognized and Stark and Johnson would travel to the center to upgrade its conduct of the trial. At regular intervals, the data monitoring committee met privately to review all safety issues, including any evidence of clinical or laboratory abnormalities that might signal some adverse reaction or danger. None were found.

Once, early in the second year of the trial, manufacturing issues arose, and there was some concern in Israel that the trial would have to be at least put on hold because there was not sufficient Cop 1 to continue the daily dosing. Fortunately, Stark had anticipated this possibility and had stockpiled surplus doses so that it was possible to continue the trial without interruption.

In the early spring of 1993, everyone involved was anticipating the end of the trial and had hopes for a positive result. Investigator meetings had been held regularly, usually in conjunction with national neurologic meetings, in Baltimore, Boston, and elsewhere. The original rules of how to conclude the trial were coming into question, however, and a decision was made to call an independent meeting at which all investigators, trial coordinators, CRO employees, and U.S. Teva leaders would have an opportunity to discuss how the trial should be completed. The meeting was held at the Sheraton Hotel in Chicago, in a lower-level conference room with windows looking out onto the Chicago River.

The primary concern was whether to end the trial as the protocol had dictated, with each patient stopping injections when they had finished 24 months in the trial. This had been intentionally designed as a way of observing if patients who were taken off medication would rebound—that is, begin exhibiting increasing MS activity once the therapy had been terminated. A lively discussion, at times heated, took place in Chicago. The final conclusion was that patients would be maintained on their assigned medication, either active drug or placebo, until the last patient had completed 24 months. This meant that patients enrolled early on in October of 1991 would extend their assigned medication throughout the winter and spring of 1994, and thus would provide useful information about Cop 1's impact well beyond 24 months.

The investigators took a firm position that Teva had a responsibility to all of the patients enrolled and that, even though the outcome of the trial was not yet known, all patients should be maintained on Cop 1, with the placebo patients being switched to active medication until the final results were known. This demand was unusual in clinical trials but Teva agreed to it, a decision that later turned out to benefit both the patients and Teva, as will be described later. Concluding the day-long meeting, at times tense but finally very productive, Bill Fletcher rolled in a large cake with multiple candles. It was Yafit Stark's 40th birthday.

The trial had gone on, month after month, visit after scheduled visit, the patients calling if they noted symptoms which might signal a new relapse. At each of the 11 study sites, the forms had been completed and placed in the patient binders, and periodically monitors would come to take them to the CRO offices, where all data were verified and entered into computers. In the spring of 1994, the final patient visits took place, all clinical and laboratory forms were collected, and the pivotal U.S. Cop 1 trial was complete.

15

From Anxiety to Euphoria

Mathematics, the queen of sciences, and its junior sibling, statistics, are essential pillars on which most science rests, and they are certainly indispensable components for all clinical drug trials. These trials, the final step and the foundation of much medical progress, rely on comparisons between the behavior of patients who receive an experimental therapy versus a placebo, or on comparisons between an experimental therapy and a standard drug already available to patients. The proper application of statistics was of critical importance for the Cop 1 (copolymer one) pivotal trial. As the analysis of the trial got under way, there was anxiety and the fear of failure, but also expectation and excitement for all of those who were involved: the Teva group, the 11 U.S. investigative centers, and all 251 patients who had contributed so much to whatever the final result would be.

Shaul Kadosh was the lead statistician for the innovative product group at Teva in Israel. Born in Israel to European immigrants, he remembers his childhood when the family was desperately poor and struggling to make a new home for themselves in the recently declared State of Israel. He was always fascinated by mathematics, and chose to become a statistician during his university years. In the spring of 1994, the voluminous data files from the U.S. pivotal trial were regularly sent to Kadosh for analysis, and he recalls those days well. To any statistician, secrecy was important until a convincing result—positive or negative, good or bad—could confidently be determined and then announced. Everyone at Teva was aware of what he was working on and watched him with almost morbid interest. Did he have a smile on his face or was he solemn? Was he holding his knife and fork differently in the cafeteria? How was he dressed? Was there some clue in his behavior to what the outcome of the pivotal trial might be? Finally, alone in his office, with just a few final keystrokes, a preliminary number appeared on his computer screen, and he was able to begin to fathom the conclusions that the trial would reveal, and what the future of Cop 1 would be.

At this critical time, most of the innovative drug development team from Teva, those who were responsible for the trial, had traveled to Kulpsville, Pennsylvania, to observe early study results. They were prepared either to begin to plan excitedly for next steps or dejectedly make reservations to go home, all based on what the data showed. Some preliminary data had been analyzed in Kulpsville, but it soon became apparent that more sophisticated statistical power and expertise had to be brought to bear. It was obvious that they needed Kadesh personally, there in Pennsylvania, to supply the best statistical techniques needed to decipher the data.

An urgent call came for him to travel to Philadelphia right away, but he was in Israel, he had a passport but no visa to enter the United States, and he had no ticket. In just hours, a ticket and visa were obtained, and he was on his way, across the Mediterranean and the Atlantic to New York. He had never been to the United States and only knew that he had to get to suburban Philadelphia, to Kulpsville. He hailed a yellow New York taxicab, gave the driver the Teva address in Kulpsville, and was off on a several-hour ride to join his anxious colleagues, who were depending on his statistical skills.

At that time, Teva still had a business partnership with W.R. Grace Co. and used the name TAG Pharmaceuticals (Teva and Grace) for their joint U.S. activity. TAG occupied a modest one-story building combining offices, a conference room, and a warehouse. It was the last building on Delp Drive, a two-lane country road just beyond a rapidly expanding suburban area north of Philadelphia. There were several offices at the front of the building, a large open warehouse space in the rear, and a modest conference room facing north, with windows looking out on a large corn field that was commonly visited by flocks of Canada geese and occasionally by a white-tailed deer. In this remote setting, the Teva internal group gathered for its first look at the trial data that would determine the success or failure of what had by now become an intense and costly 6-year effort. Just as they were about to begin, Bill Fletcher jumped up, went to the next room, came back with large sheets of paper, and taped it over the windows facing onto the rural cornfields. One could never be too careful with data this precious!

Slide after slide appeared on the screen, with Kadesh interpreting the findings for the group, from time to time adding explanatory information on a blackboard as the trial results unfolded. As the analysis rolled out, it became clear that the primary endpoint, the MS relapse rate, had been met, although not in as robust a fashion as had been seen in the smaller Bornstein trial. Nevertheless, it was a statistically significant positive outcome. Using numerous analytic methods to calculate differences in increasing disability as measured by the Expanded Disability Status Scale (EDSS) so laboriously gathered at the 11 U.S. clinical centers, an impact on slowing neurologic disability was also apparent. Finally, as the safety data were considered, it seemed very clear that, at least over 2 years, the daily injections of Cop 1 had produced no serious risks of concern. Cop 1 was on its way to becoming a commercial product, available to tens if not hundreds of thousands of people with MS.

Smiles began to appear, followed by a sense of relief that gave way to happy excitement as it became more and more obvious that the U.S. pivotal trial had confirmed the earlier positive findings published by Bornstein. Cop 1 had a good chance of becoming Teva's first innovative product, but the high hurdle of gaining U.S. Food and Drug Administration (FDA) approval still loomed on the horizon.

Shortly after this destiny-changing moment for Teva in rural Kulpsville, I was invited to meet Hurvitz on a hot July Sunday afternoon in mid-Manhattan to review the trial data for the first time. From the first moments, it seemed obvious that Hurvitz had good news, and he put his hand on my shoulder and said, "Well, Ken, we have a product." In response, I said, "Well Eli, that's great news for you and for Teva and the whole investigative team but remember, we probably now have a new therapy, a new means of lifting the hopes and futures for MS patients everywhere." These two comments captured the unique emotion of the moment, which was both a potential commercial success for Teva but also held the larger implications for improving the future for MS patients and providing an answer to the often-asked question of why clinical trial research is so important.

It was imperative that Teva get the news out, to begin informing numerous groups of the results: Teva's stockholders; the investigative groups that for over 2 years had labored to develop the data; the community of treating physicians, primarily neurologists, who would be interested in a potential new drug for MS; and the worldwide community of MS patients who needed any good news they could get that promised to improve their state.

A press release was prepared and broadcast to the investment community stating that Teva, on the basis of the recently completed U.S. trial, was going to prepare a new drug application (NDA) to submit to the FDA. The investigators came next and, on October 2 and 3, there was a joint meeting to which was invited the entire investigative group, the safety monitoring committee, Bruce Mackler, and representatives from the CRO. A large group from Teva U.S. attended, headed by Fletcher and Dr. Carol Ben-Maimon, who had assumed the role as Vice President for Medical and Regulatory Affairs. Most importantly, representatives from Israel, Pinchasi and Weiner from Teva Pharmaceuticals, and Ruth Arnon from the Weizmann Institute, were there. The agenda called for myself and Yafit Stark to present the results, followed by a discussion, urgent questions, and then the development of plans for further distribution of the data. What would become a very important decision was that new activities had to be planned for those patients who had participated. The spirit of this meeting was one of enthusiasm and satisfaction that a major new landmark in the treatment of MS was on the brink of being achieved.

Announcing the Results

Next on the list was the critical task of informing the medical community, primarily neurologists, of the positive outcome of the U.S. Cop 1 trial. In mid-October 1994, the 119th annual meeting of the American Neurological Association was scheduled at the Hyatt Regency Hotel overlooking the bay in San Francisco. The Tuesday afternoon session was to take place in the Grand Ballroom, and soon it became apparent that this was no ordinary scientific session. The large room was packed and, in the back on a raised platform were a number of video cameras to record the events. The front rows soon filled with medical reporters from various news agencies, television networks, national newspapers, and other media groups. Joining them were representatives from the financial community, ready to distribute any significant news back to Wall Street.

The third and fourth 15-minute talks of the afternoon were the reason for this extraordinary interest. At 3:10 p.m., Dr. Larry Jacobs from the University of Buffalo, New York, was scheduled to present the "Results of a Phase III Trial of Intramuscular Recombinant Beta Interferon as Treatment for Multiple Sclerosis," the drug soon to be called Avonex®. At 3:30, I would present the Cop 1 results "Copolymer 1: Positive Results from the Phase III Trial of Relapsing Remitting Multiple Sclerosis." Following these presentations, the news and financial attendees bolted from the meeting, delaying the program for several minutes. In only 30 brief minutes, two positive MS drug trials had been reported: information that would have profound implications for two commercial companies, but also would change the entire MS treatment environment and soon have direct implications for hundreds of thousands of MS patients worldwide. These two products, which would soon be marketed as Avonex and Copaxone®, would rise to the top of the sales charts and battle for over a decade for the title of market leader.

As the audience milled about in the lobby after the session, commenting on the events of the afternoon, I was approached by the editor of *Neurology*, one of the three major neurologic journals in the

United States, and asked to prepare a manuscript describing the Cop 1 trial and its implications. He also promised that if it passed peer review that he would guarantee expedited publication.

In the evening, at a festive reception attended by most persons involved in some way with the Cop 1 trial, investigators, Teva employees, and others met to congratulate each other. At midnight, I traveled by taxi with Fletcher to a commercial video studio to broadcast a message to a number of MS centers throughout Europe and the United Kingdom, further expanding the news of this never-to-be-forgotten day.

The key findings from the trial that I reported to the large audience in San Francisco were that the group who had received Cop 1 had 29% fewer relapses during the 2 years of observation than did those patients who received placebo. Statistical analysis indicated that this was a significant difference and not due to chance. Over the course of the 2 years of observation, each patient had been examined by his or her neurologist at least eight times using the EDSS described in Chapter 1. In other words, for those patients receiving either Cop 1 or placebo, there were almost 1,000 individual examinations, all recorded in the patient binders and all available to the statisticians. From this large set of raw data, it was possible to draw several types of conclusions. One straightforward question was whether patients were better or had worsened. This is what the statisticians call a *categorical analysis*, which quite simply means that, at the end of the trial, each patient is placed in one of three categories: they were worse than at entry, they were better, or—as is true in most relatively short MS trials—they were unchanged. Using this type of analysis, approximately 50% of the patients were unchanged, however, more of the Cop 1-treated patients were improved whereas more of the placebo patients had worsened, providing a statistically significant outcome in favor of Cop 1 treatment. Using other statistical probing, one could ask what percent of patients were improved or had worsened, as well as the average number of patients who had changed, and to what extent. By this test of neurologic status, the group treated with Cop 1 were better.

The symptoms of MS first appear in young adult life between the ages of 15 and 45, and approximately 70% of MS victims are women.

Defining the population in this way, it is not surprising that the effect on pregnancy is always an item of interest in any MS treatment trial. In the Cop 1 trial, in spite of the promise by the female participants that they would use an active form of contraception, three women did become pregnant. One of them chose to have a therapeutic abortion and continue in the trial, while the two others chose to drop out of the trial and maintain the pregnancy; both delivered a normal infant.

In the end, the patients had participated responsibly and with dedication, the 11 investigative sites had performed admirably, and the statisticians functioned professionally to give the sense that the trial results would be trusted and that they did in fact show a significant therapeutic benefit and comforting safety using daily injections of 20 mg of Cop 1.

Soon a manuscript was prepared, which used the time-honored format for scientific articles of Introduction, Methods, Results, and finally Discussion, backed up by a large bibliography of previously published work. The manuscript was circulated to the 11 investigative sites and to Teva for further ideas and criticisms. Once all comments had been considered, the final manuscript was sent to the editors of *Neurology* in April, approved in early May, and published in the July 1995 issue. Professional readers, neurologists, other scientists, and business leaders read and reread every word and conclusion and pondered every statistical number. All agreed that the trial had indeed shown a positive therapeutic effect by Cop 1, and that it appeared to those involved to be safer and better tolerated than the beta-interferons that were emerging as major marketplace competitors. The U.S. pivotal trial had confirmed the findings from the much smaller Bornstein trial, fulfilling the FDA requirement for two independent positive trials. Later, the article was chosen as one of seven with the most impact of all MS articles published in *Neurology* in the past 50 years.

People with MS everywhere wondered when Cop 1 would be available. For the Teva innovative group, one phase of their journey to a commercial product had ended successfully but a new phase was just beginning. In the TAG warehouse in Kulpsville, a floor-to-ceiling wire screen enclosed an area or—as it came to be called, a "cage"—to afford some security for their work. They began the monumental task of creating a new drug application, or NDA, following detailed FDA guidelines, a task new to them. The NDA had to include detailed chemical and manufacturing information of the product that Teva hoped to market, the history of the Cop 1 development process going back to the earliest days at the Weizmann Institute, a step-by-step account of all of the animal experiments, and the outcomes of all human exposures beginning with those earliest cautious Cop 1 injections in Hadassah Hospital in Jerusalem, and the German and New York preliminary dose-finding trials. The Bornstein trials were recounted in great detail. All particulars of the U.S. pivotal trial were carefully included, including every feature of how the patients were selected and observed and the final 2-year outcomes of treated versus placebo groups. When finished, the NDA document, as submitted in June 1995 to the FDA, comprised over 335 loose-leaf notebook binders and detailed every aspect of basic and clinical research and the manufacturing process. Working closely with the group from Israel was Dr. Carol Ben-Maimon, recently named Vice President for Medical and Regulatory Affairs, who had assumed a leadership role in guiding the NDA process and other activities leading, hopefully, to piloting Cop 1 to the market.

Ben-Maimon was an internist, having graduated from the University of Pennsylvania and then Jefferson Medical College in Philadelphia, where she was in one of the early classes to accept women, even though the college was well over 100 years old. Trained as a nephrologist, she had conducted clinical research in the field of oncology both at Jefferson and the University of Pennsylvania. Leaving academic life, she joined Wyeth before moving to Lemmon in 1993, 8 years after it had been acquired by Teva.

To streamline its corporate identity, Teva Pharmaceuticals USA was created, and the name of the Lemmon Company was dropped. Bill Fletcher took the position of President and CEO of the flourishing American entity, which was rapidly growing and taking its place among the world's major generic drug suppliers. He was also involved, week by week, in preparations heading toward the FDA hearing, which everyone was aware would define the future of Cop 1.

With a proactive view toward the future, it was now necessary to consider what this new product should be called. Copolymer 1 was an appropriate name when given to the agent by the Weizmann group in 1967, when they were searching for a tool to study experimental allergic encephalomyelitis (EAE), not an MS drug. The name had been commonly shortened affectionately to "Cop 1," by which it was identified in medical conversations and even in the early medical journal publications.

Copaxone®

But many amino acid polymers were being created for numerous uses in laboratories throughout the world and Cop 1, while now accepted in the neurology community, was no longer an appropriate name. First, a specific generic or chemical name was devised, *glatiramer acetate*, whose first four letters "glat" represented the four amino acids contained in the polymer: glutamic acid, lysine, alanine, and tyrosine. The next creative step was to devise an easy to remember, distinctive commercial name that could readily roll off the tongue, and differentiate Cop 1 from other marketed drugs. The word chosen was *Copaxone*, which contained the letters "cop, linking it back to Cop 1 and "axone," linking it to axon, the central component in the nervous system, which was covered with myelin, thereby bringing the whole story back to myelin basic protein, EAE, and the beginning of the tale.

The Teva team was working long hours in the screened-in "cage" in the Kulpsville warehouse putting together the massive NDA that was required by the FDA. New to the game, they relied on the expertise of several consultants, some of whom had previously been employed by the FDA. Finally, after completing the weighty document, they thought they were finished. They were disappointed in August 1995, when the NDA was rejected by the FDA because of questions concerning the chemistry section relating to certain standards or markers in the manufacturing process of the product. It was back to work, both in Kulpsville and in Israel, to revise the NDA document to the FDA's satisfaction.

A sense of relentless pressure was continuing to build for everyone connected with the Copaxone program. Betaseron®, a beta-interferon, had been the first MS drug to negotiate the difficult pathway through the FDA and had, in fact, been on the U.S. market since 1993. Avonex, also a beta-interferon, the trial results of which had been announced at the same platform session with Cop 1 in San Francisco, in October 1994, had come before the FDA Advisory Panel in December 1995 and was also recommended for approval. This created the disheartening specter that there might be two competing drugs, both interferons, on the market before Teva even had the opportunity to present the Copaxone program to an FDA Advisory Panel. The work continued, and several weeks later the NDA was accepted or "filed."

The FDA Hearing

With this positive step, the floodgates opened, stimulating a burst of new activity because of the anticipation that an Advisory Panel meeting would soon be scheduled by the FDA. If successful, this would be one of the final steps before bringing Copaxone to the U.S. markets and supplying it to MS patients in the United States. Work in the Kulpsville offices turned into frenzy, numerous meetings were scheduled in Philadelphia and in the northern suburbs of the city, and several consultants were brought in to help prepare for this critical advisory meeting. In Israel, Hurvitz, concerned with the pace of preparations for the Advisory Panel, which was costing up to $1 million a day, dispatched Israel Makov to Kulpsville to oversee all preparations.

Makov was a seasoned administrator who would, in 2002, be named the new President and CEO of Teva, replacing Hurvitz, who would become Chairman of the Teva Board. Groups and committees, Teva people, investigators from the various sites, and FDA consultants were constantly meeting. One of the critical tasks was to anticipate any possible question that either FDA officials or members of the Advisory Panel might ask, and then to prepare one or more slides to answer that question. This was before the advent of PowerPoint presentations, and every slide had to be prepared as a professional-looking 35-mm slide. These were used in the numerous rehearsals taking place in the summer and fall of 1996. When finally assembled, the enormous number of slides would be placed in several 35-mm slide carousels, which were fully indexed so that any question raised could be quickly responded to (for example, some particular answer could be found in carousel 4, slide 35 and 3).

Finally, September 19, 1996, was announced as the date when the Peripheral and Central Nervous System Drugs Advisory Committee of the FDA would meet to consider NDA 20-622 Copaxone (Copolymer 1 for Injection: Safety and Effectiveness in Use for Relapsing Remitting Multiple Sclerosis). The fateful day was marked in red on many calendars in the United States and in Israel, the day when the future of Copaxone might well be determined forever, the day that might mark the success or failure of 29 years of dedicated, single-minded focus by the Weizmann group and over 10 years of committed effort and great expense by Teva. The meeting was scheduled to take place at the ballroom of the Gaithersburg, Maryland, Holiday Inn at 8:30 a.m.

FDA Advisory Committee meetings are uniquely open and transparent, combining government, commercial, and academic expertise, often with profound, sometimes unexpected consequences. The usual setting is a large ballroom-sized room, divided roughly in half, with one side for the official activities of the day and the other half for the public. The public often includes financial analysts, the media, patients with the disease treatment under consideration, interested observers connected to the sponsor, and nonprofit organizations such as the National MS Society. The FDA Advisory Panel is composed of academic experts who, in the case of the Copaxone hearing, were mainly neurologists. A well-respected, independent statistician is always included.

The Copaxone expert panel that gathered on September 19 was composed of 11 senior professors, some of whom were chairs of neurology departments, led by Dr. Sid Gilman, Professor and Chair of the

Department of Neurology at the University of Michigan Medical Center. The charge to the committee was simple and straightforward. The Division of Neuropharmacological Drug Products of the FDA seeks the Committee's advice on two questions:

1. Teva Pharmaceuticals has provided results of two controlled clinical investigations of copolymer 1's effectiveness in exacerbating remitting MS. Are these studies adequate and well-controlled clinical investigations, and does each provide evidence that would allow an expert, knowledgeable and experienced in the management of patients with MS, to conclude that copolymer 1 is an effective treatment for MS?

2. Has the sponsor provided evidence that copolymer 1 is safe when used in the treatment of MS?

The design of the space for the panel discussions is of interest. A U-shaped table is reserved for the panel members, who face each other and can discuss issues among themselves or pose questions to various presenters during the course of the day. Space on one side is reserved for the sponsor's representatives, which included members of the Teva staff, investigators from the Weizmann Institute, investigators who conducted the trial, and various consultants hired by the sponsor. On the opposite side are members of the FDA staff, including statisticians and others who have carefully reviewed the NDA file over the last several months. A large screen allows all to view the information being presented by either the FDA or the sponsor. The entire process, questions, discussion, and the body language by the participants is open to all in the room; there are no closed sessions or opportunities for private conversations by the panel members.

The night before the Advisory Meeting, members from the 11 investigative university sites were invited by Judy Katterhenrich of Teva Marion Partners to a uniquely Baltimore-Washington evening event, a Chesapeake spiced crab dinner, a spread that probably takes place in no other region of the country. In a rough, garage-like setting, the tables, often picnic tables, are spread with newspapers or plain brown paper, and a heaping pile of local blue crabs, which have been steamed in spicy seasonings that gives them the appearance of being coated with mud, are dumped on the table. With little need for eating utensils, the crabs are attacked with a wooden mallet and the morsels of white crab meat are picked out with a plastic fork, the participants often complaining that the hot spices irritate their lips. Cole slaw or some other salad is provided, and pitchers of beer are mandatory. It was an unrivaled experience for relieving anxieties and dispelling thoughts of the events of the next day. A relaxed mood grew; probably welcome for escaping what was ahead.

The Advisory Panel meeting began promptly. Introductory remarks and the charge to the panel were made by Dr. Paul Leber, Division Director, and Dr. Russell Katz, Deputy Division Director, who had both participated in the first Cop 1 planning meeting at the University of Maryland 7 years earlier. Ben-Maimon, who would do a superb job of presenting the data, introduced Copaxone and explained the reasons why Teva felt that it was a safe and efficacious treatment for relapsing MS, presenting numerous slides from the Bornstein and U.S. pivotal trials to bolster her arguments. I briefly described the key elements of MS to what was a highly knowledgeable Advisory Panel; Wolinsky, one of the site investigators, gave a medical perspective of the usefulness of Copaxone for MS. After an FDA response, an open committee discussion was followed by invited comments from the public. Several patients volunteered their experience with MS and Copaxone treatment.

The long day moved on to a climactic close that was described by some as a roller coaster ride, especially for those connected with the long development path of Copaxone at the Weizmann and Teva. Their feelings were of relief and hope, or despair and anxiety, depending on the up-and-down course of the discussion, the questions being asked, and what the Advisory Panel's reactions or even their facial expressions conveyed. Weiner and Pinchasi, leaders of the innovative group at Teva, were seated together. They had from the onset invested enormous time, intellectual activity, and emotion into the previous 8 years. As the day drew toward its final answer, Weiner noted that Pinchasi had been tightly clutching his arm and had dug her fingernails into his forearm, drawing blood in the process. Finally, the moment of truth arrived. Chairman Gilman looked around the table, asked each Advisory

Panel member to make a closing remark or two and give his or her response to the two questions that the FDA had posed at the beginning of the morning. The tension was like a pent-up volcano as, one by one, the Advisory Panel members gave their opinion that the two questions could be answered affirmatively. In just a few minutes, a unanimous positive outcome had been reached, and the Copaxone Advisory Committee meeting had come to an emotional end.

After a stunned moment of silence, there was an outburst of energy, hugs, tears, kisses, laughter, and handshakes. All who had been connected with the long developmental process of Copaxone felt relief, joy, and profound accomplishment. For the Weizmann people, there was finally a deep sense of vindication that the scientific activities to which they had invested 29 years would indeed lead to a new drug for MS, justifying hope and a deep conviction that they had held for three decades. Only now could their long dream be developed into a reality. For the Teva team and their new partners at Teva Marion Partners, now there was a chance to bring a new commercial product to the public, and to further their goals and their vision as an important pharmaceutical company, sensing at the same time that they were contributing to new and improved welfare for those with MS, in the United States and hopefully throughout the world. For the investigators, who had with considerable interest followed the recent appearance of two beta-interferons for the treatment of MS, there was a sense of achievement. They realized that they had played a vital role in the development of the second, and perhaps even better, treatment option for managing MS in their clinics and elsewhere.

A reception bubbling with a mixture of happiness, joy, and enthusiasm followed the days' proceedings. Many of the Israeli participants had been accompanied by their spouses, making the party even more festive. After a while, I drove back to Baltimore, taking back roads through the beautiful evening countryside, considering what an incredible story had just come to a climax, and how three genius chemists and a small Israeli company led by a man of great insight and courage had brought to the MS world—a new treatment to fight the disease that shattered dreams.

16

The Competition: Beta-Interferon

As the Earth has rotated each day over years, centuries, and millennia, back through eons of prehistory, the mammalian brain has evolved through various primates to achieve our present *Homo sapiens* form. Although only a modest 3 pounds in weight, it is the most complex, creative, multifunctional, decision-making object in the known universe. Capable of countless observations, discoveries, and inventions, humans have conceived language, made the wheel and many other tools in prehistory, then—at irregular thrusts—made countless seminal advances, such as the development of gunpowder for warfare and steam power to inaugurate the Industrial Revolution. The 20th century proved to be the most intense period of discovery and invention yet. Among the most fertile of recent creative domains, pharmacology has witnessed enormous progress: multiple vaccines to revolutionize public health; antibiotics to conquer bacterial infections; improved control of strokes, cancer, and diabetes; and, more recently, monoclonal antibodies capable of destroying specific cancer cells or acting as an immunologic scalpel to inactivate circulating populations of rogue lymphocytes, the culprits now identified as critical in several autoimmune diseases.

In spite of the striking—in fact, unprecedented—advances in the treatment of human disease during the 20th century, there were few recognized improvements in MS therapy. Over the second half of the century, the National MS Society sponsored the publication "Therapeutic Claims in Multiple Sclerosis," which went through several editions, cataloging virtually every new drug discovery for human diseases. It came to the discouraging conclusion that, while hundreds of therapies had been tested, no believable evidence indicated that the course of multiple sclerosis (MS) was benefited by any of them.

As the first cautious human exposure of MS patients to Cop 1 (copolymer one) was taking place at the Hadassah Hospital in Jerusalem, another form of therapy that ultimately proved successful was entering on the long, expensive path of commercial development as well. By 1979, there was considerable interest in the possibility that MS was due to a chronic or hidden viral infection and, quite logically, this led to the idea that perhaps an antiviral therapy might benefit MS. Two decades earlier, in 1957, two innovative scientists, Isaacs and Lindenmann, had first described an antiviral protein present in all mammals, including humans, which they labeled interferon. Soon, an immense and expanding range of scientific investigations was spawned showing that interferons were actually a family of proteins, which were named alpha, beta, and gamma interferon. Hoping to expand the use of interferons into human therapeutics, in the mid-1970s, while working at the Finnish Red Cross in Helsinki, Karri Kantel found that the "buffy coat," the white blood cell component of donated human blood, could be grown in a test tube and then stimulated with a innocuous virus to make interferon which could, after purification, be used as an experimental human treatment. Infectious diseases, such as chronic hepatitis, various human cancers, and even MS, were considered as candidate diseases that might benefit from interferon therapy. However, the supply of interferon was small, and the cost was astronomical. Nevertheless, Byron Waksman, at that time Director of Research Programs at the National MS Society in the United States, thought that interferon therapy of MS should be investigated.

On a warm Saturday afternoon in the late spring of 1979, three men met at a rented conference room at the San Francisco airport: Thomas Merrigan from Stanford was a world leader in the infant field of interferon therapy, Michael Oldstone of Scripps Research institute in La

Jolla was an internationally recognized neuroimmunologist, and myself, head of the large MS research program at the University of California in San Francisco. We met to consider a potential MS treatment program using the Finnish interferon. Over a period of 3 hours, we discussed how to design a treatment trial to test this so-called natural alpha-interferon for MS. There were no precedents, no preliminary experiments, and the concept for the trial had literally to be snatched out of thin air. Ultimately, it was decided to treat MS patients daily with the highest tolerated dose known at that time, using a complex design in which they would be randomized to receive interferon or placebo, treated for 6 months, and then given a 6-month rest period, after which the treatment groups would be reversed, a so-called *cross-over trial*.

Because of the enormous cost, only 24 patients could be recruited, 12 in La Jolla and 12 in San Francisco. Many patients were eager to participate, and the trial soon got under way, showing immediately that a dose of 5 million units of natural alpha-interferon, injected subcutaneously every day, produced substantial unpleasant side effects. Nevertheless, all 24 patients continued in the demanding and rigorous study. In the end, there was little clear evidence of benefit; however, for some of the patients it seemed to take several years before they returned to their previous level of MS activity.

At almost exactly the same time, an independent group working under the leadership of Larry Jacobs, a neurologist at the University of Buffalo in New York, began a series of clinical experiments using natural beta-interferon to treat MS. Jacobs was convinced that, if a virus caused MS, it had to be in the central nervous system, and that the only hope to have a treatment effect was to inject the interferon directly into the cerebral spinal fluid through lumbar puncture. In spite of some hint of benefit, interferon side effects and the resistance of patients to repeated injections into the spinal fluid led him to abandon this line of investigation. These initial studies of MS treatment with natural interferons must be considered tenuous at best.

By 1981, the field of molecular biology had rapidly advanced. It was now possible to isolate human interferon genes that could then be inserted into either cultured bacteria or cultured mammalian cells, such as Chinese hamster kidney cells, which would then produce high concentrations of more purified human interferon. Using what seemed at the time to be molecular magic, the interferon could be isolated, purified, and made into an experimental therapy. Interest from the public was great, interferon therapy for numerous diseases was widely anticipated, and the topic was introduced to the public in an extended article in *TIME* magazine.

The improved interferons were derived through what was called *recombinant* technology. Using a recombinant alpha-interferon produced by Schering Plough Company in New Jersey, my colleagues and I (by that time I had relocated from San Francisco to the University of Maryland in Baltimore) conducted the first trial of recombinant alpha-interferon in MS, selecting a much reduced dose after recalling the unfortunate side effects experienced with the high dose chosen for the original California studies. The recombinant interferon was well tolerated in over 50 MS patients enrolled in the study, but no clear evidence of benefit could be determined. Was the idea of interferon treatment for MS wrong? Or, was the type of interferon or perhaps the dose wrong?

A small pilot trial, which would be forever remembered as a therapeutic disaster, but also as a highly informative immunologic experiment, came next. The Biogen Corporation in Cambridge, Massachusetts, approached the MS group at the University of Maryland in Baltimore with a novel new experimental direction. The alpha- and beta-interferon studies had to date been disappointing, but Biogen had succeeded in producing recombinant gamma-interferon that they hoped to test as a new MS interferon treatment. Several well-known immunologists had warned that gamma-interferon might be a potent stimulus of new MS activity, but nevertheless the decision was made to test it very cautiously, using two doses administered two times per week by intravenous infusion to MS patients with active disease. At the end of 1 month, seven of 18 patients had experienced new MS attacks. Not good! Fortunately, the MS symptoms were mild and were soon reversed. While certainly not useful as a therapy, the trial was highly informative. It showed that gamma-interferon was involved in stimulating increased MS activity, thereby cementing the idea that MS was due to aggressive and uncontrolled immunologic activity, at least in part. The underlying premise of MS was changing, focusing more on immune overactivity, rather than on a hidden virus infection. Of course, it could still be due to both in some complex manner.

The science and molecular biology of interferons continued to advance rapidly. A form of recombinant beta-interferon had been creatively engineered by the Cetus Company, a small California company that had, in turn, been purchased by the Chiron Corporation of Emoryville, California, with the prospect of using this beta-interferon as a potential therapy for numerous human diseases. The name Betaseron® had been chosen to emphasize the elegantly engineered recombinant molecule produced in the bacteria *Escherichia coli*, in which the amino acid serine was substituted for cystine at the 17th position in the string of amino acids, to improve its activity and stability.

Chiron was a small biotech company in the 1980s, and lacked the resources to support expensive human placebo-controlled trials. Therefore, it formed a partnership with the Shell Oil Company to underwrite human trials of the newly acquired recombinant beta-interferon. As Triton Biosciences, the partnership designed a series of trials targeting several human diseases, mainly cancers but also MS. After the unexpected, surprising, and potentially dangerous outcome of the previous gamma-interferon MS trial, it was wisely decided to undertake a small dose-finding and safety trial that would enroll a total of 30 patients at the University of Maryland, along with Jefferson Medical College and Temple University in Philadelphia. In this 6-month trial, the now expected, unpleasant, but tolerable side effects of interferon again appeared, but it was also apparent that no new MS activity was triggered and that there was a welcome and promising dose response trend on relapses; 8 million units injected under the skin three times a week clearly reduced the number of relapses, while lower doses were less effective, and a higher dose of 16 million units was poorly tolerated.

Based on this comforting information, a large Phase III trial was undertaken at 11 North American universities, seven in the United States and four in Canada. The trial began in 1988, and compared two doses, 1.6 and 8 million beta-interferon units versus placebo, injected subcutaneously every other day. Approximately 125 patients with relapsing MS were enrolled in each group. The trial, while planned for 2 years, was in fact carried out for over 4 years as a placebo-controlled study. This is, in itself, quite noteworthy, because most of the patients were willing to continue even though, as it finally turned out, a third of them injected placebo every other day for over 4 years. This demonstrated their compelling loyalty not only to the program, but to participating in the search for a therapy that would potentially benefit the course of MS.

During the 1980s, magnetic resonance imaging (MRI) technology had progressed at rocket speed, becoming a diagnostic standard for many diseases. This was especially true for MS, in which it was possible to see MS lesions (plaques) in the brain white matter (see Chapter 3). These increased in number and size at an unpredictable pace as the disease advanced. Would it be possible to measure a therapeutic effect of interferon by performing repeated MRIs on those groups of patients randomized to receive interferon or placebo? Dr. Stephen Marcus, who was medical director for the Betaseron trial, tells of meeting with the president of Shell Oil with the request to spend over a million dollars for yearly MRIs on all enrolled patients. When the answer came back "yes," it became possible to determine whether a positive therapeutic effect was occurring using an objective imaging test, in addition to scoring periodic neurologic examinations and counting clinical relapses.

The trial concluded in the spring of 1993, a New Drug Application (NDA) was submitted, and a U.S. Food and Drug Administration (FDA) Advisory Panel met in Rockville, Maryland. The discussion was intense, the questions penetrating, and a sense of skepticism prevailed. This was, after all, the first treatment to reach the FDA claiming that it benefited the course of MS. Also, some FDA officials were displeased, expressing the view that the mandatory rule of two independent positive trials had not been met. The MRI data was impressive, however, showing a significant treatment effect, and that evidence clearly saved the day—and Betaseron. Finally, late in the afternoon, the majority of the panel voted in favor of licensing Betaseron as an MS therapy, resulting in it becoming the first treatment to emerge as a commercial agent licensed for the control of MS.

Prior to the FDA Advisory panel, Triton Biosciences and its product Betaseron had been acquired by Schering A.G. of Berlin, Germany, which set up a North American subsidiary, Berlex Laboratories. Concerned about the outcome of the FDA hearing, Chiron, which actually manufactured Betaseron, had expanded production slowly and was overwhelmed by the clamor, the demand for the drug, that erupted with the positive FDA vote. To create a fair distribution program, a short-term national lottery was formed for MS patients if their physicians prescribed the drug.

Not long after, the Biogen Corporation brought a second beta-interferon, Avonex®, to market, with the considerable advantage that it required only once a week intramuscular injections, as compared to the every other day injections required for Betaseron. A larger needle was required, but patients or more often family members soon learned how to make the injections. Avonex was made by inserting human interferon genes into cultures of Chinese Hamster kidney cells to produce an interferon molecule similar, if not identical, to the natural beta-interferon made in the human body. The trial design for Avonex was based on retarding neurologic disability rather than inhibiting relapses, a fact that would loom large in the marketing battles that will be described in detail in Chapter 18.

A third beta-interferon product identical in molecular structure to Avonex later obtained FDA approval and came on the U.S. market in 2002. This agent, Rebif®, marketed by Serono, was injected under the skin three times weekly. Both the Avonex and Rebif trials included an MRI component that also demonstrated objective evidence of control of MS lesions in the brain. Thus, within approximately 6 years, three beta-interferon products, somewhat different in their interferon dose and frequency of injection, had successfully completed the formidable course to FDA approval and were on the market in North America, Europe, and elsewhere. They were arrayed against Copaxone as therapies that had been shown to benefit the course of MS, at least in the short term of 2+ years, the approximate length of the placebo-controlled studies.

When first defined in 1958, interferons were considered to be antiviral agents and, indeed, all interferons do have antiviral activity. They act in numerous other ways, however. As a voluminous number of published articles demonstrate, it is probably their immunologic capacity—their ability to inhibit communication between various cells in the immunologic chain of events and alter activity at that critical interface, the blood–brain barrier—that underlies their therapeutic effect in controlling MS relapses.

The emergence of the beta-interferons as a means of reducing MS activity was one of the first situations in which a whole protein molecule—human or otherwise—would require frequent injections for long periods, years or perhaps even decades. Would there be delayed negative consequences of such prolonged protein therapy? The tens of thousands of MS patients prescribed an interferon would, in fact, enter unknowingly into an extended human experiment. Only now, almost two decades later, is it becoming clear that there have been no late negative consequences of prolonged interferon exposure.

17

Challenges to Copaxone's Position as a First-line Multiple Sclerosis Treatment

Euphoria, that often unaccountable feeling of well-being or elation, is one of the most pleasant of human emotions, but also one of the briefest. Joy and happiness may last for weeks or even years, while despondence may linger for months, and anger and hatred regrettably may persist for decades.

The sense of euphoria that gripped everyone related to the Copaxone® project at the successful U.S. Food and Drug Administration (FDA) hearing on September 19, 1996—the Weizmann creators, the Teva staff, and the investigators from the 11 clinical trial centers—was well-deserved. In various ways, they had all contributed to an impressive accomplishment, a therapy for multiple sclerosis (MS) that would soon be available to patients throughout the United States and later the world.

Over the next few days, the euphoria began to fade as the reality of the situation became clearer. Because the FDA usually follows the recommendations of its Expert Advisory Panel, Teva felt quite confident that they would soon receive approval to market Copaxone in the United States if certain technical requirements were fulfilled. Among these, an agreement on a package insert was high on the list. The package insert contains the scientific and medical information supplied to physicians with every vial of Copaxone, outlining the scientific information underpinning the evidence about the drug, how the agent is to be used and at what dose, what the side effects were and—very importantly for both physicians and patients—what the drug could be expected to do. Would it reduce the risk of relapses, retard disability, or provide some other benefit? Based on the two pivotal trials, Copaxone was likely to receive an indication from the FDA for reducing MS relapses. This narrow restriction would underlie a major marketing battle over the next decade or so, with questions about its effect on neurologic disability being fiercely debated.

Since the FDA's jurisdiction extends only to the United States, there were large MS populations who could certainly benefit from Copaxone, but who could not obtain the drug: those who lived in Canada, other parts of the Western Hemisphere, Europe, and even Israel. Teva realized that regulatory approval would have to be obtained in each of these and many other countries if the market for Copaxone was to be expanded and the worldwide MS population served. While FDA approval was critical and might favorably influence decisions by other regulatory agencies, nevertheless Teva faced an extensive amount of future administrative work.

A discussion among the Teva leaders of how Copaxone would be perceived in the marketplace ensued. They reached the conclusion that its future was clouded at best, unless serious problems were addressed. Copaxone at that time was only available as a frozen product, which meant that distribution and storage would be challenging. More importantly, both trials had been conducted using daily injections under the skin, whereas one of the competitors, Betaseron®, required every other day injections, and the second interferon, Avonex®, only called for weekly injections, although with a larger, longer needle for intramuscular placement. Over time, daily injections might become a problem for patients.

The discussion turned to magnetic resonance imaging (MRI), which was conceded to be a major issue. First appearing on the medical scene during the early 1980s, MRI had evolved rapidly and by then was a common diagnostic tool in virtually every advanced hospital. It would soon be a standard technique in most community hospitals and in free-standing radiology centers. Not only was it of great diagnostic use for MS, the Betaseron trial had shown convincingly that it was an objective way to measure therapeutic effectiveness in clinical trials of MS drugs. In fact, without the MRI evidence, it is unlikely that Betaseron would have been approved. Yet neither of the Copaxone trials had employed MRI as a research measure. Would prescribing doctors recommend Copaxone for their patients if this valuable information was available only from the beta-interferon trials? Because MRI information had assumed such a central role in the diagnosis and follow-up of MS patients, the Teva group was told that, if Copaxone had little or no effect on reducing the activity of MS as demonstrated by MRI, it was unlikely to ever assume a major position in the MS treatment marketplace. This posed an immediate dilemma for Teva. Magnetic resonance imaging trials were expensive and time-consuming and, while there was ample evidence from the completed trials that Copaxone was effective in controlling relapses and had an impact on disability, its effect on changes in the brain demonstrated by MRI was unknown; if it turned out to be modest or even trivial, the future of Copaxone would be in doubt. Conducting an expensive MRI trial could be a real risk to the product, if the outcome was negative.

The development of therapies for long-term or even life-long disabling conditions such as MS has always faced the question of the duration of benefit. Not surprisingly, every pharmaceutical company wishes to conduct trials of the shortest duration, with the smallest number of participants that will provide a convincing result to gain FDA approval. Time and money are of the essence. On the other hand, any evidence that the drug has a long-term positive impact on the disease is welcome and even critical for people with MS and their physicians. Teva knew that the placebo-controlled evaluation of Betaseron had been carried out for over 4 years, while the Avonex trial had actually lasted for less than 2 years. Already, because of the manner in which the placebo-controlled phase of the Copaxone trials had been conducted, there was solid evidence for between 30 and 36 months of increasingly useful treatment for many of the participants, so at least some data of a longer duration of benefit was available. Could useful information over much longer periods of Copaxone treatment be obtained by extending the trial, with the approval of the 11 U.S. investigative sites and—more importantly—their patients? Long-term follow-up of patients would be expensive, but it might provide a new level of confidence in Copaxone that was not available for the interferon products where, in each case, the trial had been concluded and the patient groups disbanded.

As Teva anticipated approval by the FDA, new questions stimulated anxious discussion. The U.S. MS population was large—at least 350,000 known patients, being cared for mainly by the 10,000 neurologists throughout the country. What kind of sales program would be necessary to provide information to such a large market, especially in the face of active competition that was likely to be mounted by the interferon competitors? Teva had relatively little first-hand knowledge of the U.S. MS marketplace, no direct contact with U.S. neurologists, and no experience in selling any branded or innovative drug.

Teva immediately began to contact a number of U.S. pharmaceutical companies, asking about their interest in becoming partners in the commercial development and sales of Copaxone. In almost every case the response was similar: Yes, the product is interesting and the market is attractive, and each company said that it might be interested in a proposal to license Copaxone into the company for further commercial development. To all such responses, Eli Hurvitz immediately said "No," that Copaxone was not available to be licensed out but was only available in some type of a partnership arrangement in which Teva would maintain long-term control of the product.

The challenging business discussions seemed endless, and the obstacles seemed to multiply, but the faith in Copaxone was strong and the Teva group persisted.

Teva Marion Partners

By 1995, with the well-received Bornstein pilot trial results and the convincing outcome of the U.S. pivotal trial, Teva was relatively certain that it soon would gain FDA marketing approval. Once Eli Hurvitz had rejected all offers to license out Copaxone, stating that only a partnership would be satisfactory, negotiations began with Marion Merrell Dow, a Kansas City pharmaceutical company that had recently been created from a combination of Marion Laboratories and Merrell Dow Corporation. This company seemed interested in a true partnership.

The colorful history of the 1989 merger of Marion with Merrell Dow can be traced to 1950, when Ewing Marion Kauffman, a legendary name in Kansas City, started a tiny venture with $4,000 in capital. He began to manufacture a calcium supplement made from crushed oyster shells, which he produced in the basement of his home. As the company grew, Kauffman searched for new products that would be acquired exclusively by reformulating and developing already-discovered products that had been rejected or neglected by other companies. Even by 1974, after 24 years, the successful company's in-house research budget stood at zero.

Through a series of acquisitions, mergers, and partnerships, Marion's catalog of prescription and over-the-counter products grew; in time, it included Gaviscon, an antacid; the cardiac drug, Cardizem; Carafate, an ulcer drug; Ditropan, a urologic agent; and several other successful products.

Following its merger with Merrell Dow, the antihistamine Seldane, Nicorette anti-smoking gum, and the mouthwash Cepacol were added to the product line. All of these, of course, required that the expanding company hire a national sales force and develop advertising expertise throughout the United States.

In 1995, the business press announced the formation of Teva Marion Partners, which would be co-owned by Teva and Marion Merrell Dow. The business would be headquartered in Kansas City and led by

John Vandewalle, who had been an executive with Marion Merrell Dow. Soon after this partnership was formed, Marion Merrell Dow underwent several other mergers and finally was acquired by Aventis Pharmaceuticals.

As a new partnership, Teva Marion Partners (TMP) needed a Copaxone sales and marketing force and, not surprisingly, Vandewalle looked for expertise to his colleagues at Marion Merrell Dow, where he was able to convince several young, energetic, and experienced pharmaceutical managers to join him: John Hassler, Judy Katterhenrich, Marty Berndt, and others. When questioned about why they would leave secure positions to join a startup linked to an Israeli company that only produced and sold generic drugs, their uniform reply was that Copaxone seemed to be a unique and interesting product targeted at an important disease, and that the excitement and adventure that the new responsibilities would entail would be a welcome challenge. So the story of Copaxone, which had previously been known only from clinical trial reports and basic research papers, was about to be introduced to American neurologists and the hundreds of thousands of patients who were their responsibility.

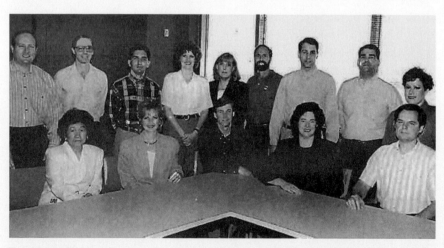

Teva Marion Partners (back row from left) Rick Mengoni, John Vandewalle, Faruk Capan, Karen Finkbiner, Judy Katterhenrich, Don Duryee, Karl Strohmeier, Bill Poikey, Vickie Peters. (Front row from left) Lillian Pardo, Cathy Kennedy, Jay Simpson, Gwen Duzenberry, John Hassler.

The pressure to proceed increased on December 23, 1996, when the welcome news from the FDA arrived with approval to market Copaxone.

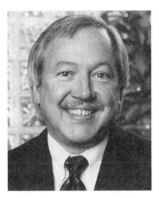

Larry Downey

Copaxone was launched on April 2, 1997, in Miami, Florida, where representatives from the Weizmann Institute, Teva in Israel, and Teva Marion Partners gathered to attend an enthusiastic, exciting, and hopeful gala dinner. The commercial product, the complex laboratory and animal science, and the multiple clinical trials had proceeded step by—at times slow—step in an incredible, hardly believable way, consuming almost exactly 30 years. It was entering a new phase, in fact a new era, which over the next 13+ years would finally position Copaxone as the most prescribed therapy for the control of relapsing-remitting MS.

Soon after the launch, Vandewalle left to pursue other opportunities, and Larry Downey, who had been active in the negotiations between Teva and Marion Merrell Dow, was named acting and then permanent CEO of TMP. He ably led the transition when Teva took full control and formed Teva Neuroscience, and has continued to this day as the highly successful head of the company. Downey recently acquired the new title of Executive Vice President, North American Brand Pharmaceuticals.

The Lack of Magnetic Resonance Imaging Data

Among the many challenges facing the Teva group in 1996, the lack of an MRI component in the U.S. pivotal trial was near the top of the list. Although the proof of clinical efficacy—that is, the ability to control MS relapses—was well established and very convincing to the FDA ad-

169

visory panel, the lack of proven effect on the disease as measured by MRI put Copaxone at a distinct disadvantage, compared to the interferons in the U.S. marketplace. This gap clearly had to be remedied. The Copaxone group at Teva began to interview prominent MRI experts and neuroradiologists, and advisory panels were gathered at major international MS and neurologic congresses to plan how to proceed.

Some preliminary information was in fact available, which was encouraging and useful in planning future MRI trials. The University of Pennsylvania Hospital in Philadelphia, one of the 11 sites for the U.S. pivotal trial, had a major, internationally recognized MRI research center that had been developed with substantial funding from the National Institutes of Health (NIH). In addition, the National MS Society had begun to appreciate the usefulness of MRI as a monitoring tool for potential MS therapies, and had provided a small grant to the University of Pennsylvania to image patients in the Cop 1 trial.

Twenty-seven of the 251 patients enrolled in the U.S. pivotal trial had been recruited there; 14 had injected glatiramer acetate and 13 had received placebo for approximately 24 months. At the beginning of the trial, all of these patients were entered into an MRI study in which regular scans were obtained each time patients returned for their neurologic visits. All of these images were available for analysis at the end of the trial, and the findings were anxiously awaited not only in Philadelphia but also in Israel.

The two patient groups had been well-matched by age, sex, and level of disease. It was welcome, in fact exciting news when it turned out that there was a significant positive MRI benefit from Copaxone therapy. The number of gadolinium-enhanced lesions—the active inflammatory lesions—was significantly less in the group of patients who had received Cop 1 and, perhaps even more interesting, the amount of brain atrophy, a known and sinister component of MS pathology, was less in the Copaxone-treated group than in those who had received placebo.

Although these results came from a very small population of patients, nevertheless they were in the right direction and were encouraging, especially because very advanced MRI techniques had been employed at the University of Pennsylvania imaging center. While certainly not adequate to counteract all the criticisms of Copaxone therapy that were being raised by many neurologists and the beta-interferon groups, nevertheless they were an early step in what would ultimately become a convincing argument for choosing Copaxone to treat relapsing MS.

Another small but informative study had been carried out in Genoa, Italy, in the mid-1990s. Exploring the MRI activity taking place in the brains of relapsing MS patients, Giovanni Luigi Mancardi and several coworkers had scanned ten patients for 9 to 27 months with monthly gadolinium-enhanced MRI. Following this pretreatment period, they then treated all ten patients with subcutaneous injections of 20 mg of Cop 1 daily for an additional 10 to 14 months, while maintaining the monthly MRI scanning. When all scans were analyzed, they found a 57% decrease in the frequency of new enhancing lesions during the treatment phase, compared with pretreatment, as well as a decrease in relapses from 42 before treatment to only three during treatment. This small study seemed to indicate that an intense monthly scanning schedule could show a therapeutic impact much more quickly than only scanning at yearly intervals.

Soon the information-gathering phase came to an end, and it became necessary to make decisions about where to go. First, it was decided that any MRI study of Copaxone should be carried out in Europe and Canada, rather than in the United States, where the pivotal trials had been conducted. In fact, the emerging study came to be known somewhat awkwardly as "The European/Canadian Multi-center Double-blind, Randomized, Placebo-controlled Study of Glatiramer Acetate on Magnetic Resonance Imaging Measured Disease Activity and Burden in Patients with Relapsing Multiple Sclerosis." Any MRI study requires a central reading center where all images are sent for uniform analysis. Yafit Stark, who had played such a central role in the day-to-day conduct of the U.S. pivotal trial, had returned to Teva in Israel and was given the responsibility of organizing the MRI study. She chose Jerry Wolinsky at the University of Texas Houston as her advisor, and together they visited many potential MRI reading centers in Europe. Major MS MRI analyses centers existed in London, Amsterdam, and Basel, but their current commitments would not permit joining Teva in what would be a major new responsibility. Finally, Stark and Wolinsky recommended that Teva partner with the Imaging Research Unit at the Department of Neuroscience, Scientific Institute Ospedale San Raffaele, University of Milan, Italy. This Center had blossomed under the leadership of Giancarlo Comi and the chief imaging scientist, Massimo Filippi, both neurologists with a longstanding interest in MS. They continued to be ably advised by Wolinsky, himself a renowned MRI expert.

The trial design was unusual—one could even say revolutionary or audacious—both in its uniqueness and in the potential for failure that was imbedded in its outline. First, it was short, only 9 months in duration, although there was a second 9-month cross-over stage; yet the entire trial lasted for only 18 months. Also, it called for the patients to undergo an MRI evaluation every month for the first 9 months, much more frequently than had ever been demanded in earlier MS MRI trials. Third, the patients not only had to demonstrate active disease by experiencing a recent MS relapse, but they also had to have active disease as measured by enhancing lesions on a screening MRI prior to being admitted to the trial. The primary endpoint was total number of enhancing lesions on the MRI.

Twenty-nine centers in six European countries and Canada participated in the trial, which enrolled patients between February and November 1997. In the end, 239 patients were selected for study, equally divided between those receiving Copaxone, 20 mg by subcutaneous injection every day, and those receiving daily subcutaneous injections of placebo. The entry criteria were identical to those used in the U.S. pivotal trial, except for the requirement for a positive pre-study MRI and, when finally analyzed, the patient groups from the two trials were remarkably similar. Most study rules for the two trials were identical; for instance, all patients who noted neurologic symptoms suggesting a new relapse had to contact their center at once and be evaluated within 7 days to establish whether they were experiencing a true relapse.

The 9 months went by quickly. The MRI reading center in Milan was exceedingly busy. A total of 1,237 MRI scans were obtained from the patients in the Copaxone group, 94.5% of the expected number, and the comparable percent of completed images in the placebo arm was 96.3%; thus, virtually every possible MRI had been captured for analysis.

It is common practice in the conduct of clinical trials to have an interim analysis, that is, a secret preliminary review of the data by an expert advisory committee before the end of the trial. Such early analyses serve one of two purposes: to determine whether there is no chance that the trial would be successful and thus should be stopped, and to determine if the trial was already showing a significant benefit, in which case it could be concluded early. A European/Canadian MRI trial interim analysis was called for when 130 of the 239 patients had completed 9 months of dosing, and the advisory committee met in Paris to review this information in the late spring of 1998. Shaul Kadosh, Teva's chief statistician, had collected all MRI reports from the trial to that point.

When he finished his presentation to the committee, it was clear that an interesting dilemma had to be resolved. The interim analysis showed a significant benefit that had just barely cleared the statistical bar to become positive. By custom, the committee should have declared the trial a success, and it should have been terminated. On the other hand, a much more convincing result might be apparent if they allowed the trial to continue for another 6 or 8 weeks. Among the five people in the Paris conference room, intense debate centered on statistics but also on ethics. When a vote was taken, three voted to continue and two voted to conclude the study at that point. The trial was allowed to continue and, in the end, the result was much more convincing when all patients had participated for the full 9 months. Also, when finally concluded, it was shown that there had been 33% fewer relapses in the group receiving Copaxone, demonstrating without doubt the double benefit of significantly reducing not only the underlying inflammation in the brain shown by MRI but also a major inhibition of MS relapses.

This little incident underlines the drama that can, at times during clinical trials, evoke ethical questions and at times anxiety, even though the effort is always to get the best information possible when developing improved MS therapies.

The conclusions from the study clearly showed that Copaxone had a highly significant and rapid effect, not only on relapses, as had been shown previously, but also on an important objective measure, MRI activity.

Further review of the large library of MRI images generated in this trial supplied other interesting and important clues about the benefit that Copaxone therapy provided. Special MRI measurements, given the esoteric name of "chronic T1 black holes," are used to detect local areas of severe MS destruction of brain tissue. When this aspect of the European/Canadian scans was analyzed, it was clear that Copaxone was capable of retarding the number of T1 black holes developing in the brain. This raised the possibility that Copaxone therapy reduced the amount of brain being damaged by MS. Also, using the most advanced MRI measurements available, it was possible to show that even in a short 9- to 18-month period, the extent of brain atrophy had been reduced in the treated patients in comparison with those who had received placebo.

All in all, this short but critical study had turned out to be highly informative for everyone interested in improving the lot of MS patients. It also benefited Copaxone's position in the marketplace, where physicians are responsible for daily decisions in choosing the appropriate therapy for their MS patients.

Long-term Studies

A question not often asked and even less often investigated is whether a treatment for a chronic illness such as MS, studied for only 2 to 4 years, will continue to be therapeutically useful for longer periods, measured over many years or decades. Can one confidently extrapolate short-term results far into the future? The beta-interferons were studied in an organized manner for relatively brief periods, Betaseron for slightly over 4 years, Rebif® for 2 years, and Avonex for less than 2 years, while Copaxone had been evaluated in a placebo-controlled trial for only about 30 months.

It is, of course, reasonable that commercial sponsors will seek FDA approval for marketable treatments in the shortest period possible. Time is money. But are long-term marketing and sales appropriate, or are they even ethical, without evidence of continuing benefit? The FDA has, after all, required proof of efficacy as well as safety, but efficacy for how long?

As the Copaxone pivotal trial approached its planned conclusion at about 30 months, the investigative group argued strongly that Teva should provide active drug to all participants, at least until the trial results were fully analyzed and announced. Without the dedicated engagement of the patients, no commercial product would be possible. After internal discussion, Teva agreed: All placebo patients should be switched to active drug and all patients would continue to be monitored in an organized manner. But soon Teva approached the investigators and participating patients with a much more generous and exciting proposal. All patients would be offered Copaxone in an ongoing program as long as they agreed to stay on Copaxone therapy exclusively. Safety monitoring would continue and, every 6 months, a neurologic examination by the study neurologists would measure their current neurologic state. No similar attempt at charting long-term benefit or safety had ever been attempted for an MS treatment. Early dropouts from the placebo-controlled phase of the pivotal trial would not continue; still, 232 patients out of the original 251 were available and agreed to continue. This bold plan was proposed and successfully achieved mainly through the efforts of David Ladkani at Teva, who had worked tirelessly on the project since the early days when Cop 1 was still being produced "at the bench" in the laboratories of Sela and Arnon at the Weizmann Institute. His superior,

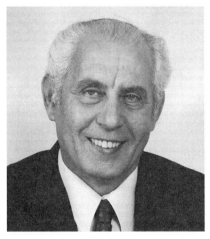

Aharon Schwartz

Dr. Aharon Schwartz, strongly advocated for this long-term plan although there was considerable concern within Teva about the cost.

At regular intervals, as data became available, detailed analysis was completed and published; two reports appeared on the 6-year progress, another at 8 years, and later at 10 and 15 years. Several conclusions of value for determining the benefit of long-term Copaxone use emerged. The drug continued to be very safe, with no late risks or negative consequences. But was treatment useful? Yes. It became clear that, even with full clinical examinations every 6 months, few patients had neurologically progressed, especially to the critical step of EDSS 6 (Chapter 1), the point at which constant walking aids were required and the quality of life began to decline more rapidly. Also of interest, those patients who had originally taken placebo for approximately 30 months had, as a group, suffered more disability; even years later, they were still worse off than the group fortunate enough to have received Copaxone from the beginning. In other words, even after being switched to Copaxone, those who had received placebo at first would never "catch up." This demonstrates a "risk" that individuals entering a clinical trial must assume to obtain the invaluable information that will later help thousands.

The long-term follow-up continued for over a decade, during which time patients took their daily injections of Copaxone. Was it worth it? Had the peril of MS worsening actually declined? The patients had a right to know, and the 11 investigative groups who had all participated in the long-term study and continued to provide data were anxious. A unique 10-year analysis was planned and announced.

To get the best information about the extended effectiveness of Copaxone, all patients still participating in the trial were compared with patients who had dropped out over the years but had agreed to come back for another hands-on evaluation 10 years after they had first joined the trial in 1991. Of the 232 patients who were eligible because they had for some period, brief or long, received injections of Copaxone, 108 or 47% were still participating 10 years later. But what had happened to the other 124? Twenty-four had been lost to follow-up, including five who had died of various causes over the decade. Others had left the trial for some negative reaction, such as pain when they made the injection or brief periods of shortness of breath and chest pain, which—while known to be benign—were still frightening to some. Of the 87 other dropouts, a few had come to the conclusion that their MS was worsening and decided to switch to another treatment, most commonly a beta-interferon. Thirty patients were unable to follow the rules of the trial, often because they had moved away from the investigative site where they had entered it. Finally, eight patients became pregnant and were dropped from the study, following the recommendation from the FDA to stop the medication, even though no evidence of danger to pregnancy from Copaxone had ever been recognized in either humans or animals. In fact, Copaxone had received a Class B (no known risk to experimental animals or humans) rating by the FDA, whereas the interferons had all been classified as Class C (demonstrated pregnancy risk in either experimental animals or humans) because of some concern about a risk to the pregnancy.

Of the 124 who had dropped out, 50 agreed to come back to their investigative sites for a final neurologic evaluation. Thus, a comparison could be made between the 108 who were still receiving Copaxone and the 50 who had dropped out.

For those who had continued, it had been possible to record the number of relapses they experienced each year. At the beginning, patients had on average experienced more than one relapse per year. The relapse rate had declined year by year for most of the 10 years, and these patients were experiencing a relapse only once every 4 or 5 years in the later years of the trial. No valid information on relapses was available for those who had dropped out.

Of the 108 continuing patients, the most striking finding was how stable their neurologic state had been over the decade. Year by year, over 60% of the patients were either stable or had actually improved from their status at entry into the study in 1991. Even more remarkable, only eight had reached EDSS 6 or beyond. Of the 50 patients who had dropped out but then came back for a 10-year evaluation, 25 (50%) had reached the serious benchmark of EDSS 6, which suggested that long-term therapy with Copaxone had a positive influence on the risk of increased disability. A valid criticism of this comparison is that many of the patients who had withdrawn from the trial were not available for reexamination.

To gain a better perspective on long-term MS therapy, some long-term follow-up has also been carried out for the beta-interferons that had reached the market by 1996 and which have been in direct competition with Copaxone. For the Avonex once-a-week form of interferon, after 2 years of therapy almost 5% of patients treated with interferon had reached EDSS 6, and after 8 years, 29% had declined to that level, although what treatments they had used after the first 2 years is unclear. Patients enrolled in the Rebif beta-interferon trial were also reevaluated after 8 years. Of those known to have received active drug for at least 4 years, 20% had advanced to the EDSS 6 level.

These percentages for Copaxone (8%), Rebif (20%), and Avonex (29%) provide a rough sense that Copaxone was more effective in delaying disability. This is rightfully subject to criticism. First, the trials were conducted somewhat differently, and the patients recruited into them were not identical, even though all tried to enroll relapsing-remitting MS patients with similar characteristics at onset. Direct comparisons between trials have been scientifically challenged because of the recognized differences in the enrollment characteristics of each group. Nevertheless, only in the Copaxone long-term study were patients known to be on a single drug over the decade and evaluated in person every 6 months.

This series of long-term follow-ups of patients who participated in various interferon trials or in the Copaxone trial are at best rough approximations of how each therapy is likely to influence the course of MS over relatively long periods of time, that is, 8 to 10 years. Comparisons at best only show trends but, nevertheless, because all three trials recruited relapsing-remitting patients thought to be relatively similar at onset, the published data would lead one to the conclusion that continuous use of Copaxone may provide long-term control of relapsing MS.

18

Battles in the Marketplace

The title of the best-selling book *The Perfect Storm*, authored by Sabastian Junger and published in 1997, has become a general, widely used descriptive phrase in the English language; it suggests that an unexpected confluence of events might produce an unlikely outcome that may often be negative or even tragic. The tale involved the coming together of extreme climactic events in the North Atlantic Ocean to create a historic storm that threatened boats and ships, resulting in the loss of a long-line swordfish trawler and its doomed crew.

In the final 4 years of the last century and the initial 6 years of the present one, the appearance of four new treatments for multiple sclerosis (MS), all somewhat similar in their effect on the disease, caused a storm of competing claims and marketing adventures, producing perplexity and doubt for treating physicians, managed care companies, and—most unfortunately—confusion for many people with MS.

The modern era of effective MS treatments began in 1993, when a U.S. Food and Drug Administration (FDA) advisory panel, in a split vote, recommended that interferon beta-1b known as Betaseron® be approved for use by MS patients with relapsing-remitting forms of the disease. While Cop 1 (copolymer one) had been the first treatment shown to improve the course of MS in 1987, Betaseron was the first drug to be marketed in the U.S., 6 years later. Even at its launch, there was considerable unrest and turmoil, especially for patients. The company selling Betaseron, Berlex Laboratories, was perhaps unprepared for the quick FDA decision, and inadequate drug supplies were available to meet the demand. Contributing to the problem, the MS population was poorly informed and often misunderstood the results from the recently completed trial, which had shown a reduction of new relapses and also benefit in controlling the development of magnetic resonance imaging (MRI) lesions in the brain. Many desperate MS patients incorrectly envisioned "a cure" or the reversal of long-term fixed disability, picturing themselves springing from their wheelchairs or throwing away their crutches to go dancing again. Not surprisingly, they wanted Betaseron *now*.

In response, Berlex announced a short-term lottery plan whereby patients with a doctor's prescription could sign up for a lottery number and those with low numbers, the "lucky ones," would receive Betaseron. The response only generated considerable anger from most patients: Why should I be denied this chance to return to normal? Great pressure was put on physicians, mainly neurologists, to write prescriptions for Betaseron, often by patients with more advanced disabling MS who were, based on the data from the trial or the information provided to the FDA, most unlikely to show benefit from Betaseron treatment. Fortunately, the supply problems were soon corrected and Betaseron became available to U.S. MS patients, both for those likely to benefit but also for those unlikely to be helped.

This period of great demand and patient clamor of course introduced Betaseron, its use, and its problems, to most treating neurologists in the United States. They began to gain personal experience with the situation in their offices and clinics, learning firsthand about the variable range of side effects that treated patients would experience. Betaseron was given by injection under the skin every other day and, especially during the first 4 to 8 weeks, most new patients experienced many unpleasant flu-like symptoms; these included low-grade fever, chills, muscle and joint aches, fatigue, headache, and stiffness, all of which could last 8 to 24 hours. Taking ibuprofen (Advil® or Motrin®) before the injection, and making the injection at bedtime helped. The patients also complained of injection site reactions, red raised areas on the skin that could last 1 to 2 weeks. During the pilot Betaseron trial in the mid-1980s, when the best-tolerated dose was being determined, the study was started during the hot summer months in Baltimore and in Philadelphia. Participating women often came to the clinic wearing shorts and sleeveless blouses. A frequent comment was that they looked like "poke a dot" ladies with their prolonged injection site reactions, leading to the requirement during the following large pivotal trial that all participants wear slacks and long-sleeved shirts or blouses to reduce the risk of unblinding the trial if examiners noted the very different injection site reactions in patients receiving interferon or placebo.

Because any long-term beta-interferon treatment might result in liver damage, it was recommended that blood tests for liver function be performed at regular intervals of every 3 months or so, even though the number of patients with this problem was very low.

The side effects of Betaseron, while common during the beginning of therapy, were highly variable as treatment continued. Some individuals reported few complaints after 3 or 4 weeks, while others were unable to tolerate the drug even after trying for several months, and were never able to become regular users. Improved education of the expected benefits from interferon therapy and careful instructions about injection technique, with regular support for the first 6 to 12 months, proved to be very helpful and have been incorporated into the educational plans for interferon treatment of MS everywhere.

The MS marketing situation in the United States settled down and was relatively calm when only Betaseron was available, but in May of 1996, a second interferon product, Avonex®, was approved by the FDA. Betaseron was known as a "re-engineered molecule" that required a substitution of one amino acid to improve its stability. Avonex, on the other hand, was made in mammalian rather than bacterial cells, and was much closer to the structure of the actual human beta-interferon.

Avonex was produced by the Cambridge, Massachusetts, biotechnology company, Biogen (later Biogen-Idec) that had sponsored the trial. The study benefited from major support from a National Institutes of Health (NIH) grant. The program called for injections of interferon once a week, using a relatively large needle that deposited the drug deep into muscle, rather than beneath the skin, as with Betaseron. Of major importance, the primary endpoint in the Avonex trial had been a reduction in neurologic disability, rather than inhibiting MS relapses. Supported by a strong, aggressive marketing campaign, Avonex quickly became the market leader, replacing Betaseron, which was reduced to supplying only 20% of the market in just a few months.

Patients and physicians soon discovered that Avonex produced the same types of side effects as Betaseron: flu-like symptoms, muscle aches, fatigue, etc. Many patients began taking the weekly intramuscular injections on Friday evening, because the unpleasant symptoms often persisted well into the next day, and patients were unwilling to lose a day of work while recovering from interferon side effects. Avonex did share with Betaseron the benefit of an MRI component in the pivotal trial, showing fewer MRI lesions in the brain, a finding that was not available to Copaxone® during this early period in 1997.

Following its launch in April 1997, Copaxone also entered the U.S. marketplace with proven claims. These included a significant reduction in relapses, the ability to stabilize Extended Disability Status Scale (EDSS) scores, and the absence of the side effects of the interferons, but with the perceived downside of requiring daily subcutaneous injections.

Between 1997 and 2002, the three products available in the United States—Betaseron, Avonex, and Copaxone, often referred to as the A, B, C drugs—all approved by the FDA, battled for the attention of prescribing physicians and for market share in the United States. Which might help MS patients the most?

The U.S. commercial scene was further scrambled by escalating competing claims when a third interferon product, Rebif®, was given FDA approval in 2002. Rebif, produced by the Italian-Swiss company Serono, had a molecular structure identical to natural beta-interferon and Avonex, but it had been tested in large European placebo-controlled clinical trials. It was administered subcutaneously three times a week. The primary claim was a reduction of MS relapses, and there was also an effect on disability and a positive effect on MRI activity. Because of its similarity to the other drugs, it had been denied entrance into the U.S. market until Serono conducted a relatively short head-to-head trial in which it was compared with Avonex and shown to be modestly superior. The FDA agreed, allowing Rebif to join the confusing mix of drugs available for U.S. doctors to consider for their MS patients.

The bewildering situation of therapeutic choices which engulfed the United States in 1997 is not too difficult to understand. Three, soon to be four, commercial products, all approved by the FDA, were available, and all required continuous injections: Copaxone daily, Betaseron every other day, Rebif three times a week, and Avonex only once a week, although it had to be given by a larger intramuscular injection, which some patients found difficult to manage. All were considered as belonging to a new class of biologics, and all were very expensive. For instance, Betaseron was priced at over $10,000 per year when introduced in 1993, and the cost—for all of them—has only increased over time.

The mandatory placebo-controlled clinical trials of each product had enrolled similar sets of patients and had shown relatively similar results. All had reduced the risk of relapses by approximately one-third, and both Copaxone and Rebif had shown a significant ability to inhibit progression of disability, although this was the primary claim only for Avonex. With the publication of the European-Canadian Copaxone MRI study in 2001, all had been observed to reduce the amount of MS activity, as demonstrated by repeated MRI scans, over relatively long periods of time. In short, there was no clearly superior drug for the continuing management of relapsing MS. Marketing veterans who had worked for a variety of companies selling drugs for cardiac disease, GI conditions, or even cancer, stated that they had never experienced the level of aggressive marketing techniques that the U.S. neurologic community was exposed to between 1997 and 2007.

In an effort to find some competitive advantage, all four companies dug back into the data collected during the various trials to find what has been called *post-hoc analysis data*, that is, data that had not been analyzed before the code of each trial was broken. Biogen published widely proclaimed MRI data showing that patients who received Avonex were less likely to suffer from brain atrophy than were placebo patients. The makers of Betaseron published data indicating that cognitive decline was less likely for patients receiving active drug. Teva showed that the destructive lesions in the brain called T1 black holes were less likely to occur in treated patients than in those receiving placebo.

A variety of head-to-head studies seemed to show benefit for one drug over the other. Serono sponsored the EVIDENCE trial in the United States, comparing Rebif and Avonex, and showed the modest increased benefit for Rebif that was enough to convince the FDA to allow the drug to enter the U.S. market. A 2-year trial in Italy, the INCOMIN study, compared the relapse and MRI changes in patients receiving Betaseron versus Avonex, and showed that Betaseron injected subcutaneously every other day resulted in improved outcomes over Avonex given intramuscularly once a week. These trials led to the general impression among treating physicians that frequent injections of beta-interferons given at higher doses were more effective and controlled MS activity better than the so-called low-dose interferon Avonex.

A number of open-label trials, without a placebo group, compared each of the interferons with Copaxone. These were studies in which the characteristics of the patients were not rigidly controlled, but more closely mirrored the broad range of MS patients in the community. In a modest-sized study from Wayne State University in Michigan, Copaxone was shown to reduce MS relapses more effectively than either Betaseron or Avonex. In a larger open-label study conducted in Berlin, Germany, Copaxone was compared with all three of the interferon products and shown to control relapses better and also to have fewer patients who stopped treatment. A study from Argentina also showed superior relapse control for Copaxone over the interferons. In general, these studies, while widely distributed to the treating physician community, tended to confuse the situation even more, although the market share of Copaxone grew slightly with each one. For every announced study there was an immediate response from competitors, pointing out any flaw, great or small, in the trial design or findings.

An impressive number of basic studies were performed in Israel, Europe, and North America. Investigations showed that Copaxone had a "neuroprotective" effect, such that less brain tissue was damaged by the experimental allergic encephalomyelitis (EAE) process in animals receiving Copaxone. This information was immediately shown to treating physicians and helped define the effects of Copaxone therapy.

It had become clear in the very earliest pilot trials of Betaseron that, in some patients exposed to interferon for a period of time, the body responded by producing neutralizing antibodies; when these appeared, the effectiveness of the drug was reduced, as measured by either clinical means or by MRI. All three interferon products were shown to stimulate neutralizing antibodies; Betaseron by approximately 33%, Rebif by approximately 20%, and Avonex by about 4% to 6%. Patients treated with an interferon probably got little benefit if they developed neutralizing antibodies. To further confuse the issue, longer-term observations showed that patients with positive neutralizing antibodies might lose them over time and that the clinical effectiveness of the drug might return. This issue was widely discussed and studied, usually in tests conducted by the commercial sponsors, leading to varying levels of distrust in the reported findings. In Denmark, only MS patients cared for in government-sponsored clinics could be prescribed any of the interferon products, and all were followed for the development of antibodies using precise laboratory measurements designated by the government. This unbiased process clarified the situation and showed that, indeed, interferon antibodies could lower benefit. Clinic investigators recommended that some antibody-positive patients should be considered for a switch to Copaxone. Neutralizing antibodies had never been shown to be a problem during Copaxone therapy.

Other studies designed to hopefully improve the drug's effectiveness soon followed. Higher doses of Betaseron were studied but, as had been shown in the very earliest pilot studies, a dose of 8 million units, the approved dose, was the highest that could be tolerated by most MS patients. Copaxone was investigated as an oral preparation in several species of laboratory animals and had been shown to be quite effective in reducing the risk of EAE. A large patient program was launched, the CORAL study, hoping to define a Copaxone "pill" that would inhibit MS and would not require injections. In spite of considerable expense, the trial failed. The search for the best of the available treatments continued.

The Clinically Isolated Syndrome Trials

Turning in a new direction, effort was made to redefine MS by searching for the earliest appearance of the disease. A new term, *clinically isolated syn-*

drome or CIS was coined to describe patients who displayed the first neurologic symptoms, such as optic neuritis (blindness in one eye), spinal cord symptoms (numbness or weakness in a leg), or other acute symptoms, accompanied by an abnormal MRI suggestive of MS. Biogen was the first, sponsoring the CHAMPS trial, which showed that the second symptoms of MS could be delayed by a number of months if patients received Avonex versus placebo. When these positive results were announced, physicians were urged to start treatment earlier, and considerable pressure was put on the manufacturers of the other interferons and on Teva to duplicate the results and show that their drug could also delay future MS symptoms. These trials cost many millions of dollars and, of course, required that many patients receive placebo for 2 or more years, undoubtedly putting some at increased risk of MS attacks. The competition in the marketplace pressured each company to add a CIS component to their labeling or package insert. Over time, all three interferon sponsors and Teva conducted CIS trials, all of which were positive; Berlex (Betaseron), Biogen (Avonex), and Teva (Copaxone) succeeded in expanded labeling for CIS.

The Battle of the *P*-values

The 12 years between 1996 and 2008 have been called "the battle of the *p*-values." This refers to the fact that significant clinical trial findings have a positive *p*-value, a statistical evaluation demonstrating that there was a less than 5% chance that an outcome or claim, whatever it might be, could be due to chance alone. The multiple findings from all of the trials, the post-hoc analysis of information from each trial, the conduct of other trials such as the CIS placebo-controlled trials, all provided the opportunity to determine dozens if not hundreds of comparisons with a positive *p*-value that might give a competitive marketing advantage to one product over another. But how to get this mass of information to treating physicians and even to patients in this crowded and clouded competitive and confusing market?

Each of the drug companies or sponsors began to develop a staff of pharmaceutical drug sales representatives who were assigned to regions throughout the United States and Canada. These "drug reps," who tend to be well-educated, well-spoken, and well-groomed individuals, were given extensive education about not only MS but about the various drugs and the advantages that one drug had shown in some fashion over its competitors. Each representative was supplied with a new automobile to allow them to cover their territory, and it soon became customary for physicians' offices to expect visits from the drug reps of various companies who would seek to meet with the prescribing physician and leave educational materials, which usually would contain some slant toward the products that they were "detailing" or selling. The same information would commonly appear in medical journal ads. (The companies had to be careful with the material they distributed, because the FDA monitors print material for accuracy and sends warning letters if material is too biased.)

Gifts and Food

The drug reps did not come empty-handed. Soon physicians' offices would reap the benefit of labeled pens, coffee cups, desk clocks, sticky pads, lotion, calendars, and other relatively inexpensive but useful items with the product name printed in bold letters. The p-value arguments also led to marketing battles, which became a weekly experience in physicians' offices, not only for doctors but also for nurses, receptionists, and others.

Food always gets attention, and it became commonplace for drug reps to provide lunches for the doctors and office staff. This meant that many physicians' offices could expect a visit from one of the competing drug company drug reps at least once a month; since there were four or even five drug reps marketing products, that could lead to office lunches at least one day of every week, month after month.

Searching for more focused venues, the pharmaceutical companies offered to provide speakers to hospital and medical school grand rounds sessions, and a group of well-known national MS experts soon were "on the circuits," traveling to cities throughout the U.S. to give lectures, often followed by meetings with the resident staff to discuss issues related to MS patient care. Depending on the speaker, this could be a somewhat-biased presentation, and some of the companies demanded that only a set of slides produced by that company could be used in these presentations. Most MS experts refused to be restricted to this extent and viewed their role as providing an important educational service that would ultimately improve MS care.

Another educational activity was to host dinner meetings, during which the expert would present a talk on MS treatment at a well-known, often quite expensive, local restaurant. At the beginning of the decade, local physicians were able to bring their spouses; for many practicing physicians, this meant that they and their spouses could dine at an exclusive restaurant monthly if not more often. Reaction to this practice was of course bound to occur, and soon nonphysicians were not permitted to attend. A national organization, Pharmaceutical Research and Manufacturers of America (PhRMA) began to form guidelines that called for increasingly severe restrictions on what was allowed. These practices were, of course, not limited to only MS drugs but were widely employed and then increasingly restricted over time.

Regional and National Meetings

To better understand the treatment decision-making process, and the reasons why certain MS drugs were prescribed by practicing neurologists, each of the companies scheduled regional and in some cases national advisory meetings, to which they invited physicians with a strong interest in and practice of MS care for 2- or 3-day discussions. Experts provided information about topics such as the newer clinical trials, the basic mechanism of action of each product, and the importance of MRI and other diagnostic tools. Following lectures, there was a question-and-answer period or break-out sessions in which the sponsor could gain better insight into the understanding or perspective of the treating neurologist and MS care in general, as well as about the position of their product in the marketplace. In the beginning of the decade, spouses or children were invited to such regional meetings, but in time this was prohibited by PhRMA rules and the attending physician had to pay for his or her family to attend.

Physicians look forward to attending national meetings, and the companies recognized that the national and international neurologic meetings were an important avenue to promote their product and gain new information from the treatment community. The American Academy of Neurology meeting, held every spring and recognized as the largest neurology meeting in the world, is attended by over 10,000 physicians. All major pharmaceutical companies brought large displays that provided information about their product. For several years, between 1997 and 2008, often the largest displays at these meetings were provided by the various manufacturers of MS treatments, and each one attracted a constant stream of physicians, mainly neurologists, eager to learn more.

International Meetings

These activities were not restricted to the United States and North America. In the early 1980s, an organization was developed in Europe, the European Committee for Treatment and Research in MS (ECTRIMS). It holds yearly meetings that rotate throughout major European cities; these venues provide information about the progress of research and treatment of MS. This organization grew slowly and attracted only a few MS experts from the United States and Canada. Attendance expanded rapidly after 1993, when Betaseron arrived on the market, and many European physicians were invited to come, sponsored by Schering AG, the European manufacturer of Betaseron. In 1995, a new organization, developed to mirror ECTRIMS, conducted its first meeting in Miami as the Americas Committee for Treatment and Research in MS, or ACTRIMS. The plan was to have a combined ECTRIMS-ACTRIMS meeting at 3-year intervals on one side of the Atlantic or the other. The first such joint meeting was held in Basel, Switzerland, in 1999, the second one in Baltimore, Maryland, and the third in Thessalonica, Greece. Each grew larger than the last. The 2008 combined meeting in Montreal, Canada, attracted 5,500 MS physicians and researchers from around the world.

These meetings have, without doubt, substantially improved the understanding of MS and the care of MS patients everywhere. It is very unlikely that this rapid expansion of international meetings and the distribution of new and useful information about MS and its treatment would have occurred without the appearance and support of the commercial drug companies, and the expectations that other new and perhaps even more effective treatments for MS would soon be on the way. Teva and Copaxone have been well represented at these meetings.

Patient Support Programs

The perfect storm of competing claims and market confusion was not always a negative thing. Multiple sclerosis, as repeatedly noted, is a highly variable disease, and the use of the ABCR drugs, the three interferons and Copaxone, certainly improved the course of the disease, but their use often brought new challenges for patients. Side effects were always an issue, but there were also insurance concerns and other questions that complicated the patient's life. Each of the sponsors developed a nationwide patient support program, one of the most successful of them being Shared Solutions, a Teva initiative. A corps of well-trained nurses at Teva Neuroscience headquarters in Kansas City receives over 32,000 incoming calls per month to answer disease and treatment questions and give useful aid to patients. Insurance coverage was a major early issue for the 2,000-plus patients beginning Copaxone therapy each month. Depending on the type of insurance, drug shipments must be arranged and other logistical problems eased. Long-term compliance with treatment is the only way to ensure long-term disease control, and the Shared Solutions nurses provide frequent support for enrolled patients. These nurses help with any concerns or problems with the daily Copaxone injections.

Improving Copaxone

When first approved for marketing by the FDA, Copaxone was only available as a frozen product, the form of drug used in the U.S. pivotal trial. With the demand for a daily injection, this required that patients thaw the drug, mix it with a sterile diluent, and then inject the liquid. Soon, evaluation at Teva found that a refrigerated form of Copaxone was just as effective; the FDA agreed, allowing distribution of refrigerated Copaxone. A major advance in patient convenience was announced in early 2002, when a Copaxone prefilled syringe was approved, which did away with the need to mix the medication prior to each injection. Patients could simply take that day's dose from the refrigerator, warm the syringe slightly, and inject, a process that required less than a minute and, because of the lack of interferon-related side effects, one that could be done at any time of the day.

Copaxone continued to be used more widely year after year, eventually gaining the number one position in the U.S. Even though new information continues to be published about its long-term effectiveness, its favorable mechanism of action, and its clear ability to improve the MRI, many physicians continued to rank it as a less-effective MS treatment than the interferons. The enormous number of publications and the intense educational and marketing efforts mounted by the interferon competitors and Teva prompted physicians to make difficult treatment decisions. While most conceded that Avonex was less effective than the alternative therapies, the once-a-week injection has been a common choice, often requested or even demanded by patients. Despite evidence to the contrary, physicians said they thought of Copaxone as less effective because of its lack of side effects. The interferons made patients sick, at least in the first weeks of therapy, and there was little doubt something was happening. Physicians tended to misinterpret this as a therapeutic effect; the treatment had to be "stronger." This is, of course, contrary to long-term medical experience. Antibiotics are powerful and clearly effective, yet have few side effects, at least for most acute infections. The family of statin drugs has clear-cut endocrine benefits, lowering cholesterol for years with few adverse problems. Increased side effects do not equate with increased effectiveness, yet Copaxone had to confront this misguided perception.

Expanding to Europe

The FDA approval in 1996 only allowed for Copaxone sales in the United States. This was soon followed by approval in Canada. Europe has a large MS population; both physicians and patients demanded that Copaxone be made available, as the interferons already were. Teva decided to apply to regulators in the United Kingdom; if approved there, sales would be allowed throughout the European Union under the Mutual Recognition Procedure. For a number of reasons, the U.K. process was slow, requiring a formal hearing and other appeals. Finally, in August 2000, approval was granted and Copaxone was launched in December. Germany, with the largest MS population in Europe, was among the first to distribute Copaxone, but only in 2003 did France permit its use.

Slowly, Copaxone was becoming available to MS patients everywhere.

19

Unraveling the Mysteries
of Copaxone

Almost all of the drugs used to treat human diseases have a specific chemical structure that consists of a molecular spine, often with well-defined side chains. Diagrams of the drug's structure are frequently found in textbooks of pharmacology and are included in the package insert of information accompanying most prescription drugs. Not only is the structure of small-molecule oral drugs well known, but large, complex, injected drugs also have a well-defined chemical structure. In Chapter 16, we described how a single amino acid in the immense protein structure of beta-interferon was substituted with the amino acid serine to improve Betaseron®'s stability. This molecular magic, of course, relied on complete knowledge of the amino acid-by-amino acid makeup of the interferon, a large human protein.

No such specific chemical structure exists for glatiramer acetate (Copaxone®). Each syringe used for its daily subcutaneous injections contains tens, thousands, or perhaps tens of thousands of peptides or strings of amino acids of undetermined length, all of which result from the carefully designed proprietary manufacturing process first developed at the Weizmann laboratories and then refined by Teva to the satisfaction of the U.S. Food and Drug Administration (FDA). These huge numbers of synthetic peptides are all composed of four amino acids,

L-glutamic acid, L-alanine, L-lysine, and L-tyrosine, the four amino acids originally chosen by Sela and Arnon in their early creative work in 1967.

The fact that glatiramer acetate is not a single molecular entity or structure but rather a heterogeneous mixture that contains a huge, perhaps incalculable number of active amino acid sequences, has long been appreciated. The FDA has always recognized that copolymer 1 (Copaxone) is not a conventional drug, neither in chemical composition nor in its presumed mechanism of action. This was stated in a letter from Paul Leber, M.D., then Director of the Division of Neuropharmacological Drug Products, to Teva's FDA consultant, Bruce Mackler, on December 10, 1992, just as the U.S. pivotal trial was getting under way. The most remarkable outcome of this unusual drug development history is that this mixture of uncountable numbers of synthetic peptides or strings of amino acids, employed as a drug, has proven to be very safe, even with prolonged treatment of thousands, and has risen to become the most widely prescribed therapy worldwide for the early stages of MS.

The pharmacological genius of glatiramer acetate (Copaxone) may well lie in the very fact that it is composed of large numbers of synthetic peptides. Investigators and governmental regulators have questioned whether a specific peptide in this immense mixture might be the single active ingredient. Pursuing this line of reasoning, and relying on modern immunologic theory, single altered peptide ligands or a precise string of a few amino acids have been created and tested in mice and even in small human MS trials. In one, the altered peptide ligand seemed to have some immunologic activity similar to glatiramer acetate but, in another, serious safety concerns arose when at least one participating patient developed an acute immunologic reaction that appeared to be similar, if not identical to experimental allergic encephalomyelitis (EAE). Unlike inbred laboratory mice, people with MS have a broad genetic and immunologic makeup, and individuals may respond differently to various peptides contained in glatiramer acetate. Other peptide mixtures have been considered for development as MS drugs but, thus far, Teva has successfully argued that glatiramer acetate is unique and that other similar peptide mixtures cannot be considered either safe or effective without long-term clinical trials, thus for the time being preserving Copaxone's sole position as a commercial peptide-based MS treatment.

Most drugs, either oral or injected, can be detected in the blood for various periods of time, either as the intact drug molecule or as breakdown products. The drug or its breakdown products are usually eliminated through either the liver or kidney, allowing detection in the stool or urine. No similar process exists for glatiramer acetate, which is rapidly broken down close to the site of its injection. Rather than persisting either intact or in fragments, to accomplish its therapeutic purpose, glatiramer acetate initiates an immunologic process by changing the nature of nearby lymphocytes.

The immune system depends on a complex series of steps, engaging several cell types to work what almost seems to be magic. An antigen-presenting cell that is capable of breaking down a foreign protein into smaller fragments or peptides begins the process. These peptides, usually called *antigens*, are then presented, in a complex process, to a noncommitted lymphocyte, thereby "teaching" or stimulating the lymphocyte to recognize that protein or antigen. For example, during an infection with measles virus, an antigen-presenting cell will fragment one or more of the measles virus proteins, and then present them to a lymphocyte that then becomes capable of recognizing and later attacking and inactivating the measles virus. Some of these lymphocytes are destined to become long-lived memory cells that are capable of destroying measles virus even decades later. A similar process occurs with measles virus vaccine; the measles antigen is presented by the antigen-presenting cell to the naïve or uncommitted lymphocyte, thus creating a population of committed memory lymphocytes capable of recognizing and deactivating measles virus during any future episode of virus exposure.

The immunologic events taking place for an unfortunate victim of MS have been the subject of intense study for over 60 years and much progress has been made, even though many issues are still unclear. In a genetically susceptible individual, some protein fragments or peptides from the central nervous system (CNS)—perhaps a fragment of myelin basic protein (MBP)—are taken up by a circulating antigen-presenting cell, which then presents it to a naïve or uncommitted lymphocyte, thus initiating the complicated process that leads to MS. Alternatively, in a theoretical process known as *molecular mimicry*, a small fragment of a virus protein that has a string of amino acids or a peptide identical to a fragment of MBP is taken up by the antigen-presenting cell and likewise presented to the uncommitted lymphocyte. In this unfortunate situation, the newly "trained" lymphocyte may migrate across the blood–brain barrier into the CNS and, when confronted with a fragment of MBP, misidentifies it as a component of a virus and begins an immunologic attack. This acute attack may expand, recruiting other lymphocytes and inflammatory cells to produce the acute MS lesion or plaque that can often be recognized on a magnetic resonance imaging (MRI) scan. Immunologic control factors finally arrive as inhibiting "firemen" to put out the fire, so to speak, or reduce the inflammatory activity, but often only after serious damage has been done both to the myelin surrounding local axons or the axon itself has been damaged or destroyed.

In the case of Copaxone or glatiramer acetate treatment of MS, an antigen-presenting cell incorporates peptides of glatiramer acetate and presents them to a lymphocyte, similar to the process with a vaccine, thereby creating a unique population of lymphocytes responsive to glatiramer acetate circulating in the blood. Because this complex process probably occurs at the site of the Copaxone injection each day, it is possible to determine that an immunologic process is taking place not by detecting a fragment of a drug, but rather by detecting a population of lymphocytes with new therapeutic powers, as explained later in the chapter.

After the discovery that Cop 1 was capable of inhibiting EAE in many species of animals, there was, of course, considerable interest by Sela, Arnon, and Teitelbaum about how this immunologic process might be occurring. Following a number of creative studies in animals, in 1991, Teitelbaum and her colleagues reported that Cop 1 inhibited the multiplication of those human lymphocytes that were capable of reacting to MBP. Three years later, the Weizmann group was able to show that Cop 1 bound directly to the portion of the antigen-presenting cell that is required to stimulate or educate the T-lymphocyte, thus blocking the direct immunologic attack.

In the same time period—that is from the late 1980s through 1995—immunologic knowledge in general was rapidly expanding and the concept of *pro-inflammatory* (Th1) and *anti-inflammatory* (Th2) lymphocytes was gaining momentum. These two populations of lymphocytes can be identified by the chemicals or products that they manufacture and then secrete. These products are called *cytokines* and, in general, can also be divided into pro-inflammatory and anti-inflammatory populations. The Weizmann program continued to attract other talented immunologists, including Rina Aharoni, who was the lead author in a May 1997 paper that described how Copaxone could stimulate the production of Th2 cells, anti-inflammatory cells that inhibited the inflammatory response by secreting anti-inflammatory cytokines. This major finding was rapidly confirmed by numerous independent laboratories in Europe and North America. This fundamental immunologic principle, the anti-inflammatory activity of Cop 1, by now known as glatiramer acetate, was soon solidly established.

By the late 1990s, with the completion of two successful MS pivotal trials of Copaxone, FDA approval of the drug as a first-line MS therapy, and the increasing body of knowledge of the composition of the drug and how it worked, considerable interest and excitement were generated in major neuroimmunologic laboratories around the world. Notable among the investigators who were drawn to the scientific questions surrounding Copaxone's mechanism of action were Suhayl Dhib-Jalbut, in the Department of Neurology, University of Maryland School of Medicine in Baltimore and more recently the Robert Wood Johnson School of Medicine in New Brunswick, New Jersey; Rinehart Hohlfeld and several of his laboratory fellows at the Department of Neuroimmunology, Max Planck Institute of Neurobiology in Martinsried, Germany; David A. Hafler at the Laboratory for Molecular Immunology at the Brigham and Woman's Hospital, and the Harvard Medical School in Boston; Amit Bar-Or at the Neuroimmunology Unit,

Montreal Neurological Institute, McGill University, Montreal; Roland Martin of the Neuroimmunology Branch at the National Institutes of Health (NIH), Bethesda, Maryland; and Scott Zamvil, Department of Neurology, University of California, San Francisco. While it is impossible here to describe in detail all of the discoveries and reports by these and many other investigators, a clearly established sequence of events, confirmed independently in numerous laboratories, provides a clear roadmap of how glatiramer acetate affects the immune system to benefit the course of MS.

Our current understanding of Copaxone's effect begins with the generation in peripheral tissues of a population of glatiramer acetate-specific lymphocytes, which circulate in the blood and are capable of migrating into the CNS tissue by crossing the blood–brain barrier. Once there, these cells encounter fragments of several myelin proteins that stimulate the glatiramer cells to multiply and begin to produce anti-inflammatory cytokines or products. This process has been given the name *bystander suppression*, indicating that the population of glatiramer lymphocytes products can suppress the inflammation under way in the local area of diseased CNS tissue. Recent reports indicate that these cells also have an immunologic regulatory function and are capable of providing enhanced regulation or control of the immune system in a beneficial way.

This therapeutic process initiated by the glatiramer lymphocytes begins early, certainly within 1 month of starting therapy, and continues to have a long-term therapeutic effect, which has now been shown to last well beyond 12 years.

During the early years of the 21st century, a new element in the mechanism of glatiramer acetate began to emerge, the concept of *neuroprotection*. This is a process by which a treatment can prevent or slow injury to brain tissue. It was shown that glatiramer acetate cells were capable of producing another product, known as *brain derived neurotrophic factor* or BDNF, which protects both neurons and nerve fibers, in addition to inhibiting inflammation. Thus, glatiramer acetate therapy may have dual activity, both as an anti-inflammatory agent but also as a neuroprotective form of treatment, acting within the brain tissue itself. This well-established dual mechanism of action in animals explains how many of the clinical benefits of daily Copaxone therapy can now be accounted for. The anti-inflammatory activity is responsible for reducing the number of clinical relapses and the way in which foci of disease activity seen on MRI are inhibited. The neuroprotective effect helps to explain how glatiramer acetate therapy may slow the worrisome process of neurologic disability and even impact the ominous concern of brain atrophy.

As important as this long historical series of immunologic discoveries is, and as beneficial as Copaxone therapy has become to tens of thousands of people with MS, it still must be recognized as a partial therapy. It does not cure the disease, and it does not seem to be effective in every patient. A critical question being investigated in several laboratories is how to define responders and non-responders, and determine who will be the most appropriate MS patients to begin on Copaxone therapy. The answer to this burning question will be of great aid to patients and also to their concerned doctors.

Perhaps most remarkable is that this leading MS therapy was discovered by accident, and that its immunologic principles were not understood when its early positive effects on EAE and then MS were recognized.

20

Becoming Number One

Over the long history of multiple sclerosis (MS), from the first clear description of its features in the mid-1860s, through decades of hopeless despair for its victims, a lightning strike of genius in Rehovot when a useful treatment was first contemplated, and now continuing throughout the first decade of the 21st century, hope has finally arrived for victims of the disease that shatters dreams. From the first clear description of MS by Charcot in 1866, to the surprising and unexpected announcement by Bornstein in 1987 that Cop 1 (copolymer one) was an effective treatment—a span of 119 years—many false hopes and long periods of dark struggle that had been the daily lot for those with MS began to melt away.

Why, one may ask, did it take so long to discover a treatment for MS? Of many likely reasons, two stand out. First, there was little understanding of the underlying causes of the disease. In fact, one of the three approved drug classes, beta-interferon, was first investigated on the false premise that MS was due to a hidden virus that would yield to the antiviral potential of interferon; in fact, interferon's positive action appears to be due instead to its control of dangerous, poorly regulated immunologic activity. Second, there was little understanding of how to search for an MS treatment. Some major human therapies, such as antibiotics for bacterial infections or narcotics to control pain, were of obvious benefit as soon as they were discovered. Identifying effective

MS therapies was more difficult, requiring long periods of observation of large groups of patients, and comparing the effect of a potential treatment versus placebo. Such experiments or trials required a massive monetary investment available to only a few organizations, such as governmental agencies like the National Institutes of Health (NIH) or large, profitable pharmaceutical companies.

The experience of the two decades between 1987 and 2008 illustrates how difficult the search for MS treatment has been. Of over 18 potential therapies that have been considered as rational and sure bets to succeed—that is, they showed positive results in animal experiments and appeared safe enough to test in human MS trials only three, the beta-interferons (Betaseron®, Avonex®, and Rebif®), glatiramer acetate (Copaxone®), and natalizumab (Tysabri®) received U.S. Food and Drug Administration (FDA) approval through 2009 and have been widely prescribed for relapsing MS. All the others failed, some stimulating increased MS symptoms, some causing unacceptable and sometimes fatal side effects, while others simply didn't work. Tysabri, while now approved for MS treatment, has been related to several fatal viral infections in the brain and can only be prescribed by precertified physicians who must monitor patients monthly.

While the total dollar investment in this long string of drug failures is not known, it surely exceeds several billion dollars in direct clinical trial costs alone. In spite of the enormous monetary burden and despite the human cost in dedicated time and risk to patients participating in failed MS trials, there is no doubt that the three approved therapies now available have produced monumental improvements in the MS landscape. They have significantly reduced measurable disease activity, and have undoubtedly improved the quality of life for hundreds of thousands of treated patients.

By 2004–2005, 8 or 9 years after the various therapies first became widely available, a peculiar pattern of use in the United States had become apparent. Avonex, which had been the most widely prescribed agent, was declining in market share and Copaxone was slowly gaining ground. The two high-dose interferons, Betaseron and Rebif, continued to limp along, capturing only 15% to 20% of the market. Why was this?

Expert advisory panels of neurologists routinely rated the higher-dose interferons as "stronger" or more effective. While Avonex was always considered a less effective drug, as was Copaxone, treating physicians seemed unable to make a clear choice as to which of the available preparations was most effective or best suited to their patients.

Several comments may help explain the dilemma that had emerged in the MS marketplace. The various interferons had been compared to each other in two well-regarded and published head-to-head studies. One, the EVIDENCE trial, had revealed the superiority of high-dose Rebif over lower-dose Avonex; the other, the Italian INCOMIN trial, had confirmed that high-dose Betaseron was also more effective than Avonex. Why then did Avonex maintain its substantial lead among the interferons in the market? Marketing strategies may have had an influence—perhaps drug reps from Biogen were simply more convincing in their arguments. Or, perhaps many physicians had gotten into the habit of prescribing Avonex when it first became available and simply continued their practice. More likely, the marketing lead was the result of its being a once-a-week injection and that, when patients heard about the alternatives, they made the decision to choose Avonex treatment. For whatever reason, the battle for the lead in the market seemed to be shaping up between Avonex and Copaxone.

The question of which of the available agents to prescribe was not simply a commercial one, a contest between pharmaceutical companies. More importantly, it was a question of which of the available products was not only most convenient, safest, or best tolerated, but also which one was most effective. How would patients best be served in their daily battles with MS? How could that thorny question be sorted out? The obvious business strategy that might answer these questions in favor of the high-dose interferon companies was to take aim at Copaxone, which by 2006 had just about caught up with Avonex as the market leader. They set out to prove to physicians that their interferon product was superior to Copaxone in controlling MS symptoms, even if it caused more side effects and might stimulate neutralizing antibodies, which had been shown to decrease its effectiveness in as much as 20% to 33% for the high-dose interferons.

Head-to-Head Trials

Well-designed head-to-head comparisons between each of the high-dose interferons versus Copaxone had begun to be organized by 2004. The manufacturer of Betaseron, Schering AG of Berlin (now Bayer), sought to answer two questions. First, would it be possible to improve MS control by increasing the dose of Betaseron? This was not a new question; in fact, the small dose-finding trial of Betaseron, conducted almost 20 years earlier, had shown that the commercial dose of 250 micrograms (µg) was the highest that most patients could tolerate. Nevertheless, the decision was made to compare the commercial dose of Betaseron with a higher one, 500 µg. The trial would also compare both doses of Betaseron with Copaxone to determine once and for all whether either dose was more effective in controlling MS symptoms (relapses) than Copaxone.

EMD Serono, the manufacturer of Rebif, also announced a well-designed direct head-to-head trial comparing the FDA-approved dose of three times a week injections of high-dose Rebif with daily injections of Copaxone.

Each trial used the approved dose of Copaxone, 20 mg injected daily. The contest to eliminate Copaxone was on.

The two head-to-head trials were enormous. The Betaseron trial, called the BEYOND study, finally enrolled 2,244 patients, divided into three groups that would receive regular or high-dose interferon or Copaxone. The Rebif head-to-head trial, the REGARD study, enrolled 764 patients, equally divided between Rebif and Copaxone at their approved doses. Several magnetic resonance imaging (MRI) scans were scheduled during the 2-year course of each trial. Because of the staggering number of early relapsing MS patients—more than 3,000 for the two trials—patients were enrolled at MS centers in North and South America, throughout Western Europe, and also in countries such as Russia and other Eastern European countries. The cost to the sponsoring companies was also huge, estimated at well over $100 million.

Both trials were enrolled fairly rapidly, and suspense began to build throughout the worldwide MS community. Finally, there would be an answer. After over a decade of uncertainty, argument, and marketing activity, physicians would be able to confidently select the best therapy for their patients. Each trial was concluded during 2007, and the expectation was that there would be a triumphant unveiling of the results with press conferences, news releases, and presentations at international conferences. Instead there was silence. Statisticians from both companies looked at the results and applied one statistical technique after another. Finally, in late 2007, the results began to emerge. The Rebif versus Copaxone comparison, the REGARD study, was published in the journal *Lancet Neurology* in October 2008. The comparison of Copaxone versus two doses of Betaseron was announced by press release but not published until late 2009.

To the surprise of the sponsoring interferon companies and many physicians, there was virtually no difference between treatments in these two massive head-to-head trials. In the case of Betaseron versus Copaxone, the two doses of interferon—the commercial dose and the higher dose—all showed precisely the same effect on controlling relapses. In the head-to-head comparison between Rebif and Copaxone, the clinical results were identical: In each comparison patients had approximately 80% fewer relapses than they had experienced prior to entering the studies. When the MRI scans were analyzed, some measurements favored the interferon, whereas others favored Copaxone.

By late 2008, the status of the available MS drugs had changed considerably. By clinical and MRI measurements, the higher-dose interferons Betaseron and Rebif, and also Copaxone, had proved to be approximately equal in well-run, randomized, head-to-head controlled trials. Of course, earlier, the high-dose interferons had been shown to be more effective than Avonex. The interferons posed different side effects for patients, and there was the risk of developing neutralizing antibodies that interfered with treatment. The one challenge for Copaxone patients would still be the daily injection routine.

In the two decades that had elapsed since 1987, since Cop 1 had emerged as the first therapy ever shown to benefit the course of MS and long before it was called Copaxone or given the scientific name of glatiramer acetate, the drug had met all challenges as Teva Pharmaceuticals guided it to the number one position as an MS therapy. The interferon competitors had been persistent, and the marketing battles had often been bruising, but finally the proven benefit and the safety profile of Copaxone became increasingly recognized by therapists worldwide, who were always seeking the best choice for their patients.

To achieve this position as Number One, even if only temporarily, was an enormous accomplishment for the two Israeli organizations, the Weizmann Institute of Science and Teva Pharmaceuticals, who together had created this monumental success. The many thousands of MS patients who have benefited—with fewer relapses, a reduced risk of increasing EDSS score, and few side effects—were undoubtedly the ultimate winners in Copaxone's success.

But physicians were left with the perplexing situation in which the high-dose interferons and Copaxone were judged more or less equal. The evidence that a drug has value can be measured in multiple ways; one scientifically valid way is to compare similar groups of patients treated with active drug versus placebo in a double-blind trial. Such an exercise is known as an *efficacy trial* and has been the "gold standard" method for obtaining evidence that is convincing not only to regulators such as the FDA but also to treating physicians. Such clinical experiments are the scientific foundation for the large number of drugs now approved for hundreds if not thousands of human diseases. Placebo-controlled efficacy trials or head-to-head double-blind comparisons are the essential experiments that govern physicians' treatment choices in their unending quest to provide the best for those patients who depend on them.

Efficacy Versus Effectiveness

A question often not even considered is whether it is scientifically correct to extrapolate or extend the results obtained in a placebo-controlled trial to the larger, much more diverse MS population suffering from the disease. It is simply assumed that a short (2-year) trial will provide answers to the treatment of a life-long disease. Placebo-controlled trials are, by design, narrowly defined: that is, they seek to recruit a population of similar patients with very specific characteristics and then randomize or divide them into two groups, one of which receives the treatment in question and the other a placebo or some other comparator treatment. Such controlled studies evaluating Copaxone, as described in this book, rely on the careful selection of alike or very similar patients. As an example, in the U.S. Copaxone pivotal trial, patients had to be between the ages of 18 and 45 and had to be in the relatively early relapsing stage of disease, with little evidence of fixed disability, and they must have experienced a relapse in the previous year. In the subsequent European/Canadian MRI trial, the patients also had to have very specific MRI characteristics to gain entry. The confounding question that arises is whether these narrowly defined groups of MS patients are really representative of the broad population of patients scattered throughout the community who might and should be considered for MS therapy by their personal physician, even though their condition differed from the narrow definition used in a trial.

This question of how to determine the effectiveness of a drug for the large, broadly defined population of MS patients in the community has been intensely studied, debated, and written about by a large school of practitioners in the field of pharmacoeconomics. They have been interested in not only the restricted medical benefits of treatment, but also the broader consequences to the whole population of MS patients, as well as the financial benefit or worth of a therapy. The techniques they use are different, primarily statistical rather than medical, and the populations involved in their analysis are frequently much larger and more diverse than those involved in a randomized trial. Even the word "trial" is probably inappropriate; rather, they measure long-term outcomes experienced by a population, searching for both medical and economic benefits of a treatment. Since several treatments may be available, they may be able to compare them and judge on which is best.

How might it be possible to measure the benefit or merit of an MS therapy for the large eligible community population, hopefully identifying the most effective treatment for MS patients? Was a comparison of Copaxone versus each of the interferon products possible? The patient populations to be compared should, first of all, come from the entire MS population, from all regions of the country. They should have received prescribed treatment from their local physician, hopefully unbiased by commercial influences other than the marketing efforts of sponsors. In addition, would it be possible to determine all of the direct medical costs, including costs of hospitalization, physician visits, drug costs, insurance co-pays, and other patient expenses? It turns out that such information can be obtained in the United States by analyzing databases developed by national health insurance companies, at least for the managed care component of their insured populations. Such data are available for the treatment outcomes from large populations, treated over defined periods of time, as for instance, between the years 2001 and 2006. The patients are "de-identified," that is their names, residence, and other specific identification is excluded; however, other important demographics are available, such as their age, sex, and additional disease diagnoses—for instance, diabetes, hypertension, or elevated cholesterol. Distribution of the patients by regions also can be determined.

Each patient in such a database is linked to a specific diagnostic code, such as MS, so it is possible to determine which of the tens of thousands of patients in the database have MS. It is possible to determine which patients were started on one of the MS drugs, either Copaxone or one of the interferons, as a result of a decision made by their personal physician, and it is also possible to determine how long the patient continued to receive a specific therapy: Did they start and then stop, or were they continuous users for some duration of time, for example, at least 2 years? Finally, what were the total health care expenses during the defined period?

It has in fact been possible to analyze such a managed care database for MS therapy in the United States between 2001 and 2006, when all three interferon products and Copaxone were commercially available. Of the millions of patients in the database receiving managed care, 51,000 had been diagnosed with MS. From this group, over 9,000 had been started on therapy with one of the interferons or Copaxone during these 5 years. Statisticians call such a group the *intent to treat* (ITT) group, indicating that they had been started on one of the four MS treatments. Perhaps it would be easier to call them the "started treatment" group. From this ITT population a smaller group, the *continuous use group*, numbered almost 1,000 and were known to have stayed on the same drug, one of the interferons or Copaxone, for at least 2 years.

It is possible to determine several things from this real-life analysis of treatment effects on the MS population. First, and most importantly, the MS activity experienced by these groups could be determined. If a person was hospitalized with a primary diagnosis of MS, it was counted as a disease event or relapse. Also, if the patient was seen in a doctor's office and given a primary diagnosis of MS, and then within 7 days given a prescription for high-dose steroids, the common treatment for MS relapses, that was also counted as a new MS event or relapse. While this is an indirect way of defining MS disease activity, it is valid because the same definition for MS activity was used for all of the treatments being compared. Also, the total cost of medical care could be determined for each patient. This method does not allow for measurement of disability, however.

Experienced health care statisticians pored over this huge data collection in what is called a *naturalistic disease study*, rather than a clinical trial study. Like many other moments of critical discovery in this age of theories and statistics, a eureka moment came, probably with a single final keystroke. The completed analysis showed that Copaxone was significantly more effective in controlling MS-related clinical events or relapses than any of the interferons, but also that the total medical care costs of the patients with MS using Copaxone were less than for those on interferon therapy. The same pattern of improved clinical effectiveness and lower cost was true whether the ITT population was analyzed or the smaller population of 2-year continuous users was the study focus.

What this effectiveness (rather than efficacy) analysis cannot do is to determine the broad consensus of the treating community during the period of the data collection. If most treating doctors had the opinion during that time that Copaxone was less effective, they might have only prescribed it for those of their patients with milder MS, who may have experienced fewer relapses. Therefore, this type of effectiveness analysis will probably have to be repeated as new information (such as the head-to-head trials) is available to the community-wide treating physician group.

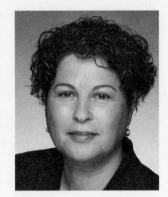

Rivka Kreitman

Slowly, in fits and starts, using information from several clinical trials, MRI analysis of patients receiving Copaxone or placebo, countless hours of laboratory investigation, and the analysis of larger populations of patients in the community, Copaxone was proving to be a highly effective drug, with proven safety in the control and management of MS patients in the early stages of their life-defining disease. Science and experience had proven that Copaxone deserved its position as the bedrock, the number one prescribed treatment for MS.

A key Teva executive overseeing much of this progress was Dr. Rivka Kreitman, who had patiently guided the long-term series of studies that were necessary to project the sense of confidence in the scientific underpinning of glatiramer acetate and in the marketplace. Kreitman was born in Rehovot and had received her degree at the Weizmann Institute, followed by postdoctoral studies at Princeton University in New Jersey. She joined Teva in 1992, and so was participating in the development of Copaxone from its earliest years. Needing to have a strong voice in North America, she relocated to the United States in 2001, and has risen to become Senior Vice President, Head of Global Innovative Research and Development, Teva Pharmaceutical Industries.

21

Multiple Sclerosis Heroes Revisited

Volunteering for a clinical trial of a new multiple sclerosis (MS) drug is risky. Patients randomized to the placebo group risk getting worse as their disease continues unchecked, while patients randomized to active treatment risk possibly serious drug side effects. If the final outcome is positive, not only the participants in the trial but everyone with the diagnosis if MS will potentially benefit, hence the title of hero is appropriate and deserved for all those patients who were involved in the trials.

In Chapter 2, two volunteers to the U.S. pivotal Copaxone® trial were introduced. In the 18 or so years that have passed, what has happened to them, both in their lives and in the course of their disease? Both, as time would tell, had been randomized to receive Copaxone, so its possible benefit began immediately.

Case 1 was a 20-year-old college student who was appropriately concerned and readily admitted that he was frightened and depressed when given the diagnosis of MS. In spite of a great fear of needles, he was an early participant in the trial starting in late 1991. The daily injection, while unpleasant, soon became routine.

In September 1992, about 6 months into the trial, he developed an episode of optic neuritis that was treated with a high dose of intravenous steroids and his vision soon cleared. It was the last MS relapse he has experienced.

Receiving daily Copaxone shots has not been entirely without side effects, however. A few months into the trial, while at his parent's home, he made his injection and almost immediately felt hot, developed a flushed face, and was frightened by pressure and some pain in his chest that lasted for about 10 minutes and was in his words, "horrifying." Fortunately, he had been given his trial neurologist's home phone number and by the time he reached Dr. Hillel Panitch, the symptoms were subsiding. Panitch recognized the symptoms as a well-known, frightening, but benign side effect of Copaxone, and was able to reassure the distressed patient and his parents that nothing serious was happening. During the almost 3 years of the trial, the patient experienced nine similar attacks and—even now, over 18 years later—still notes an occasional one, although they tend to be much milder and are no longer a cause for panic or worry. They require no treatment.

Living what he describes as a normal, happy life, he finished college and now works in the optical department of a large ophthalmology practice in Baltimore. He married and is the proud father of two daughters, ages 6 and 2.

One may ask: Does he really have MS? His early attacks are typical and his MRI, while mildly abnormal, shows the lesions one expects with MS. On neurologic examination, a mild increase in deep tendon reflexes in the left leg is the only abnormality now evident. He describes a recent experience while vacationing at the Maryland shore. During a long jog of several miles on the beach in 90°F weather, he noted weakness of the left leg and had a noticeable limp when returning to his family. The symptoms rapidly faded when he cooled down and had a cold drink. This so-called heat intolerance is a well-known characteristic of MS. He has experienced no short-term symptoms during his twice-a-week workouts at the local gym. He considers himself a well person.

The second MS hero (Case 2) was 28 years old when, in 1987, she noted her first MS symptom, numbness in her right hand. Other attacks, at times following pregnancies, were often severe. In September 1991, a major episode she described as "stroke-like" came on, but resolved with steroid therapy and physical therapy. She began active treatment with Copaxone on January 31, 1992, and has not had an MS attack since.

Her neurologic examination is now normal, but she notes faint numbness in her left arm and has had some fatigue, which may be due either to MS or to hypothyroidism, for which she is being treated. Similar to Case 1, she has experienced two immediate post-injection episodes of flushing and a "heavy chest" lasting about 5 minutes. She developed some dimples or areas of localized atrophy in her thighs and no longer uses these areas to make injections.

Considering herself a well person, she works full time as an accountant. Her children, now ages 20 and 18, have a hard time accepting that she has MS.

Both of these cases with well-established MS that was very active during their young adult years have, with continuing Copaxone therapy, been almost free of symptoms for almost two decades. Many patients with a similarly benign pattern have been observed in the large number of participants who entered the U.S. Copaxone trial in 1991–1992 and who have faithfully taken their injections, not used other MS drugs, and have been examined regularly. A few, but not many, have not done nearly as well and have followed a course more typical of untreated MS, with increasing disability.

What has the experience been for the large group of patients who have been followed closely, still numbering over 100, even after a decade? Teva and the 11 U.S. Copaxone investigative sites agreed at the end of the pivotal trial to offer all participants continuing supplies of drug for some period into the future; all of the placebo recipients would be switched to Copaxone. This program has now continued for over 15 years, clearly the longest and most informative extended MS trial ever carried out and probably one of the most interesting long-term treatment studies for any disease.

A total of 231 patients who received Copaxone in the trial were eligible, and were reported on after approximately 10 years of exclusive Copaxone therapy. They have returned to the clinics regularly for neurologic evaluation. After 10 years, 108 were still under regular observation and 123 had at some point dropped out for one of a number of reasons. Some moved away from the investigative site, some wanted to try another MS treatment, some had or wanted to become pregnant, and so forth. The two heroes described earlier were among the 108 continuing participants.

Of the 123 dropouts, most could be identified and were invited to return to their investigative site about 10 years after entering the trial; 50 agreed to return for an examination.

So, what was learned? While on Copaxone therapy, the average relapse rate dropped from almost 1.2 attacks per year to an average of 1 relapse every 5 years. Multiple sclerosis patients all fear relapses, but they fear increasing neurologic disability even more. "Will I end up in a wheelchair?" is a common question. After 10 years, over 60% were either the same or had improved while taking Copaxone injections. The Expanded Disability Status Score (EDSS) examination scale described in Chapter 1 was very valuable because it could be used at every clinic visit to measure or gauge how patients were performing, and how they were faring in their daily lives. The EDSS grade 6 is especially informative because it is the point at which MS patients decline to the level of requiring some form of walking assistance: a cane, a crutch, or even a walker. Of the group of participants still in the trial after a decade, only eight of the 108 had reached EDSS 6 or beyond. In contrast, of the dropouts who volunteered to return for an examination after a decade, 50% had progressed or declined to EDSS 6.

While this is a striking difference, 8% always on drug versus 50% among the dropouts, still the fact that 73 patients had dropped out but not returned for reexamination raises some question about just how powerful daily Copaxone injections are in slowing long-term neurologic disability.

Attempts have also been made to determine the effect of the three beta-interferon products on slowing disability. Unlike the Copaxone experience, these studies have been hampered by the fact that none of the patients in the various trials was maintained exclusively on interferon treatment, but may have used other treatments or none at all. Nevertheless, at least 20% or more of the patients in these trials had declined to EDSS 6 or greater when they were rechecked at 8 years or beyond.

The confusing debate over the role that neutralizing antibodies may play in limiting the usefulness of the various beta-interferons seems to have been solved by recent studies. If neutralizing antibodies do appear in the blood of patients taking interferon (4%–5% with Avonex®, 20+% with Rebif®, and over 33% with Betaseron®), the usefulness of the interferon injections is lost even if the patient is free of relapses. In one financial comment, over $1.25 billion each year of interferon is wasted because the benefit is lost due to neutralizing antibody formation. No evidence of neutralizing antibodies has been detected in Copaxone users despite intense search.

Comparing the benefits of a MS treatment from one trial to another and one drug to another is always questionable, because the groups of patients in various trials will never be identical and the duration needed to measure a benefit may vary. Also, benefit may decrease or even disappear over time. All one can finally say is, given the long-term data available (over 8 years), Copaxone appears to be better at managing disability than any available interferons.

22

Postscript

The course of medical discovery is seldom straight, but is usually marked by plateaus followed by rapid advances that are often dependent on new insights and occasionally on frank serendipity. So it was with the path leading to Copaxone® as the first successful treatment for multiple sclerosis (MS). Soon after Charcot's clear description of the disease in 1867, Pasteur's revolutionary vaccine for post-exposure rabies set the stage for the recognition that the immune system could attack and damage the central nervous system, even though the link was unclear at that time. The observation that repeated injections of mammalian nervous tissue, the vehicle for the vaccine, could lead to the previously unknown acute neurological disease that we now know as post-vaccinial encephalomyelitis, was of critical importance. Proceeding into the 20th century, Rivers ignited an explosion of discovery with his description of experimental allergic encephalomyelitis (EAE), echoes of which continue unabated to the present day. Experimental allergic encephalomyelitis is often considered an experimental model for many features of MS.

Armed with sophisticated knowledge of protein structure, Sela, Arnon, and Teitelbaum set out to unravel the mystery of EAE using their advancing mastery of immunology. They created several small peptides, including Cop 1, to use as tools to study EAE. What might have been regarded as failure by many was, with their genius for recognizing and expanding on unexpected outcomes, the first step on the pathway to Copaxone. From consistent inhibition of EAE by Cop 1 in many animal species, to careful and expanding exposure of patients with MS, the journey accelerated, culminating in the startling report by Bornstein, Miller, and co-workers in 1987 of substantial control of relapsing MS with safe, well-tolerated daily injections of Cop 1.

Taking a giant step from being a small regional Israeli company to operating on the world stage, Teva undertook sponsorship of the expensive U.S. pivotal trial of Copaxone (Cop 1 or copolymer one), which led to the positive and very emotional U.S. Food and Drug Administration (FDA) hearing on September 19, 1996, in suburban Maryland. Copaxone had arrived as an MS drug, but numerous challenges clouded the future. Joining with a Kansas City company to form Teva Marion Partners allowed marketing of Copaxone to patients in North America. Later, the drug was made available worldwide. The concurrent appearance of various beta-interferons, also approved by the FDA for MS, led to an era of intense competition and considerable confusion as to how best to manage the early stages of MS. Only in the final years of the first decade of the 21st century have new head-to-head studies established the equality of Copaxone as a first-line treatment, without the interferon-related safety issues and complications of persistent neutralizing antibodies that diminish the effectiveness and value of interferon therapy.

A new era has emerged. With expanded knowledge of the immunologic underpinning of MS, and with the development of powerful new pharmacological weapons to control the errant immune system, a number of new drugs have entered into the final stages of clinical testing. They certainly are scientifically logical, and several have shown benefit in treating MS in early trials. The major new question, not encountered with Copaxone, is: Are they safe? Can MS patients with a life expectancy of 20 to 40 years after diagnosis risk being exposed long-term to their use? The daunting question, well-known to physicians is: Is the benefit worth the risk? These questions have become a central issue in this complex new treatment era.

The remarkable journey of Copaxone continues.

Index

Note: Boldface numbers indicate illustrations.

Index

Index

love fully, be peace, drink in beauty, offer your heart, seek truth, shine out, savor bliss, step into your presence, connect to your essence, embrace diversity, honor your light, do your duty, sit in the darkness, awaken to courage, revel in community, offer compassion, nurture kindness, cultivate skillful engagement in the world, take time to calm, breathe, relax, feel, watch, allow, welcome experience, climb a mountain, befriend life, soar into your dreams, tend to real intimacy, open to grace, hug into your power, be the goodness, connect, fill up with joy, embody your ideals, dance in the splendor, cradle creativity, sing with zest, unearth your potential, release tension, delight in chocolate, build strength, stay dynamic, take in the alchemy of nature, flourish, extend your heart into the world, attend to your needs, remember it is all already inside, be yourself, sparkle with brightness, smile just for fun, speak your truth, laugh because you want to, play and make noise, scream loudly, sing with determination, discover something new each day, speak your mind, aspire to your highest, live the future now, pick wild berries, revel in kindness, heal through touch, trust your intuition, nurture your body, be present with loved ones, soften, bask in your luster, grow sweetness, savor a treat, reach for something greater, step into love, root into your foundation, feel the internal fire, attune to the universal, awaken your passions, accept yourself wholeheartedly, embrace the ordinary, stay flexible, be extraordinary, make peace, honor the gift of life, explore complementary contrasts, get crushed out, affirm your values, ride the waves of your breath, receive love, stand up for your beliefs, stay in the inquiry, give love, delve into the wonder, acknowledge the little things, fine-tune your focus, cultivate dedication, offer your gifts, celebrate beginnings, honor endings, flow with life, open to transformation, explore your sensuality, hug a tree, eat close to the source, practice yoga, foster your spirit...

... nourish your light.

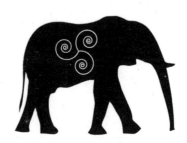

i

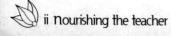

nourishing
the
teacher

inquiries, contemplations, & insights on the path of yoga

by danny arguetty

with anjali budreski
& kelli adams

editing: *kelli adams*
illustration: *bella arguetty, cody drasser*
design: *danny arguetty*

This text is geared towards yoga practitioners with at least one year of consistent practice experience and teachers of yoga. It is not intended to teach the specifics of asana, pranayama, or meditation techniques. Guidence of a qualified instructor is strongly recommended. Before embarking on any asana or pranayama practice, consult with a qualified professional regarding any health issues, injuries, or physical limitations.

ISBN 978-0-615-24596-6

Printed in Canada

For every 5000 number of books printed the following resources have been saved :

71 Trees
4525 pounds of solid waste
42 707 gallons of water
9936 pounds of air emissions

It's the equivalent of:
Trees: 1.4 American football fields
Water: a shower of 9.0 days
Air emissions: emissions of 0.9 cars per year

 Recycled
Supporting responsible use
of forest resources
www.fsc.org Cert no. SW-COC-000952
© 1996 Forest Stewardship Council
FSC

 100%

ECOLOGICAL STATEMENT:

This text has been produced with the welfare of our planet in mind. It exists as a testament to our ability to economically produce high quality products with minimal impact on the environment, preserving the well-being of the Earth for generations to come.

 Done using this book? Please pass it on, recycle, or compost.

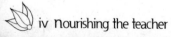

teachers
by danna faulds

We are teachers, yes and also listeners, healers, lovers of truth.
    Conduits of energy, we create opportunities for
        body,
        mind &
        breath
to coincide in the same place and time.

We point the way to inner experience, see past fears
    and limiting beliefs to the free expression of all beings.

We nurture the seed of self-acceptance, respecting each soul's
    unique qualities and depth.

We are awake, alive, diving into the unknown over and over
    until
    we barely know ourselves.

We open the doors so Spirit can soar, and more important
    than this, we bring the sacred with us into the world,
    letting actions speak our prayers.

We are teachers, yes,
    and students too,
    daring to be fully human,
    choosing to embrace the all of this existence as divine[1].

Om saha navavatu
Saha nau bhunaktu
Saha viryam karavavahai
Tejasvi navadhitam astu
Ma vidvishavahai
Om shantih, shantih, shantih

May we be protected together
May we be nourished together
May we work together with great vigor
May our study be enlightening
May no obstacle arise between us
Om peace, peace, peace.

Gurave Sarvalokanam
Bhisaje Bhavaroganam Nityaye Sarvavijnanam
Tasmai Srigurave Namah

To the teacher of all the worlds,
to the healer of all misfortune, to the eternal presence of wisdom,
to that essence our salutations.

הנני עושה את עצמי מרכבה לשכינה
Hineni ose(a)h et atzmi merkavah lashchinah

I make myself a chariot/vessel to be and see the divine in the world.

on the inside

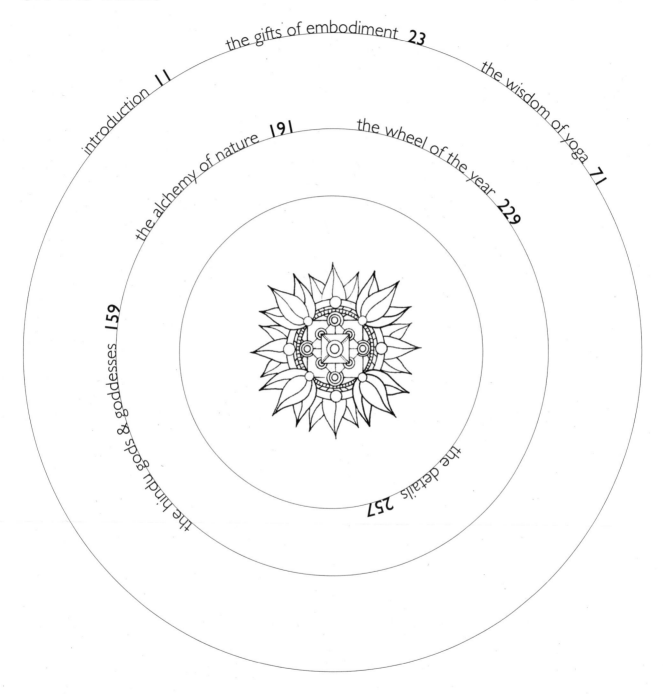

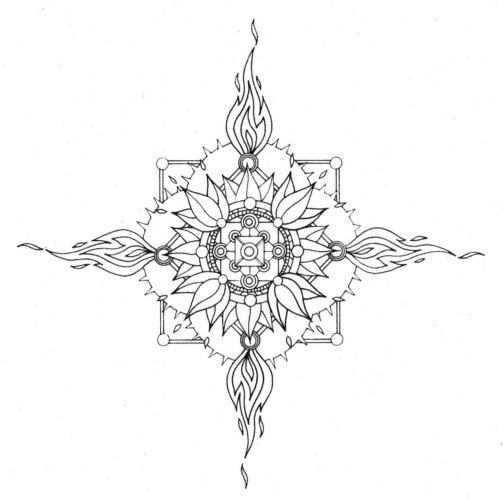

introduction

*"If I am not for myself, who will be for me?
If I am for myself only, what am I?
And if not now, when?"*

-Rabbi Hillel

Jai Lakshmi: *Gratitude from Danny*

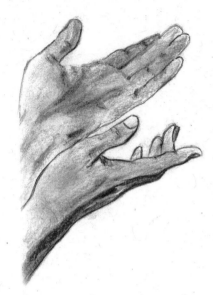

Shri Vidya philosophy states that the divine wanted to experience her radiance through the reflection of existence in order to know herself more fully. For this reason, divine consciousness manifested herself as all of creation—becoming the stars, the elements, nature, and living creatures—solely for the delight of basking in her own magnificence. We are likewise blessed to have mirrors all around us in the form of family, friends, co-workers, and even strangers to serve as reminders of the splendor that is life. As we learn and grow with every interaction, we can gain more insight into the brightest and darkest parts of ourselves. I am extremely blessed to have encountered many remarkable people on my path who have provided me with numerous opportunities to know myself more deeply and to acknowledge the diversity that makes my life so rich and rewarding.

First and foremost, I would like to acknowledge the members of my family, who have remained steadfast as I have explored my diverse and wandering passions. Thank you, Mom *(Bella)*, for your softness, multifaceted wisdom, and creative spark; Dad *(Isaac)*, for always believing in me and helping me stay motivated; & Mihal, for being a constant friend and the best sister ever. I offer immense gratitude to my teacher Douglas Brooks. Douglas is a profoundly insightful guide who has contributed immensely to my knowledge and practice of Tantra yoga philosophy and ritual. His deep comprehension of Sanskrit, his grasp of Hinduism as well as other religions, and his humble spirit are truly remarkable. Douglas' ability to share yoga from both his personal experience and his scholarly point of view creates an atmosphere for learning that is captivating and exquisitely rich. Warm thanks to Ann Greene, a shakti-infused woman who has the ability to teach complex Anusara® principles in clear and creative ways. Ann is quick on her feet and knows how to impart accessible structure to complicated information. She continually inspires me to expand my teaching practice to address a variety of learning styles. My sincere appreciation goes to Devarshi Steven Hartman for his passionate and insightful love of yoga. Devarshi is incredibly talented at fostering safe, sacred space for rich transformations while embodying the beauty and grace of inquiry-based learning. For me, he has always modeled deep courage and the ability to ride the waves of life with resilient spirit. I feel a profound sense of gratitude to Todd Norian for the many teachings he has shared which have allowed me to live more authentically. It was Todd who first introduced me to the teachings of Tantra, Anusara Yoga® and the tools of dynamic language, inspirational themes, and heartfelt expression. He is a truly astute teacher and brings the various components of yoga teaching to life with elegance and skill. His sensitivity, strength, and ability to constantly adapt and learn inspire me to reach for my highest. Loving thanks to Sudha Carolyn Lundeen, an astonishing yoga teacher and friend who lives her life with utmost authenticity and grace. She has taught me how to stay open to new ideas, how to lead classes that accommodate all types of students, and how to laugh even in the midst of intense sensation. I offer my gratitude to PremShakti Stout, who models tremendous courage and shares her wisdom of the yogic path with genuine passion and delight. I am extremely grateful for all of my Kripalu teachers: Dinabandhu Garrett Sarley & Ila Sarley, Jairaj Randal Williams, Kaviraj Stephen Cope, Priti Robyn Ross, Rashmi Sue Jenkins, Vidya Carolyn Dell'uomo, and Yoganand Michael Carroll. All of these phenomenal beings have supported me and so many others in rich transformations. I hold immense appreciation for the teachings and wisdom of Swami Kripalu, who was the inspiration for Kripalu Center and has had a powerful influence on the way I lead my life. Finally, I extend genuine thanks to John Friend, the founder of Anusara Yoga®. He has fused profound philosophical teachings with an intuitive and refined approach to asana, which has reinvigorated my personal study and practice of yoga.

I express my unending appreciation to Anjali Budreski for inspiration, creative ideas, and indispensable support. Anjali is a genius at bringing all of the elements of a yoga class together with intelligence and charm. She draws on her intuitive connection to nature, her knowledge of various philosophies, and her sincere love for people as she crafts. She supported me in fine-tuning these insights, brainstorming visual meditations, creating the overall structure of this text, and refining my writing. She also wrote several contemplations that convey her rich love for yoga. I will cherish our experiences of virtual meetings, belly laughs, and conscious conversations throughout the writing process. Anjali is a dedicated friend, a masterful teacher, and a bona fide baked-goods goddess. I feel blessed to know her and look forward to continued exploration of our shared passions and creative visions. I offer much gratitude to Kelli Adams, a talented yoga teacher and artist who brings her creative energy to the art of editing. She spent many, many hours enhancing my writing and remained steadfast even in the most challenging moments of our work. Kelli is adept at reworking words and sentences to make them flow cohesively, giving them deeper meaning and purpose. She is an amazing friend and a wonderful listener and is always in search of new learning as she engages wholeheartedly with life. These remarkable women are my partners in bringing this work to fruition, pouring in countless hours with dedication and heart; I can't thank them enough! I offer immense thanks to my mom Bella, who worked long hours in the final two months of this project to infuse life into this book through her elegant illustrations. I extend many thanks to Cody Drasser for sharing his heartfelt illustrations. His art has always made me pause in admiration, and his strong yet gentle spirit is a true gift. Many thanks to Derek Hansen for valuable graphic design support and Heidi Spear for exquisite copy editing. Finally, I feel deep appreciation for the employees of Recycled Paper Printing, who helped me fulfill my desire to produce an ecologically conscious book.

Indeed teachers arrive in many forms and under varying circumstances, and I am grateful for the ways in which my life has been touched by: Bruce McCormick, Caroline Boyce, Dahlia Dawood, Doug Keller, Elizabeth Brown, Galit, Eli, Ori, Gaya, & Roee Bina, Georgia Kerr, Jyoti Danika Kuhl, Kajal Dhabalia, Kathy Budreski, Knavin, Leonie, Arianna, Itai & Alina Arguetty, Lina & Leon Arguetty, Maya Weintraub, Miriam Arguetty, Nava & Yoram Weintraub, Paul Muller-Ortega, Roger McKeever, Shiva Rea, Susan Maier-Moul, Yael & Israel Milikovski, volunteers at Kripalu, and fellow students from my own yoga teacher training as well as those from the trainings I have had the privilege of assisting at Kripalu & with Todd. Much gratitude to all the creative and heartfelt poets that gave me permission to reprint their work, their inspiration through words is truly profound. Finally, a special note of thanks to the nature that surrounds me in the Berkshires and to my collection of lively dance music, both of which have served to renew and revitalize my energy during the lengthy writing and editing process.

Jai Lakshmi: *Gratitude from Anjali*

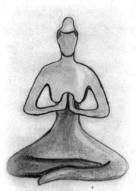

Gratitude first and foremost to this embodied life, the incredible teacher that can invoke the greatest joys and the deepest challenges and every flavor in between. I am grateful for the rolling Green Mountains of Vermont, which I call home; for the rivers, lakes, and oceans; and for the sweet birdsong that brings me into the present moment. I am grateful also to the blue sky, the swirling snowflakes, and darkness of winter and to the brilliant green and aliveness of summer. The earth is my inspiration and my home.

Unending gratitude to all of my spiritual teachers: my Mother, Kathy Budreski, who took me to an ashram in Scituate, Massachusetts, when I was a little girl and taught me to have compassion and to value the many diverse ways of connecting with spirit; my Father, Fred Budreski, who taught me that nature is the greatest sanctuary and gave me a deep appreciation for the ocean and the mountains of New England; Lisa Limoge, who welcomed me into her yoga studio in Burlington, Vermont; Todd Norian, who taught me to open my heart in a yoga class and what it means to teach yoga from a place of love, playfulness, and authenticity; Deb Neubauer, who opened my eyes to the service of teaching and encouraged me even when I was afraid; Douglas Brooks, who turns my world upside down and always reminds me that "I am the point the Universe is trying to make"; Sara Rose Page, for guiding me along the path of owning a yoga studio; and the many other teachers who have inspired me: Mitchel Bleier, Darren Rhodes, Paul Muller-Ortega, Shiva Rea, Angela Farmer, Ann Greene, and Eric Schiffmann.

Gratitude to my Vermont Family! Lisa Masé, for her ever-faithful shining love and self-full service; Jyotidhara, for her positive support and friendship; Fearn Lickfield, whose powerful presence is a true gift; Lydia Russell, my companion in bringing Anusara Yoga to our community; Molly Rose for her depth and fragrant beauty; Nina Shoenthal, for her incredible art and potent strength; and Devon Byers, Sandy Lory, and Sarika Tandon for being my other guiding stars in the sky. I extend many thanks to the Yoga Mountain family for constantly inviting me to clarify, expand, and stand more firmly rooted in myself: Lindsay Armstrong, Ellen Fein, Katie Harrington, Patrick McAndrew, Danielle Murphy, and Cettina Costagliola. Special, thanks to my friend and bookkeeper Jason Pugliese. Gratitude to my extended Kula, Lucy D'Aponte, Carolyn Connor, and Arica Bronze. Gratitude to my dear new and old friends: Kirstin Edelglass, Wendy Teller-Elsberg, Rachel Jolly, Elizabeth Brown, Chris Ellingwood, and the Burlington/ Montpelier Kirtan community. Gratitude to my birth family who are the very foundation on which I stand: my brothers Mark and Jon, little Max and Teddy, and all of the many amazing and wonderful cousins, aunts, and uncles whom I feel so blessed to be close to.

A Meeting Of Souls:

It is truly rare and precious when one soul finds in another a light of recognition reflected back as a spark of remembrance and homecoming. It is a gift to find in another human being the blessing of true friendship, which Celtic poet/mystic John O'Donohue refers to as "Anam Cara," or soul friend. These encounters of connection can happen at any time or place; it's as if our own intentions, combined with the play of the universe, merge to create an opportunity for each spirit to be nurtured by the other and for each person to become more of who he or she already is. Such an encounter occurred the day I met Danny Arguetty. There had been other connections that brought us together, which of course were revealed to us later, but it was on the day when we shared a beautiful harvest meal at my home in Montpelier that the warmth between us glowed and creative ideas regarding yoga, meditation, and life began to spin out like a brilliant spider's web. Being with Danny felt like coming home.

Since that first meeting, our connection has continued to deepen like a vibrant Vermont woodland in autumn, and for this, I am eternally grateful. Danny has offered the sweetness of unconditional love and friendship, never-ending support through life transitions and difficult times, and inspiration for me as a yoga teacher. It seems only natural that we would collaborate on a project as enormous and demanding as writing a book. I can't think of anyone as committed, dedicated, and able to take on this seemingly daunting task of gathering many ideas and churning them into a beautiful offering to share with the world. Countless hours have gone into this project, and I feel absolutely blessed to have had the opportunity to play a part in it.

Through working with my Virgoan/Israeli Bubby (as I affectionately refer to Danny), I have learned much about steadfastness and the willpower necessary to realize a dream. Yes, my Piscean spirit might still be stuck in the watery world of dreams and ideas if it weren't for his gentle (and sometimes not so gentle!) prodding. With a sharp mind and humble heart, Danny assembled a wonderful kula (community) of collaborators, kept the ship of his vision afloat and on course, and weathered the storms and rode the waves with faith and determination. When he would occasionally email me with sentiments like, "You have to help me, I'm soooo over this book," I would just smile to myself, secretly knowing that even the lila (play) of challenge fed and delighted him in a deep way.

To this end, Danny created even greater challenge for himself by setting rigorous standards around the publishing of Nourishing The Teacher. From the outset, he was concerned with the environmental impact of the publishing industry and spent hours on the phone and Internet educating himself about recycling labels and standards, learning the subtleties of printing an eco-conscious text. Danny clearly walks his talk and is bringing the teachings of yoga to life through his commitment to the environment and awareness of his own impact. I have been continuously amazed and heartened by his efforts to add to the beauty of this world through actions steeped in integrity and in optimal alignment with nature.

Thank you Danny, for being a soul-friend, for trusting me to help steer the boat of your wildest dreams, and for offering the deep-seated treasure of your heart as a gift in the form of this book. May we share many more back-porch meals together, and may the creative strands of our unique webs continue to entwine in support of the larger whole.
Blessings to the space between us!

Sankalpa: *Intention*

When I walk into my home, I sometimes pause to wonder, "Is this really my life?" Pictures of Hindu deities, altars, a harmonium, images of Jesus and Buddha, a Jewish menorah, and elements of nature pepper the environment of my living space. What began as a physical inquiry confined to a rubber mat has now blossomed into an endeavor to live life with deeper consciousness, greater openness, and a desire to constantly grow. One of the most meaningful lessons I have learned from my teacher Douglas Brooks is that rituals and practices require our participation; while we can respect the guidelines and structures of tradition, it is our choice to adopt and activate them in our own lives that is ultimately of greatest value and can become a catalyst for truly savoring the gift of life. The intention of this book is to make an offering of seed concepts that have transformed my day-to-day existence. Although I have chosen to create this book and have deepened my own connection to yoga in the process, I wish to state clearly that I am still very much a student on the infinite path of expansion. The ideas in this book are intended to serve as appetizers of sorts, providing tastes of the vast intelligence of yoga philosophy and the remarkable alchemy of nature. This text is by no means intended to be an authoritative voice on what is right or wrong, and each concept requires your participation and inquiry to fully come to life and be shared. Yoga is a lifelong endeavor, and the subjects broached in this book will hopefully provide inspiration and direction for further contemplation and study along the way.

Asana: *A Seat of Perspective*

With regard to any piece of writing, an understanding of the author's perspective—as well as the history underpinning that viewpoint—is vital. My relationship with yoga began with Ashtanga, and I later transitioned to a more vigorous vinyasa style of movement. Although these were the forms of yoga I practiced in the physical sense, none of the philosophy or more esoteric traditions of the practice made any sense to me for the first few years of my journey. Over the course of three months spent volunteering at Kripalu Center for Yoga and Health, I began to better understand that the practice far transcends the physical forms of asana. I was introduced to the various strands of yoga such as bhakti (*devotional*), jnana (*knowledge*), karma (*service/action*), mantra (*sound*), and raja (*deep states of meditation*), and this led me to realize that yoga could apply to any aspect of my life. I came to value Kripalu's focus on breath awareness, recognition of the inherent intelligence of life, and process of awakening the heart through cultivation of witness consciousness. By stepping more fully into the role of conscious and compassionate observer, I began to respond to my life instead of reacting to it. I felt newly empowered to choose my course rather than fall victim to every word, action, and disturbance that came into my life. Swami Kripalu writes, "Growth allows a portion of the mind to remain an objective witness even in a disturbed state. The witness is always there, if one can keep a wakeful attitude in one's self[1]." Through this practice, I learned how to truly honor my body, accept myself with all of my imperfections, and step into the resulting wonder manifested within. After my time at Kripalu, I traveled to India to see firsthand how spiritual practice was enacted in the land that gave birth to yoga. I was humbled by my trip and treasured my interactions with the people of major cities and small towns alike. I continue to be thankful for the various spiritual communities that gave me food, housing, and an opportunity to experience their lives for a few days. My time in India encouraged me to take my practice into the world while at the same time applying it to my daily life. When standing on a bus made for fifty passengers but packed with eighty, I began to underst___ the benefits of deep, mindful breath. When I passed hungry people living on the streets, I was ___ ___el sincere gratitude for the abundance I had known in life. When I looked into the eyes of ___ ___uls I encountered, I was able to see myself as worthy of their offerings. I didn't pu___ ___gs away, but instead embraced the discomfort and drank in the full spectrum ___umans are privileged to encounter. My time in this foreign land opened me ___erconnected, and although I live my life thousands of miles away, I am now ___d thoughts influence even those beyond my small circle. After my time ___ke my first yoga teacher training, which was deeply transformative. The ___ional tools for teaching yoga and helped me see all parts of myself ___e program, I taught in Boston and Vermont for a few years before ___er and workshop leader. Working at a large yoga center has been ___d me to meet a wide range of yoga practitioners, deepen my ___lvement with our volunteer and teacher training programs.

___een immersed in study of Anusara Yoga®, a system founded b___ ___orted me in expanding my teaching through its practices of ___ ___and integrating ingenious class elements. In addition to spec___ ___a has enhanced my knowledge of Tantra philosophy, which ___ ___and is essentially rooted in the belief that everything is imbue___ ___yoga traditions that preceded it and encompasses the full sp___ ___t to note here that even under the umbrella of Tantra, there ___ ___hich continue to evolve. The Tantric lineage to which I am m___ ___in the teachings of Professor Douglas Brooks and his teacher ___ ___eminent scholar of Hinduism and a Master of the Tantric Go___ ___m, or Shri Vidya. For me, the essence of yoga has become ___ ___tradition, which encourages practices of learning to savor eac___ ___etimes this translates to dancing with the light, while in other ___ ___Occasionally, the practice becomes one of simply pausing at ___ ___overies at the edge of my existing truths. The exploration of Ta___ ___y revealing process that is unconcerned with arrival at a fixed destina___ ___s offered in this book are written with this point of view in mind—that th___ ___o transcend the potential suffering of the human voyage, but rather to swim in th___ ___e are privileged to know. This perspective is seeded in the recognition of ourselves as pa___ ___eater whole, interconnected and yet each positively unique. Rooted in these principles, we can ___ our power of discrimination to practice skilled engagement in life.

Matrika Shakti: *The Power of Dynamic Language*

The more I have immersed myself in yoga, the more I have become aware of my language and its potential to influence both my internal state and my external reality. "Matrika" is a Sanksrit word meaning "little wombs," and "shakti" is the word for creative power. Together, they convey the ideas that everything carries vibration and that we can ultimately birth our reality. As forms of vibration in our daily life, words and verbal communication offer us a ready portal for shifting the context of our lives. Although this notion has its origins in Sanskrit, this inherent power of words carries into every spoken language. The way we speak both externally to others and internally to ourselves can serve as a mirror enabling us to see ourselves more fully. Internal conversation and external dialogue are inextricably linked. If, for example, we grow up in an environment characterized by negative media bombardment, violent speech, and unsupportive words, we might be more apt to internalize those particular vibrations. These "contra-mantras," as dubbed by Priti Robyn Ross, can become the very foundation of our experience of life. As our internal speech becomes more negative, unloving, and full of disbelief, our external life begins to reflect this internal reality. A vicious cycle is thus initiated that can lead to feelings of unworthiness, lack of interest in life, and inability to tap into inner potential. Often this occurs at such a subtle level that we might not even be aware of these vibrations seeping into the crevasses of our inner being. Luckily the brain, body, and cells are malleable, and we can rewrite our patterns by entering new data. Through a renewed internal dialogue and more vibrationally affirming interactions, we can craft a more positive self-image, align with our deepest desires, and motivate to serve not only ourselves but also the world at large.

Words empower us to communicate our experience of life, allowing us to share internal states that might otherwise only remain accessible to us. Through language we can share joy, invoke emotions, and tap into the fabric of creation itself in order to shift the universe from the inside out. Verbal communication is extremely powerful and can strongly impact our relationships with ourselves, loved ones, and even strangers. Models of conscious communication from the Kripalu tradition include "I" statements, reflective listening, and whole messages. Nonviolent Communication, or NVC, is a well-respected and powerful modality for creating clear dialogue based on feelings and needs. If you are not familiar with these instruments of speech, you may want to seek resources for further study. If you are a yoga teacher, you have the added opportunity to intensify your inquiry of dynamic language since so much of the teaching experience is expressed through words. Visit www.nourishingtheteacher.com to download continually updated resource files on common language habits, Stage I, Stage II, and Stage III Kripalu Yoga leading words and phrases, and a growing yoga-related thesaurus to spice up your database of expressive vocabulary.

Hrdayya: *Heart-Opening Themes*

As a natural progression on my path as a student of yoga, I came to realize that I wanted to offer others the possibility to tap into the insights that have uplifted and changed my life. After personal inquiry and contemplation of the concepts offered in this book, you might find yourself called to infuse your classes with what you have experienced and learned. When we as teachers begin to weave focused contemplations into our classes, we open the door for the hearts and minds of our students—as well as our own—to blossom and awaken. I find this to be true in my own experience as a yoga teacher, which indeed served as my inspiration to continue expanding my knowledge and refining the way I guide yoga experiences.

When I first started teaching yoga, I taught the physical form of asana with excitement and zeal. After a while, though, I sought to give more in my interactions with students, and I had the urge to delve more deeply into the practice of teaching. I began to seek sources of inspiration that would facilitate the journey to this next level, both for myself and for my students. I researched sacred words, studied various topics in yoga writings, and began to pepper my classes with inspirational readings. The first manifestation of this work was a lesson plan in which I read a quote at the outset of class, taught the physical asana practice, and then revisited the quote at the culmination of practice. After many classes utilizing this model, I was hungry again. I wanted to offer a richer experience that would encourage students to explore their inner landscapes through the vehicle of asana practice. Inspired by Anjali Budreski, who was studying Anusara Yoga®, I started a teaching journal and began to read exhaustively on yoga philosophy and concepts from nature. I invested more time in planning my classes and started incorporating elements of everyday life that truly sparked my interest. When I embarked on my own Anusara® Teacher Training with Todd Norian, I learned the refined methodology and techniques for teaching yoga classes infused with one central concept throughout. Teaching now, I feel inspired and energized as I step into the flow of class and guide students through a practice crafted with unique imagery, gracious heart, and heightened sensitivity. I feel the vivacity in the room, the depth of the breath, and the radiant splendor emerging for students both within and without. Visit the book's website to download exciting resources on class themes.

Inquiries, Contemplations, and Insights:

Nourishing the Teacher is divided into five sections: The Gifts of Embodiment, The Wisdom of Yoga, The Hindu Gods and Goddesses, The Alchemy of Nature, and The Wheel of the Year. To fully engage with each concept, I recommend reading the topic fully and then choosing at least one of the inquiries, practices, or rituals related to the subject matter. This will help facilitate a deeper exploration of the ideas that will permeate every part of your being. Please note that this text is not intended as an instructional manual on how to do physical postures, breath exercises, or sequence a personal practice. If there are postures, breaths, or practices listed with which you are not familiar, take time to explore them through qualified class instruction and/or personal investigation.

After each contemplation in the text, inquiries and practices are offered to support you in deepening your personal experience. Note that every category will not necessarily appear every time, and remember that less is more; avoid doing all of these each time you step on your mat.

Inquiries:

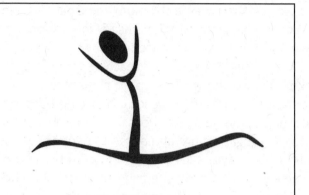

On the Mat: These are ideas and suggestions for how you might approach a particular contemplation in your personal practice. Note that for most insights, there are specific poses suggested which embody the energy of the principal concept.

Off the Mat: Here you will find suggestions for investigating a given idea or concept in the context of your daily life.

Practices:

In the technology of yoga, we are comprised of more than merely the physical being. The following categories utilized throughout the text offer ways to engage a specific idea on the various planes of existence, such as the verbal, visual, energetic, and emotional. We can tap into the practices of mantra (*power of words*), yantra (*visual instruments*), pranayama (*breath practices*) and puja (*celebratory rituals*) to fully embody a particular contemplation.

Supportive Words
By having multiple ways to describe the same concept, we can come to understand it more fully. Use these words as meditations to simply ponder, as mantra for repetition, as source ideas for journaling, or to inspire a creative collage.

Visualizations
Images stimulate a different part of the psyche than words. Utilize these visual representations as focal points for meditation or as inspiration for art.

Complementary Breath
The breath carries vitality in the form of oxygen and the life force of prana. Explore

Words create our reality. Repeat these specific breath practices as means of feeling and integrating a particular contemplation.

Closing Ritual
Rituals have the potential to restore joy and vitality to the core of our being through a sense of heightened participation. Exercise creative freedom as you enact these nourishing customs and cultivate your own.

Teacher's Note
Here you will find creative suggestions to support you in the process of teaching a particular concept once you have spent ample time in your own personal inquiry.

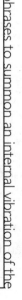

phrases to summon an internal vibration of the contemplation

Inspired by:

Following the title of each contemplation, a particular individual is credited with having inspired the thoughts and inquiries presented. This person is either a formal teacher with whom I have studied or a loved one who has embodied a particular quality I address.

Madhura: *Sweetness*

As a practitioner and guide of yoga, each and every one of these inquiries, contemplations, and insights has enriched my life for the better. These unique representations from yoga philosophy, nature, and daily living have given me access to the various facets, both constant and changing, that make up my complete being. As a result, I feel more prepared and more excited to step into the fire of life, embracing with open arms the full spectrum of emotions that have been gifted to me in this human experience. As Swami Kripalvanandaji writes, "To perform every action artfully is yoga[2]." I wish you love and blessings as you embark on this continuously evolving journey, making art, sharing love, and nourishing the teacher within.

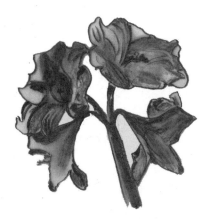

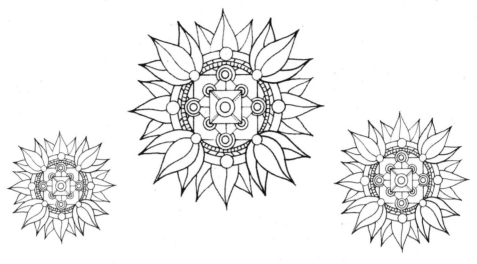

the gifts
of
embodiment

*"I think the real miracle is not to walk either on water or in thin air,
but to walk on earth."*
-Thich Nhat Hanh

Graceful Beginnings: {inspired by The Sun}

I have lived most of my life in urban environments, but I have spent the past few years living in Vermont and in the Berkshire Mountains of Western Massachusetts. Through living in these more rural places, I have become more attuned to the rhythms of nature. One of the most prominent shifts that has occurred as a result of this attunement is my early hour of waking. As the morning light blooms slowly from the darkness of night, I feel a renewed sense of joy in pausing to acknowledge the beginning of a new day. Because of this awareness, I find that I make more space to notice new chapters in my life and in the lives of others.

Beginnings tend to have a sweetness that uplifts the spirit with feelings of grace and ease. Through the gift of embodiment, we as humans get to taste the diverse flavors of life, and among the most precious of these is the celebration of new beginnings. The initial moment of any given situation is one that can set the tone for what will transpire for hours, days, or years to come. With intention and heart, we can welcome these moments and treasure them as gifts to inspire and fuel us at our deepest core. This might take the form of a mindful breath, a brief moment of marveling at a garden, a seated meditation, or a pause to acknowledge a new meal before us. By doing something small to honor the commencement of the various episodes of the day, our whole being has a chance to refocus, and the ensuing experience is received in a much different way. This simple yet profound practice can thus infuse us with a greater sense of ease and vitality as we advance through the dance of life. As Byrd Baylor writes:

> Some people say there is a new sun every day, that it begins its life at dawn and lives for one day only. They say you have to welcome it. You have to make the sun happy. You have to make a good day for it. You have to make a good world for it to live its one-day life in. And the way to start, they say, is just by looking east at dawn. When they look east tomorrow, you can too. Your song will be an offering—and you'll be one more person in one more place at one more time in the world saying hello to the sun, letting it know you are there. If the sky turns a color sky it never was before, just watch it. That's part of the magic. That's the way to start a day[1].

Inquiries

On the Mat: Bring special awareness to the initial moments of your practice, focusing attention first on the body, then on the mind, and finally on the breath. Use this transition to retreat from the events of your day, land fully in the moment, and link to the vibrations of your practice. As you chant the sound "aum," sense how it serves as a ritual of commencement, imparting your intentions to the task at hand and further aligning the rhythm of your heart to the greater flow of the universe. In addition to inviting a graceful beginning at the outset of your practice, be mindful of honoring each transition into various segments of your sadhana (warm-ups, breath exercises, standing poses, floor postures, etc.) by way of subtly pausing to welcome each new chapter of the practice. Furthermore, explore each subsequent posture as a unique opportunity to focus on the breath and the first moments of a particular movement or position of the body.

Off the Mat: In the span of a week, commit to four specific occasions when you will intentionally honor a beginning—be it great or small. Notice the effects of this exercise.

Practices

Supportive Words
commencement, dawn, onset, spring,
starting point

Visualization
Savoring the first few moments of a beautiful sunrise, the subtle light intensifying and becoming brighter as the day reveals itself.

Complementary Breath
viloma *(inhale)*
Focus on the first moments of each cycle of breath.

Closing Ritual
During meditation, hold one word in your mind's eye to invoke a graceful beginning for the next segment of your day.

of each day with delight

along my path

I make

I meet the initial moments

space for opening rituals that help me thrive

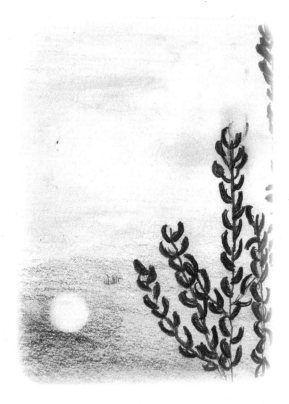

The Inquiry: {inspired by Kripalu Yoga}

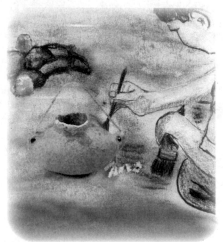

Given that I am now in my third decade on the planet, I am thankful to have never had chronic pain or serious bodily injuries. Good fortune and the practice of yoga have supported me in staying strong, open, and injury-free. One day, though, I was helping my dog Knavin into the car while standing on a sidewalk that was higher than the norm. I failed to bend my knees properly, and I suddenly felt a jarring pain in my back. I rushed home as the pain intensified, and a short while later I was lying on the living room floor, unable to move. After some time, I was able to crawl around, and I began a treatment of herbs, arnica cream, and ice. I had to find subs for my yoga classes, and I spent much of the day in bed. As I slumped around indoors, I was surprised by the thoughts that entered my mind. The thoughts of "Oh, no," "This sucks," and "Why me?" only lasted for a few brief moments. What prevailed instead were thoughts of how this was an opportunity not only to feel something new, but also to relate to others who have had a back injury or live with chronic back pain. It was rather startling but positively refreshing to find myself in this space of inquiry and appreciation as opposed to one of unrelenting self-pity.

As children, our mode of operation is rooted in inquiry; random objects find their way into the mouth as a means of exploring and understanding them, unfamiliar smells and textures pique our curiosity, and new flavors elicit genuine, definitive responses. As we grow older, though, most of us lose this sense of fascination with the world around us. How would life be different if we chose to meet our present experiences with this childlike sense of inquiry? Instead of directing significant attention towards what we find frustrating about a situation, we can better utilize our energy to study the circumstances from a new angle. Engaging in genuine examination allows us to remain immersed in the conversation of our lives, and we begin to realize the point is not to get a concrete answer and end the dialogue. Rather, we see that the more we probe, the more content we have to enrich and inform our experience. Living in this state of study enables a sense of fluidity that allows us to ride the currents of life fully and authentically. In a challenging moment, our first inclination might be to run away, or we might get caught up in the labels of "good" or "bad". If we look beyond this, though, we can contemplate what is of value in any given set of circumstances. How will staying in the question of what is unfolding support further expansion and learning? As a specific example, consider how this concept is central to the field of archaeology, which is founded on the premise of inquiry. The exact way in which historical events unfolded will never be fully known, but archaeologists are constantly digging through layers, dusting off ancient relics, and putting pieces together to construct a story. This narrative of proposed events is ever-evolving, as each subsequent round of investigation illuminates new ideas and perspectives regarding what may have occurred. As Michel de Montaigne writes, "the world is but a school of inquiry".

Inquiries

On the Mat: Step into an inquiry of your practice and become an explorer, continually developing your own personal story based on educated guesses, heartfelt assumptions, and actual encounters. Utilize your mat space to analyze what comes to the surface, bracketing your doubt and fear to simply honor the process before you. Approach your practice like an archaeologist who is dusting off clues and discovering elements of an emerging story, thus remaining open as each subsequent chapter unfurls. Sense whether this process of examination supports you in deepening your relationship to self. Note how this endeavor spans the physical, emotional, and subtle realms of your being, as your process of questioning permeates all three.

Use downward dog as a pose of focused inquiry, pinpointing different elements of the posture as you play. Begin by exploring the spacing of your hands and feet. In your first iteration of the pose, have the hands close together and the feet similarly spaced. Notice how this feels. Next, investigate the opposite extreme by making ample space between the hands as well as the feet, and compare this sensation with that of the first position. Finally, bring your feet to hip-width distance apart and hands a little wider than shoulder width, and take note of how this feels in the body. Also experiment with various angles of the pelvis, observing the resulting impact on the torso and low back curve. Ideally there should be a little dip in the lumbar so that it is not overly swayed or overly flat. If the hamstrings are tight, try to bend your knees and see what occurs. For wrist support, roll up the front of your mat, placing your palms on the roll with fingers spreading onto the floor. Notice whether this provides more support. With a firm foundation rooted in these principles, expand your study to include three-legged dog, twisted leg in three-legged dog, or one arm twist in down dog.

Off the Mat: The next time you encounter a challenging situation, engage in the practice of inquiry. Connect to your breath, witness what emotions are coming up, and simply practice compassionate curiosity in lieu of trying to change things. Note whether the spirit of exploration gives rise to a solution or deeper understanding.

Practices

Supportive Words
examine, explore, inspect, investigate, probe, question, study, survey

Visualization
Archaeologist dusting off an ancient relic, putting the pieces together to construct a story through ongoing examination.

Complementary Breath
ujjayi

Closing Ritual
seated meditation

Teacher's Note
Pair students up for one of the rounds of downward dog, and encourage them to support one another in their explorations. Although this is a common posture, many students find it challenging and will appreciate the time to fully investigate the structural details and subtle nuances of the pose.

I examine my life with mindfulness. I investigate the ways in which I interact with those around me. Like a dedicated archaeologist, I build my story through ongoing inquiry.

The Path of Compassion: {*inspired by High School Friendship*}

One day, I was having a heated conversation with a friend over religion, the existence of God, and the theories of science. After we had finished our roué, I could not stop thinking about how deeply wrong she was and how profoundly right I was. After several days of stewing in my frustration with her, I suddenly had a vision of her in my mind's eye with a multitude of silhouetted figures standing behind her. In that instant, it hit me: my friend's convictions, as well as my own, were made up of so much more than merely what was apparent in the moment. I understood that both of us had been influenced by each and every person, instance, and interaction that had colored the pages of our lives until then, including our parents, teachers, cultures, religious or nonreligious upbringings, traumas, and joys. I felt myself soften as this realization coalesced. I finally understood how people, whom I believe to be essentially embodied love, can take part in insidious acts and hold seemingly narrow beliefs. I remember realizing then that even if someone walked up to me and yelled hateful profanities, I would still be able to find compassion for that person. I would not condone such an action, but I would understand that one's accumulated layers are largely responsible for his views and consequently his behavior in the world. Since that day, I always envision this backdrop of silhouettes behind those with whom I converse.

Compassion is one of the fundamental elements of yoga practice both on and off the mat. Leading our lives from a place of tenderness and empathy, we are not only less violent with ourselves, but we can also perceive and connect with the divine in those around us. As we live our lives, strong reactions to others are bound to arise. When such a reaction does manifest, we have an opportunity to soften and contemplate what has shaped another's position. Slowing down in this way allows us to recognize the light that exists in others' hearts even though their views may be at the opposite end of the spectrum from our own. It is this ability to recognize our shared humanity that creates space in our interactions and allows us to respond to any situation as we ourselves would want to be treated. Compassion is by no means easy to cultivate, but as we recommit to the practice on a daily basis, we can begin to source it even for those who trigger us most strongly. As Thich Nhat Hanh beautifully writes in *Please Call Me by My True Names*:

> Don't say that I will depart tomorrow—
> even today I am still arriving.
>
> Look deeply: every second I am arriving
> to be a bud on a Spring branch,
> to be a tiny bird, with still-fragile wings,
> learning to sing in my new nest,
> to be a caterpillar in the heart of a flower,
> to be a jewel hiding itself in a stone.
>
> I still arrive, in order to laugh and to cry,
> to fear and to hope.
> The rhythm of my heart is the birth and death
> of all that is alive.

I am a mayfly metamorphosing
on the surface of the river.
And I am the bird
that swoops down to swallow the mayfly.

I am a frog swimming happily
in the clear water of a pond.
And I am the grass-snake
that silently feeds itself on the frog.

I am the child in Uganda, all skin and bones,
my legs as thin as bamboo sticks.
And I am the arms merchant,
selling deadly weapons to Uganda.

I am the twelve year-old girl,
refugee on a small boat,
who throws herself into the ocean
after being raped by a sea pirate.
And I am the pirate,
my heart not yet capable
of seeing and loving.

I am a member of the politburo,
with plenty of power in my hands.
And I am the man who has to pay
his "debt of blood" to my people
dying slowly in a forced-labor camp.

My joy is like Spring, so warm
it makes flowers bloom all over the Earth.
My pain is like a river of tears,
so vast it fills the four oceans.

Please call me by my true names,
so I can hear all my cries and laughter at once,
so I can see that my joy and pain are one.

Please call me by my true names,
so I can wake up
and the door of my heart
could be left open,
the door of compassion[2].

Inquiries

On the Mat: Make space to source compassion for the way your body looks, feels, moves, and doesn't move. Utilize the laboratory of your yoga practice to slow down, move inside, become a more astute observer of ready triggers, and meet the experience residing beneath the surface with deep understanding. Dedicate your yoga to someone with whom you struggle or to a part of the body you have always berated. Make space for the full range of your experience, and acknowledge everything emerging in the course of your sadhana. Source kindness for even the darkest thoughts and sensations that arise. Remember that through cultivating deeper understanding of your own views, feelings, and internal dialogue, you can stretch your capacity to hold space for the differences you perceive in others. To support the experience of inner empathy, utilize the power of forward folds like standing forward fold, bound angle, head to knee, seated forward fold, and seated wide-angle forward fold.

Off the Mat: Pick one person in your life with whom you have consistently struggled. Journal about how you might offer them compassion. Where do their beliefs and actions originate?

Practices

Supportive Words
empathy, kindness, softness, tenderness, understanding

Visualization
Hands in lotus mudra in front of the heart, literally holding and extending the space of compassion.

Complementary Breath
ujjayi
Utilize the ocean sound to soothe, soften, and connect to your heart space.

Closing Ritual
metta meditation

I feel the shared humanity between myself and others. I utilize skillful empathy in situations that provoke me. I step into each moment with a silent prayer of kindness and compassion.

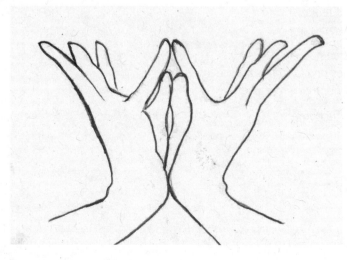

Go In and In: {inspired by Danna Faulds}

Danna Faulds is a former Kripalu resident and a long-time yoga teacher who has published several books of poetry sourced from the heart of her personal yoga practice. One of her most inspiring books is the collection entitled *Go In and In*, which offers countless treasures of wisdom and insight.

Go in and in.
    Be the space
between two cells,
    the vast, resounding
silence in which
    spirit dwells.
Be sugar dissolving
    on the tongue of life.
Dive in and in,
    as deep as you can dive.
Be infinite, ecstatic truth.
    Be love conceived and born in union.
Be exactly what you seek,
    the Beloved, singing Yes,
tasting Yes, embracing Yes,
    until there is only essence;
the All of Everything
    expressing through you
as you. Go in and in
    and turn away from
nothing that you find[3].

Because most of daily life transpires at the external layer of experience, the invitation of yoga and other mindfulness practices to explore our innermost realms beckons us into unfamiliar territory. Often, we assume that this process of going in and in will be a daunting journey involving finding something dark in the wilderness of our hearts. We believe we'll have to don our proverbial armor and fight terrifying battles as we confront our personal demons. Yet, the journey of turning inward needn't be a fight; instead, it can be a subtle, gradual exploration. By taking steps towards reconnecting with our innermost self, we are able to bring forgotten elements of our spirit to the surface and reignite them to enrich our lives. Living life in this way empowers us to welcome all that shows up in our lives—whether dark or light—as we move into closer relationship with the diverse aspects of ourselves.

This poem invites the recognition that dark and light are comprised of the same material that is "All of Everything" and that by embracing one, we welcome the other. The last line is particularly striking, as it invites us to turn away from nothing that we find. Whatever may surface from within or come at us from the outside, all is part of the greater whole and contributes to developing character and enhancing strength. Douglas Brooks writes: "The universe *(and consequently us as well)* grows itself by consuming itself as it evolves.by what it takes in. Nourishment and toxicity go hand-in-hand, and our process is one of radical affirmation, saying 'yes' first to all experience. Even if it is toxic, we can say 'yes,' because by taking it in we can digest it and offer it back as beauty and light[4]." As we journey inside, we can assume the stance of curious investigator as we encounter the various layers of our being. Instead of getting sucked into the drama of "What if this weren't here?" and "Why is this part of me so prominent?", we can simply be in the inquiry of what a particular facet has to offer. How will each specific landmark enable our words, thoughts, and actions to be more fully expressed? The journey of going in and in is a never-ending adventure, and one that guarantees limitless food for thought and personal growth. By delving into our innermost dimensions, we can cultivate a stronger relationship to self and offer the fruits of this process to those around us.

Inquiries

On the Mat: In yoga, the breath and the poses provide us with means of focusing our attention as we hone our ability to skillfully probe within. The majority of our daily activity transpires with an outward focus, but our sadhana carves out precious time to retreat from this as we replenish our energy from the inside. Begin your practice with an extended experience of viloma pranayama, which will aid you in transitioning into an inquisitive state. As your practice progresses, notice textures, feelings, and questions you find as you go in and in. Hold on to these offerings from within, noticing any resistance that manifests and allowing it to surface and possibly dissipate with the release of each pose. Soften, embrace the pauses, and honor spaces as they arise in your experience. Investigate standing forward fold, knee-down lunge, runner's stretch, goddess, warrior two, lateral angle, triangle, tree, standing wind-relieving; standing hand to big toe, head to knee, pigeon, bound angle, and seated wide-angle forward fold.

Off the Mat: Identify an area of your life in which you are functioning merely at the most superficial level (*such as relationships, eating habits, professional pursuits, or movement practice*). Take one week to dive as deeply as you can into this particular facet of your life. At the end of the week, write in your journal about what you learned by plunging purposefully into this realm.

Practices

I open to the place where spirit dwells inside of me

Supportive Words
inner, inside, internal, inward, within

Complementary Breath
viloma *(inhale)*

Visualization
Diving into the spaces between the cells, finding treasures and honoring the diversity that thrives there.

Closing Ritual
Sit and take a few deep breaths. Allow each inhalation to serve as a pathway to the innermost realm of your being.

I journey inside, extract my inner treasures, and share them with the world

dive more deeply into who I am

With each exhale

Mystery & Wonder: {inspired by Devarshi Steven Hartman}

Walking out of Kripalu one evening after a long day of work, I looked up at the night sky as I always do. On this particular night, I was rendered motionless as I experienced a moment of pure wonder and awe. There was a crescent moon, and the brightly lit slice was resting softly against the backdrop of its barely visible, shadowed round wholeness. The stars surrounding this natural masterpiece sparkled brilliantly, and the intense darkness of the night sky tinged the whole scene with crispness and elegance. Adbhuta[5], the Sanskrit word for wonder, curiosity, and mystery, came to mind as I continued to walk, relishing the splendid nature of this instant.

Adbhuta is often recognizable in the eyes and facial expressions of little children as they explore the infinite fascinations of the world around them. Often, the simplest things lead them into the ecstasy of mystery, such as seeing someone make a funny face, tasting a new food for the first time, or being introduced to other soft and cuddly living creatures. As adults, many of us have lost this sense of curiosity and awe for the lives we lead. Instead, days and weeks become one long to-do list, and we forget to pause and mingle with astonishment or marvel at the many gifts of our existence. Without a sense of wonder, our experience of the world can quickly become tedious and bland. One of my teachers, Devarshi Steven Hartman, led our teacher-training group in an exercise in which we pretended to be aliens who had just landed on a new planet. He encouraged us to fully embody this role and explore our outdoor surroundings as the mystery they would be if they weren't so familiar to us. One of the primary teachings of this exercise was that quality of life could be drastically enhanced if we approached more of our daily experiences with this sense of awe.

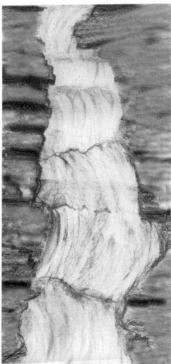

In addition to this association with the greater majesty of life, adbhuta can also be inspired by moments of unfathomable coincidence thus imbued with a magical quality. Turning a corner in Providence, Rhode Island, to see a friend from Vermont on the other side of the street, going on a blind date to discover you both grew up in the same small town, or choosing a tarot card that reflects exactly what is manifesting in your life at present; in these special moments, we are reminded of the incredible and delightful randomness which characterizes our existence. These magical instances can actually become more frequent as we learn to actively seek adbhuta in daily life, and the natural environment is likewise an ever-abundant source of this sense of awe. After watching an episode of the BBC's *Planet Earth*, a friend commented on her amazement at the remarkable mélange of vital energy apparent in our world. The lively nocturnal life of the world's deserts, the grand waterfalls that inspire us to pause in reverence, and the intricate social structures and behaviors of millions of planetary species are all true marvels. Indeed, we live our lives as walking marvel machines, as demonstrated by the following facts: the left lung is smaller than the right to make room for the heart; every person has a unique tongue print; the liver performs over 500 different functions; the body is made up of over 600 muscles and over

200 bones; bones are four times stronger than concrete; on an average day, we engage more than 26,000 cycles of breath; the heart pumps 4,000 gallons of blood daily; the small intestine is 22 feet long[6]. Living in a corresponding state of fascination requires not only that we attune our awareness to receiving these qualities, but also that we continuously cultivate deeper connection with our intuition and hearts. At these levels of our being, we recognize that we are indeed manifestations of this same miraculous energy and that not everything need be rationalized with our logical, cause-and-effect reasoning. As Edward Abbey writes:

How strange and wonderful is our home, our earth, with its swirling vaporous atmosphere. Its flowering and frozen climbing creatures. The croaking things with wings that hang on rocks, and soar through fog, the furry grass, the scaly seas… To see our world as a space traveler might see it for the first time, through Venusian eyes or Martian antennae, how utterly rich and wild it would seem[7].

Inquiries

On the Mat: Over time, we may lose the sense of mystery that infused our practice when we first discovered this form of movement and breath. Take time to notice how your sadhana differs when you explore the body's motion with a sense of awe, concentrating, feeling, and observing as each arm extends and each toe spreads to make contact with the earth. Explore an arm-balancing sequence, which has the potential to create truly wondrous shapes. Move through plank, side plank, firefly, eka hasta bhujasana and visvamitrasana.

Off the Mat: To reignite a sense of wonder, take time to contemplate things you don't understand. Spend time in nature admiring the iridescence of a hummingbird's feathers, or gaze up at the Milky Way on a clear night. Look around your seemingly ordinary surroundings to find rich sources of astonishment residing in plain sight, be open to surprise and randomness in your life, and ask questions without always seeking concrete answers.

Practices

I welcome surprise and randomness as gifts of the universe

Supportive Words
astonishment, awe, bewilderment, fascination, marvel, surprise

Visualization
The splendor of a huge cascading waterfall.

Complementary Breath
kapalabhati
Note how a few rounds of this powerful breath can stimulate a sense of wonder and surprise from the inside out.

Closing Ritual
As you meditate, take time to do a body scan as an act of consciously honoring the many marvels of your body.

abilities of my own body

I allow my

self to be astonished by the breathtaking power of nature   I marvel at the intricate and subtle

Welcoming: {written by Anjali Budreski}

While vacationing on Cape Cod, one of my favorite things to do is take long walks on the beach to collect unique treasures. As I walk along picking up pieces of broken shells, smooth round pebbles, and sea glass, I am reminded that everything is precious and possesses its own splendor. Everything is welcomed into my palm! Sometimes, it is the imperfections that make a rock or shell even more interesting and exquisite. The jagged edges tell the story of a shiny, white-washed clamshell and all it has weathered. In much the same way, our own rough edges and sharp points tell our stories and become an integral part of us. The question, therefore, becomes whether we can welcome everything to the table of our consciousness as readily and unconditionally as we would welcome these one-of-a-kind beach gems into our palms. As the seventeenth century mystic poet Rumi says, "...even if they are a crowd of sorrows, who want to sweep your house clean...can you welcome them in for tea and conversation?" Welcoming is the spirit of inviting all the guests to the table, beckoning even the unwanted ones such as sorrow, despair, pain, and grief to sit alongside the joy, love, peace, and openness we so desire. Yoga teacher Richard Miller talks about allowing these "bubbles" *(the guests)* to rise to the surface of our consciousness, rather than continually pushing them back down. Bubbles naturally want to rise and pop, and when we allow them to ascend to the surface, they miraculously reintegrate into the waters from whence they came. It is only when we truly welcome the full spectrum of our experience, rather than suppress or deny it, that the bubbles can rise, be acknowledged, and then dissolve back into the vastness of consciousness. In this way, a welcoming disposition can help facilitate the deepest healing and transformation, leading us to right action and skillful intent. As Rumi eloquently describes:

This being human is a guest house.
Every morning a new arrival.

A joy, a depression, a meanness,
some momentary awareness comes
as an unexpected visitor.

Welcome and entertain them all!
Even if they're a crowd of sorrows,
who violently sweep your house
empty of its furniture,
still, treat each guest honorably.
He may be clearing you out
for some new delight.

The dark thought, the shame, the malice,
meet them at the door laughing,
and invite them in.

Be grateful for whoever comes,
because each has been sent
as a guide from beyond[8].

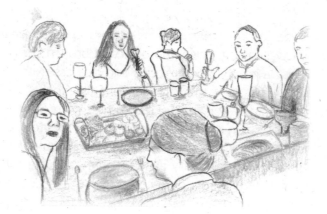

Inquiries

On the Mat: Take note of when bubbles begin to form during your practice. Do they float to the surface when you are in a challenging, vigorous, or simple yet deep pose? As you stand strong in warrior pose, what bubbles up? As you fold forward in seated forward bend, what emotions arise? In an intense chair pose or a full bow, notice how the inquiry becomes not only what rises to the surface, but also whether you can linger there to experience the many bubbles that emerge. Can you remain present long enough for them to break the surface and dissolve? In essence, can you welcome all of the guests to the table of your heart? Remember that something you think should be profound may not be, and something you might not expect to could open a floodgate. When these various guests arrive, the practice turns to welcoming them in all their diversity and opening to what they have to offer, knowing each is a treasure and, as Rumi says, "a guide from beyond" perhaps "clearing you out for some new delight¹." In this practice, investigate chair, lateral angle, down dog, bridge, one arm stretched overhead in camel, and one-armed little thunderbolt.

Off the Mat: As you move through a single day, consciously welcome all of the experiences that show up. At the end of the day, write in your journal about any insights that surfaced.

Practices

Supportive Words
embrace, greet, meet, receive, take in

Visualization
A colorful array of guests welcomed and seated at a dining room table.

Complementary Breath
dirgha
The ability of the breath to make space for all

I give myself permission to slow down and truly welcome that is arising.

Closing Ritual
Spend a few minutes at the end of your practice in a seated meditation. Envision any thoughts that arise as bubbles, and simply allow them to float to the surface of the mind and disperse.

valuable teachings to share

all that arises

With each

breath, I partake in the conversation of my practice

I embrace each guest as a guide with

Little Gems: {inspired by Knavin the Three-Legged Dog}

Working with clients on topics of nutrition and well-being is a constant reminder of how the little things in life can have the most transformative impact. Drinking water, breathing deeply, sleeping soundly, finding time for relaxation, and cultivating joy can all affect profound changes in health. Once when I returned home from a five-day retreat, my dog, Knavin, met me with bursting enthusiasm. We played together nonstop for a full hour, chasing one another, dancing with sticks, and laughing and barking. There was such sweetness in the air as time flew by, and my heart was buoyed by this simple yet genuine joy. Such reunions with our loved ones are an example of the little gems of our lives, as these moments leave us with a sense of fullness within. Moving through our days, it can be so easy to dwell on all that isn't working and overlook the power of the small things. If every day is spent in worry, distress, and mental confusion, we literally fill up with negativity and crowd out any opportunity to recognize the glimmering jewels available to us in a given situation.

Traditionally, gems are objects imbued with great importance and revered due to their rarity and preciousness. What in your life can you identify as sacred and appreciate in the same manner? As you cultivate this awareness and make yourself increasingly more available to life, these moments can reveal themselves in the smile of a neighbor, a card from a friend, the brisk caress of the wind, or the simple delight of an avocado on whole grain toast. Feelings of disconnection usually arise when we have been rushing through our days and missing the many small gifts that contribute to a sense of wholeness. All it takes is a brief moment of acknowledgement to tap into the profound sense of well-being these treasures foster. The same holds true for actual gems, each of which is associated with specific qualities and characteristics; we can only absorb these benefits if we take the time to consciously recognize them. As Mary Jean Iron writes:

Normal day, let me be aware of the treasure you are. Let me learn from you, love you, bless you before you depart. Let me not pass you by in quest of some rare and perfect tomorrow. Let me hold you while I may, for it may not always be so. One day I shall dig my nails into the earth, or bury my face in the pillow, or stretch myself taut, or raise my hands to the sky and want, more than all the world, your return[9].

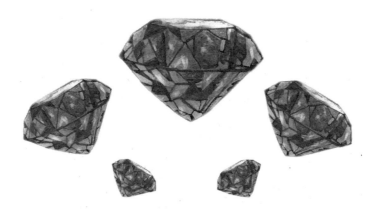

Inquiries

On the Mat: Instead of focusing solely on the big picture of each posture and rushing to achieve a particular form, take time to notice the various details supporting you in the expression of the pose. Each of these details of alignment is like one tiny facet of a glorious gem reflecting its light. Take note of other little gems that arise before, during, or after a practice, perhaps manifesting as a moment of meditation, spaciousness between one pose and the next, or being wholly present to a luxurious stretch. Sense what shifts within as you pause to appreciate even the simplest aspects of your yoga. Flow through a potpourri practice, seeking hidden jewels in plank, three-legged dog with optional twist, one-legged king pigeon, cow face, bound angle, seated wide-angle forward fold, and supine twist.

Off the Mat: Cultivate the practice of offering little modest treasures to a loved one.

Practices

I acknowledge the countless little gems that populate my day   I notice how the minor details enhance the greater whole   I embrace the glimmer of a single breath, the fleeting smell of luscious food, or a hug from someone dear

Supportive Words
Little: *minor, miniscule, minute, modest;*
Gems: *jewels, precious items, treasures, valuables*

Visualization
A revered gemstone reflecting its color brilliantly in the light.

Complementary Breath
viloma *(inhale & exhale)*
Focus on the brief pause following each segment of the breath, appreciating the gems available in this space.

Closing Ritual
Spend time writing about three precious moments that graced your day.

Where Do the Mermaids Stand: {*inspired by Roger McKeever*}

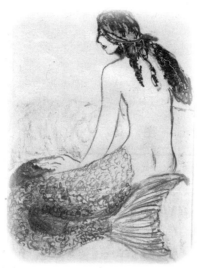

One of my favorite inspirational stories is called "Where Do the Mermaids Stand?" and is found in the book *Everything I Ever Needed to Know I Learned in Kindergarten* by Robert Fulghum. Though I am unable to reprint the whole story here for copyright reasons, both this excerpt and the book can be found online. To summarize, though, the story is about a schoolteacher who gathers his students to play the game Giants, Wizards, and Dwarfs. He explains the rules of the game and then arrives at the critical point when the kids must choose whether to embody a giant, wizard, or dwarf. In this moment, one little girl comes up to him and asks, "Where do the mermaids stand?" The teacher explains that there is no such thing as a mermaid, but she remains true to herself and claims that she is one, not relating to the other categories offered by the game. The teacher is thus inspired to consider, "Well, where do the Mermaids stand? All the Mermaids—all those who are different, who do not fit the norm, and who do not accept the available boxes and pigeonholes?" "Answer that question and you can build a school, a nation, or a kingdom on it," he realizes[10]. He then declares that mermaids stand right beside him, the King of the Sea. The last line of the story is my favorite, as the teacher says, "It is not true, by the way, that Mermaids do not exist. I know at least one personally. I have held her hand[11]."

Each time I read this story, I have the same reaction. Goose bumps emerge, and I feel profound softness in my heart. I know it resonates so deeply for me because for much of my life I have felt like I am on the fringe, an outsider in traditional society. I feel estranged because my beliefs and ways of seeing the world are often different from those of the majority. It has been challenging and yet unbelievably rewarding to hold my ground and learn to trust that I am not the only one who vibrates on this particular wavelength. This story serves to remind me of the power manifested when we honor our uniqueness and beauty. Macy Gray says it best in her song *Sexual Revolution* when she sings, "Time to be free amongst yourselves; your mama told you to be discreet and keep your freak to yourself, but your mama lied to you all this time; she knows as well as you and I; you've got to express what is taboo in you, and share your freak with the rest of us cause it's a beautiful thang[12]." Although we are all extensions of the same source energy, each and every one of us is a distinctive, beaming individual. This inner "mermaid" is revealed in the structure and intricacy of our very own face, as there has never and will never be anyone with the same exact features. Even identical twins are not exact duplicates. They share the same genotype, but the DNA is expressed in a completely different manner in each twin[13].

Inquiries

On the Mat: Use this time on your mat as an opportunity to be wholly in your own skin and awaken to the freakiness, wonder, and delight of your unique being. Generate an internal revolution of sorts to love yourself more fully even with all of the quirks and idiosyncrasies that color your personality. Find the mermaid within by connecting to your silliest, most outrageous self. Invite a friend to practice with you for double the fun, and experiment together with playful arm balances, freeing yourselves to make noise and be irreverent. Embody the spirit of the mermaid through plank, side plank, upward boat, core strengtheners, mermaid pose, L at the wall, bhujapidasana, and firefly.

Off the Mat: Contemplate where your inner mermaid stands in the game of life, and consider the negative connotations of the word "freak" in our culture. Take one day to honor a quirky part of yourself that you don't typically reveal. Whether in the solitude of your own home or out in the world, give yourself permission to explore your inner mermaid, if only for a single day.

Practices

Supportive Words
bizarre, fantastic, taboo, quirky, unconventional, wacky, whimsical

Visualization
A glittery mermaid in her splendid uniqueness of being half human and half fish. She is truly extraordinary and moves between two worlds; she can linger on land by breathing air, but she can also roam freely in deep waters to explore what exists beneath the surface.

Complementary Breath
bramari
Do three rounds of the bumblebee breath. Express a unique sound in each round.

Closing Ritual
Before beginning your cool down sequence, play a lively song (*such as Sexual Revolution by Macy Gray*), and set your inner mermaid free by dancing with total abandon.

Teacher's Note
Begin the practice with a few cat and cow warm-ups, having students face each other, and then transition to lion's breath, inviting them to playfully frighten one another. Ask them to pretend they are mermaids, and encourage them to leave their mats to frolic with other mermaids. In a few of the poses, guide students to introduce their own variations, individuating their class experience and making it a personal creation. Invite students to allow their inner mermaid to swim playfully as they honor their freakiness without inhibition.

the parts of myself that long to be set free

I honor the freak within, liberating

I embrace the many gifts of my own unique spirit

I express what is taboo in me because it is a beautiful thing!

Please Change: {*inspired by Isaac Arguetty*}

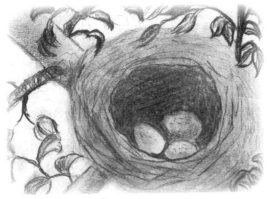

Have you ever wanted to change someone in your life? Perhaps you feel life would be calmer, happier, or more exciting if only this person would shift. When I visit my dad, I arrive with the same intention each visit: to avoid criticizing him and practice acceptance of his lifestyle even though it is not in line with my ideals of sustainability. I usually remain strong in this intention for the first three or four days, and then I meet my edge and end up crossing the line. During one of my visits, my dad was in the kitchen unpacking the groceries. When he was done, he bunched up all of the plastic bags and threw them in the trash. My frustration peaked instantaneously, and my blood began to boil. Armed with a disparaging tone, I began my verbal assault. As I concluded my righteous remarks, my dad remained quiet, but his whole body was communicating a sense of defeat. His physical form deflated, his energy field clouded, and it was easy to see that his heart had closed. In this moment, I realized that although my message was extremely important to me, my dad could not receive it because of my browbeating approach.

Susan Page, author of *If We're So In Love, Why Aren't We Happy*, advises us to avoid trying to fix and change the people in our lives. When we try to change others, we are essentially communicating they are not enough as they are and implying we would love them more if they were different. The other person is left feeling criticized, assaulted, and misunderstood. Page suggests that instead of trying to fix someone else, we instead turn our attention inward and explore our own response to the situation. We can ask ourselves, "Where is this big charge coming from?" or ponder whether our reaction might be related to something lingering unresolved inside of us. Page proposes we work on shifting our reaction to a specific situation and seeking nonviolent and life-enhancing ways to honor where others are in any given moment. The content doesn't really change, but the way we choose to respond to our own internal triggers and to those around us can make a world of difference. When we stop trying to fix people and instead create an atmosphere of love and acceptance, they sometimes begin to shift from within, first and foremost for their own benefit. Often, what we wanted to change in them actually morphs as a result of the safe space, love, and consistent modeling we offer. Even if the shifts aren't immediately evident, by not criticizing we enable access to conscious and nonviolent dialogue. It all boils down to the approach we utilize in engaging with the world; aggressive equals defensive, as nature clearly demonstrates. When we first walk into the forest, the animals quiet their chatter and song because they feel threatened or unsure of our intentions. If we choose to be loud or violent in their environment, the animals run away in search of refuge. When we take a seat, soften, and move about the space in a respectful way, the animals return to their natural state of ease and comfort. It is through this same kind of gentle interaction that people in our lives begin to open up, become able to hear and honor our perspective, and—if they choose—initiate a shift motivated by their own internal calling.

Inquiries

On the Mat: Notice moments when your focus moves from the breath to the desire to change or fix a part of yourself you don't fully accept. Just as with relationships, approaching your sadhana this way creates an atmosphere of deficiency and lack. Mentally and energetically, you are telling your body and mind they would be more loved if they were different. Instead of lingering in this critical stance, you can probe more deeply and use your reactions to explore these shunned parts of your being. From this place, the natural wisdom of your body can take over, creating the shift you are seeking in a kinder, gentler way. Practice both simple acceptance and determination to hold sacred space for your process, and begin to move in a new direction. Culminate this practice in restorative bound angle, feeling how it serves as a safe container holding all your perceived imperfections while simultaneously allowing you to soften. Go into inverted postures such as standing yoga mudra, dolphin dog, standing forward fold, downward facing dog, headstand, shoulderstand, and restorative bridge with a block under the sacrum.

Off the Mat: Over the course of three days, take note of two or three people whom you constantly attempt to change. Notice how you communicate this to them. Is it overt? Subtle? Do you send this message through passive-aggressive words or body language? For the three days that follow, consciously shift your habitual behavior towards these individuals. Give them space to be exactly who they are, and affirm one aspect of their personality you appreciate. Note any changes in your interactions with them as a result of this exercise.

Practices

With intention, I explore the aspects of myself I seek to change. I allow

Supportive Words
change: *alter, convert, modify*
allow: *accommodate, bolster, consider, hold, regard*

Visualization
A nest woven together with feathers, twigs, twine, and little bits of trash to create a safe haven for growth and development. Even the trash (*symbolic of the part we may try to change in another*) is essential to the structural integrity and beauty of the nest.

Complementary Breath
natural
Simply notice the breath to honor exactly where you are, and trust that conscious change is taking root deep inside.

Closing Ritual
Place both hands onto your heart center. For ten breaths, utilize every exhalation as an opportunity to affirm a specific aspect of your being, honoring each facet exactly as it is.

my various imperfections

others to be fully themselves with

I honor my perfect nature even as I acknowledge

out trying to change or fix them in any way.

The Next Logical Step: {*inspired by the Teachings of Abraham*}

My friend in Vermont decided she wanted to move her yoga studio to a larger space, but she knew it would require additional funds. Instead of rushing headlong into this massive undertaking, she chose to progress mindfully and build step-by-step. Her first move was to commit to a weekly meeting with her business advisor to brainstorm and clarify her intentions and ideas. Together, they began preparing a business plan and researched the actual costs of upgrading the business. When the plan was complete, they met with a loan consultant at the bank, and after making slight edits and providing some additional information, they were approved for a loan. One phase at a time, their vision inched towards fruition. "The next logical step" is one of the concepts offered in the teachings of Abraham as described by Esther Hicks. This particular teaching explains that reaching a goal is not always an instantaneous achievement. Instead, from a foundation of connection to our deepest intention, we simply have to take the next logical step, followed by the next logical step, followed by the next. Before we know it, the next logical move is the one that brings us to our desired destination. Often, people try to fast-track right to a goal and become overwhelmed in the process, losing their focus or will. An important part of any undertaking is recognizing exactly the right time for taking each subsequent step and seizing these opportune moments to move ahead. How would our lives shift if we could utilize this tool of bearing the end goal in mind while remaining so open that we can easily identify the next best decision even if the road swerves in an unexpected direction? As Lester Long writes:

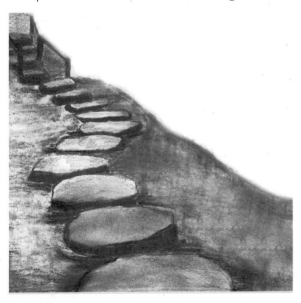

*Journeys to the Sacred City
begin with a single step*

*Exist not for the future
nor revel in the past*

*Walk at dawn,
the Sacred City lies obscure*

*Continue, resolute
Your target Enlightens.*

*The goal is not the
Sacred City in the distance,*

*But the Sacred City
Under the foot*

Of the Next Step[14].

Inquiries

On the Mat: Instead of becoming fixated on the end result of each pose, focus on the intelligent phases involved in receiving the full experience of the asana. Explore the natural order (*i.e. building from the ground up*) that aids you in moving into each pose, especially those postures that present added challenge. In this practice, investigate upward-facing bow. Open your quadriceps, hamstrings, and hips, as the legs govern the openness of the spine. When you feel warm and ready, attempt the posture, pausing to experiment at each stepping stone as you move towards the full expression of the pose. Explore urdvha dhanurasana in several rounds, and build the posture in slow, progressive steps to counter the common tendency of rushing to press up. In the first round, focus on firm clawing of the fingers and parallel placement of the feet (*put a block lengthwise between your feet*) as you lift the pelvis skyward, hold, and then release. In the second round, align your hands and feet, lift the pelvis, and then curl to pause on the top of the head. Holding here, bring awareness to drawing your shoulder blades onto the back and propelling the heart forward; linger here for a few breaths, and then release. In the third round, build all of the previous alignment details, and press into the full pose from this stable positioning of the shoulders, anchoring the gaze at the fingers. If the inquiry of upward bow doesn't fully serve you, experiment with proprioceptive neuromuscular facilitation (*also known as PNF*), which involves contracting and then relaxing a particular muscle several times. Do this throughout your practice, and sense the effects of each next logical step leading to more openness in the landscape of the body. Explore back extensions with high lunge, knee-down lunge, down dog, half frog, cobra, locust, hands inside the foot in knee-down lunge, quad stretch in knee-down lunge, twisting lunge, bow, pigeon, quad stretch in pigeon, camel, runner's stretch, one-legged reclining hero, bridge, and upward-facing bow.

Off the Mat: Envision an ideal day. What little steps would be necessary to reach that ideal? On a piece of paper, draw five stepping stones. On each stone, write one small act that serves your final goal. As you engage this inquiry throughout the course of your day, honor each stepping stone in turn, taking time to savor each stage of the process. At the end of the day, reflect on your experiment.

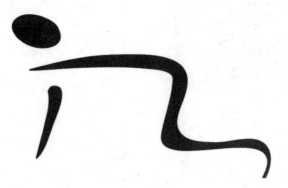

I move towards the next logical step that will lead me in the direction of my goal. I honor each phase and all of the possibility contained therein. I place each stepping stone with intention as I edge forward, relishing the process.

Supportive Words
logical: *clear, coherent, consequent, perceptive, rational, sensible*
step: *degree, level, phase, stage*

Visualization
Stepping stones creating a continuous path that serves as a bridge to your goal.

Complementary Breath
dirgha
Focus on the way the breath builds one step at a time to awaken belly, then rib cage, and finally collar bones to expand the torso in all directions.

Closing Ritual
journal contemplation
What effects did the step-by-step sequencing of the practice have on your posture, breath, and heart?

Teacher's Note
Invite students to feel how each detail towards upward facing bow, like a stepping stone, supports the final variation of the pose best suited for their unique body on this particular day.

Will & Surrender: {*inspired by Kripalu Yoga*}

Food is one of my greatest passions in life. One of the most valuable lessons I learned in nutrition school at the Institute for Integrative Nutrition was to "burn the rice" or, in other words, experiment in the kitchen. One day when I was feeling ambitious, I decided to try my hand at baking bread. Little did I know that this most ancient human tradition would teach me a great deal about the partnership of effort and surrender. The first step in the process of bread making involves mixing all of the ingredients together. The water has to be just the right temperature for the mixture to become the proper consistency. Once the dough is ready, it is kneaded to stimulate the gluten, which potentiates the bread. At this point in the process comes the first act of letting go, as the dough requires time to sit and rise. It then gets punched down and left to rise a second time. Next, the dough is placed in pans and allowed to rise for a third and final time. Finally, the moment arrives to put the loaves in the oven and bake them at just the right temperature for a specified duration. Ultimately, much of the wonder of making bread is the silent, bubbling alchemy that transpires when the bread is left alone in warmth and darkness without human interference.

This pulsation of effort and surrender is likewise evidenced through numerous examples in nature. Squirrels diligently collect food during the warmer months so they can rest and nourish themselves during the winter. Birds expend much effort in their migration, at times flying thousands of miles per season, then when the time comes to land and give their wings a break, they bask in the beauty of simply being. As humans, we get to explore being both willful creators who channel energy into the world and gracious receivers who soften and trust in the intelligent functioning of the universe. Iccha, or will, describes the actions we initiate once we are fully clear regarding what we are willing to do to make something happen.

Niradh, or surrender, is the equally essential practice we engage when we feel the time has come to sit back, incubate, and trust the process. Once we become well acquainted with both of these energies, we access the ability to customize the degree to which we utilize each one in a given situation. As John Friend writes:

> Intertwined with attitude and intention is willpower—a deep inner force that is a balance between self-effort and the ability to surrender. This dynamic balance is like a bird in flight, flapping its wings but also riding and working with the wind. You must use both effort and surrender in order to align your intention with the flow of Grace. Effort and surrender are like two wings of a bird—both are equally important for a smooth and joyful flight[15].

Inquiries

On the Mat: Consider whether you are either expending so much effort that you end up exhausting yourself or whether you are so receptive that you ultimately block the benefits of a more awakened practice. Notice when you approach a pose with too much effort. Does your physical frame lock up in resistance as it registers the onset of an unsafe state? Now identify the instances wherein opening to a posture allows you to ease in, make more sense of the pose, and offer yourself up to it more fully. What shifts when you back off a little but remain evenly engaged? Often the body finds room to soften, and the stretch can actualize more benefit as the belly of the muscle is activated. At the other end of the spectrum, feel how too much surrender—especially in an active pose—affects your nervous system. Either of these extremes can communicate an unsafe state and thus activate fight-or-flight protocols in the body. To enable deeper understanding of these two complementary ideas, engage one posture overly willfully, and then explore another with too little effort. Notice what shows up. Explore a practice focused on back extensions utilizing poses like warrior one and two, lateral angle, reclining hero, baby cobra, half locust, locust, half frog, and crocodile.

Off the Mat: List the primary activities that populate your typical week. Assess your level of engagement with these different aspects of your life. Highlight one area in which you may be efforting too much and another in which it might benefit you to engage more fully. Use the coming week to adjust the level of effort and surrender in each of these realms and observe the results.

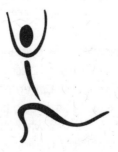

Practices

Supportive Words
will: *effort, exertion, labor, muscle*
surrender: *back down, soften, yield*

Visualization
Hiking up a steep mountain on a summer day, utilizing moments of exertion and moments of rest to savor the delights of being out in nature.

Complementary Breath
ujjayi
Focus on the ability of the ocean sound to foster clarity of action and simultaneously encourage softness.

Closing Ritual
In a seated position, contract all of the muscles of the body at once and then release with an audible sigh. Repeat three times.

Mirrors of Consciousness: {*inspired by the Kripalu Volunteer Community*}

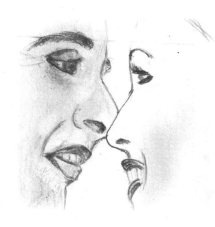

While volunteering at Kripalu, I was immersed in a community of people who were there to serve and learn. It was the first time in my life I had to communicate clearly and work intimately with so many individuals. Prior to this experience, my tactic had always been to simply ignore those who agitated me and shut them out of my life. Luckily, I learned to take a different approach while volunteering, exploring these feelings and asking myself probing questions: What is this person showing me? How could I shift within to soften this particular trigger? What do I need to learn here? Through these inquiries, I learned how to cradle my inner critic, hold space for the stubborn little boy, and dismantle the self-generated stories leading me to states of intense frustration. My experience taught me to observe my reactions more skillfully and refrain from immediately shutting down and withdrawing from the world at the first tinge of discomfort. As a result of my observations, I began to slow down, recognize my role in emerging situations, and more consciously choose my responses. Every interaction in our lives—especially those that have the potential to ignite us—can serve as an opportunity for intensive self-study. It is up to us whether we choose to engage this learning by pausing to observe our inner workings in a given interaction instead of immediately projecting our frustrations outward.

In Shri Vidya Philosophy, the divine chose to reflect herself in all of creation so as to experience her own luminous splendor. Just as Grace is reflected, we, too, are seeing reflections of ourselves through our relationships with others and with our surroundings. In reality, we will never be able to see our own face with our own two eyes; although a mirror brings us close, we are ultimately seeing only an inverted image of our true form. One of the remarkable gifts offered up by those with whom we interact—

whether for a moment or a lifetime—is their capacity for revealing to us our most beautiful qualities as well as our darkest patterns. If we lived in isolation and solitude, we wouldn't have these opportunities for getting to know ourselves more fully. It is through our active participation in relationships that we can discern who we truly are and experience abundant growth. In my first yoga teacher training, my teacher Yoganand Michael Carroll said, "If you think you are enlightened, go visit your family." With these words, he was referencing this idea that relationships can be one of life's greatest teachers. Through examining our interactions with those around us, we can identify the varied layers of our conditioning and our belief systems. Relationships with family members, co-workers, and intimate partners have tremendous potential to yield profound learning. In addition to providing support in the exploration of our darkness, our interactions with others serve as reminders of our own inherent radiance. Teachers wouldn't be able to share their light without the commitment and enthusiasm of students, and conversely students wouldn't have openings and breakthroughs without the guidance of teachers. Each role mirrors the brilliance and authenticity being offered by the other. As Krishnamurti shares:

> Understanding of the self only arises in relationship, in watching yourself in relationship to people, ideas, and things, to trees, the earth, and the world around you and within you. Relationship is the mirror in which the self is revealed[16].

Inquiries

On the Mat: Utilize your body, breath, thoughts, and inner wisdom as mirrors in your personal practice. When you attune to what is revealed through these reflections, you can pause to investigate whether your ways of interacting with yourself and consequently the world are enhancing or detracting from your vitality. As these awarenesses surface, you may initially ignore them in favor of holding on to more comfortable patterns and established beliefs. As you continue to practice and probe more deeply, though, you will become increasingly aware and conscious. Eventually, you may decide to engage these observations and examine your anchored attitudes. Remember that just as our practice aids us in expansion and growth with regard to our blind spots, the mirror of yoga also reminds us of our inner and outer beauty, our inherent strength, and our capacity for abundant joy. Explore an arm-balancing practice with side plank, crane, side crane, and eka pada koundinyasana.

Off the Mat: Choose someone in your life who serves as your mirror. Over the course of a week, consider how this person mirrors your beauty. Likewise, notice what you learn about your less refined elements by means of the reflection they offer.

Practices

Supportive Words

depict, echo, emulate, exemplify, illustrate, personify, represent, show

Visualization

Two people looking into each other's eyes and seeing themselves reflected in one another's gaze.

Complementary Breath

anulom vilom
One side mirroring the other.

Closing Ritual

Meditation facing a mirror or partner, absorbing the reflection you or they offer.

Teacher's Note

To highlight the power of others to mirror both our beauty and our blind spots, have students line up in rows opposite a partner while they practice. Rotate partners several times during the class to exemplify how each source of reflection has something different to offer.

revealing new understanding

I acknowledge the reflections

I recognize each pose as a potential reflection

offered by others as teachers on my path

Perceiving the World: {*inspired by Galit Bina & Douglas Brooks*}

On one of my trips to Israel, I went for a walk with my cousin, and we started talking about the state of the environment in Israel. At one point, she said that perhaps Israelis would have more energy to care for their natural environment were they not surrounded by enemies. I felt compassion for my cousin because I understood how she had arrived at this deeply held belief. The first Jews who arrived in modern Israel came directly from the concentration camps of the Holocaust, where they had been severely victimized. Understandably, they carried this imprint with them as they settled in their new land. Sadly, historical events in Israel unfolded in ways that served to reinforce this victim consciousness. Because of the past conflict and present-day reciprocal violence, many people in Israel perceive their lives as under constant threat, which serves to further perpetuate their role as victims. Statistically, though, Israeli civilians are more likely to be killed in a car accident than in a terrorist attack[17]. What fascinated me most about my conversation with my cousin was the realization that every person sees a given situation through his or her own unique lens. Our inner world of beliefs and convictions wields more power over our perception than the actual facts evident in the world. The word asana means "seat"; in our lives, each of us takes our own individual seat, and we look out at the world from this particular vantage point. One seat is not necessarily better or worse than another; the view from each offers a clear perspective that is one among many. Our individual perception of the world is indeed powerful, as it generates a vibration that ultimately makes what we see on the inside a reality on the outside. "We can't change the world, but we can change the way we perceive the world[18]"; as such, this work begins within.

The situation in this region of the world is and always has been challenging. Indeed there are many Palestinian and Israeli extremists who are channeling their efforts towards the ruin of the other, but there are also plenty of Palestinians and Israelis who simply want to move on, improve their respective economies, establish peace, and enrich their daily experience of life. Certainly, political efforts at the national and international levels must continue, but what would happen if the citizens of both countries employed a new tactic alongside them? Instead of only trying to affect change on the outside, what if people began turning within to inquire, "What is the true source of the anger I carry? Is it wholly mine, or is it an accumulation of the views of extreme media, polarized family members, and historical propaganda? Could I step into others' shoes and perceive the world from their point of view? Could I move in the direction of forgiveness, acknowledging the incredible difficulty of the situation but also recognizing the fundamental similarities we all share as human beings?" Luckily many people and organizations in the Middle East are asking these questions and taking concrete steps to move towards seeing their counterparts in a new way. The power of shifting perception internally is that the outside world begins to mirror the new reality incubating within. Humans are vibrational beings, and shifts in our moods can be evoked through the simplest change of music or through a brief moment of drama or comedy on the screen. Thoughts serve as catalysts in the same way, as they carry potent vibrations. As such, it is essential to identify whether our thoughts are exacerbating an unhealthy situation or moving us towards a new realm of possibility. If we allow them to feed the notion of being in danger, the futility of peace, or victim consciousness, our reality will surely mirror these beliefs. Challenging yet potentially meaningful is the endeavor to acknowledge a thorny situation and simultaneously work towards its resolution on both the subtle and concrete levels of existence.

As an example of the power of perception, think about the first definition that comes to mind when you contemplate the word darkness. Most of us would say that darkness is the absence of light, as this is what we have been taught or have commonly observed. Yet, in scientific terms, darkness is actually defined as a relatively low level of light. A darkened object simply echoes a smaller amount of observable photons than other objects and therefore seems dim in comparison. Since this definition of light encompasses the whole of the electromagnetic spectrum, in reality it is impossible to create absolute darkness[19]. This example thus reinforces that everything is a matter of perception. The shifts that can occur in the way we see the world can be profound as we gather new information and access the ability to view a situation from an alternate vantage point. As the Dalai Lama states:

> *A new way of thinking has become the necessary condition for responsible living and acting. If we maintain obsolete values and beliefs, a fragmented consciousness, and self-centered spirit, we will continue to hold on to outdated goals and behaviours[20].*

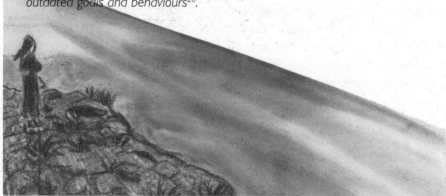

Inquiries

On the Mat: Take note of what perceptions are forming your current reality. Are the thoughts of "I'm not flexible," "I'll never be able to do that pose," "I'm too old for yoga," or "This yoga style is the best" coming up? Instead of blindly moving through your practice with these prevailing beliefs, simply recognize where you position yourself. Investigate the layers of why and how you adhere to a particular point of view, and contemplate whether this stance is truly serving you. Note whether limiting patterns of belief surface in your sadhana. Create a sequence to repeat four to five times, and be aware of how your perceptions morph or stay the same with each repetition of the postures. End your sadhana with ample time seated in half or full lotus to integrate your experience. To serve this particular inquiry, utilize head to knee, cow face, baby cradle, fire log, heron, bound angle, reclining hero, seated wide-angle forward fold, and half or full lotus.

Off the Mat: Choose someone in your life with whom you have a difficult relationship. Take time to metaphorically step into this person's shoes and attempt to see the world through his or her eyes. Notice what becomes illuminated through this effort to understand another's perception of the world.

Practices

Supportive Words
angle, belief, notion, outlook, perspective, slant, vantage, viewpoint

Visualization
Looking out from a mountain peak, appreciating your current vantage point while also acknowledging what you can't see *(even on a clear day, there is a limit to how far we can see)*, and then shifting the gaze in another direction to experience a different view.

Complementary Breath
alternate-nostril kapalabhati
The power of the breath shifts our perceptions.

Closing Ritual
Take two minutes to engage in a slow walking meditation. Next, sit in meditation with your eyes open for two minutes. Soften your gaze until your eyes are half open, and sit for another two minutes. Finally, sit for a few minutes with your eyes fully closed. Afterwards, reflect on how these varying states of perception affected each experience.

Teacher's Note
End class in a circle, inviting students to take in a different view of their classmates.

I recognize the view I habitually choose and consider the one I could potentially adopt. I sense the power of my inner world of beliefs and convictions. I breathe into the areas in which my perceptions of the world create constriction.

Sacred Sabbath: {*inspired by Jay Michelson & Adam Lavitt*}

Contemplation and learning surfaced during a trip to New York City to celebrate a friend's birthday in Central Park. I arrived on Friday afternoon to find my friend preparing dinner, and at first I was confused about why he was cooking so early. After a few moments, I remembered he practices the ritual of the Sabbath. Once the sun goes down on Friday, he enters a twenty-four hour period of rest. The observances of Shabbat (*the Hebrew word for Sabbath*) vary depending upon how strictly one chooses to practice. In general, people don't use electricity, walk instead of drive, and get together with family or friends for meals and prayers. Common rituals include lighting candles, blessing wine, breaking bread, studying and discussing scripture, going to synagogue, and singing zemirot (*special songs*). One of the most striking prayer songs to welcome Shabbat is called "L'Cha Dodi" by sixteenth century Kabbalist Shlomo Halevi Alkabetz. It states, "Beloved, come to meet the bride; Beloved, come to greet Shabbat. Shabbat peace and blessing…in fame and splendor and song. Towards Shabbat let's go, let's travel…for she is the wellspring of blessing[21]." As implied here, this notion of respite from the typical day-to-day is indeed a conduit for increased vitality and well-being.

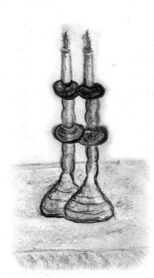

Shabbat can be practiced in many different ways, but the essential focus of the day is rest and rejuvenation. When we take the time to recharge and nourish ourselves, we can be more effective in our various routine tasks and avoid getting burned-out. How often do we give ourselves a day to turn off the computer and phone, be fully present with family and friends, or spend uninterrupted time in the majesty of nature? What shifts within when we do take the time to bring a ritual like the Sabbath into our lives? As my weekend in New York came to an end and I began my journey home on the train, I had a sudden revelation. I realized the ritual in which I had just participated was similar to what I do and teach in my yoga practice every week. Yoga is often the only opportunity for people to have Shabbat-like time in the course of a hectic day. In yoga, we begin our practice with a centering and opening "aum", which parallels the opening meal of Shabbat as an act of welcoming sacred time. Afterwards, we flow through our practice with a deeper sense of mindfulness, focusing on our thoughts, breath, and body movements. We have an opportunity to rejuvenate, release anxiety, and open to our innate nature. We gather in community to share this experience with others, and as class comes to a close, we take repose in savasana to bathe in the effects of our dedication; this window of time is the ultimate expression of rest. After relaxation, we sometimes join together as a group to meditate. At other times, we chant or take a moment to share a final "aum" with delicate intention to bring closure to the ritual of the practice. After a yoga class, people often report feeling more relaxed and energized and thus more effective at working and managing their time.

Both in yoga (*through various yoga styles*) and in observing the Sabbath (*in the diverse methods used to do so*), the rituals can be customized to meet individual needs while preserving the fundamental tenets of rest, mindfulness, and renewal. Essentially, both of these practices invite a sense of reverence through connecting with loved ones, spending time outside, or sourcing the will and dedication to turn off the computer, take a break from the phone, and resist the allure of unfinished work. Consciously establishing a boundary around routine tasks to make space for rest, reverence, and renewal recharges us from the core in the same way that savasana after yoga sends us back into our daily lives feeling more whole and refreshed. The parallels I have observed between the Sabbath and yoga inspire me to cultivate more spaciousness in my life and to hold these unfettered moments, hours, and days as sacred. As the United Nations Sabbath program proclaims

> We who have lost our sense and our senses—our touch, our smell, our vision of who we are; we who frantically force and press all things, without rest for body or spirit, hurting our earth and injuring ourselves: we call a halt. We want to rest. We need to rest and allow the earth to rest. We need to reflect and to rediscover the mystery that lives in us, that is the ground of every unique expression of life, the source of the fascination that calls all things to communion. We declare a Sabbath, a space of quiet: for simple being and letting be; for recovering the great, forgotten truths; for learning how to live again[22].

Inquiries

On the Mat: Make time to slow your practice down and offer yourself forward folds, twists, and inversions that will support deep rejuvenation from the inside out. Step into the inquiry of softer forward folds, twists, and inversions with: easy pose twist, seated yoga mudra, bound angle, standing forward fold, standing yoga mudra, supported bridge with block, legs up the wall and/or shoulderstand.

Off the Mat: Choose a week in the near future when you can commit to one day of Sabbath. Turn off the TV, computer, and phone, and nourish yourself by cooking a fresh meal, journaling, making art, and spending time in nature. If taking a full day off is not possible for you, try dedicating half a day or even just one hour to creating some sacred space for rest and rejuvenation.

Practices

With each inhale, I breathe in the freshness of the Sabbath pause

Supportive Words
break, cease, pause, rest, suspend

Visualization
Brightly lit candles marking the transition into the Sabbath.

Complementary Breath
chandra bhedana
Breathing through just the left side activates the ida nadi cooling and calming the body.

Closing Ritual
candle-gazing meditation

authentic self

I customize my life to

In the sanctuary of rest I reconnect to my

create a sense of the sacred, both inside and out.

Present Moment, Wonderful Moment: {inspired by Thich Nhat Hanh}

Thich Nhat Hanh is a profound spiritual teacher and one of the first people who influenced my spiritual journey. His teaching sparked my initial interest in mindfulness and present-moment awareness, which set the foundation for my current practices. With profound wisdom, he writes of the present moment, "Waking up this morning, I smile. Twenty-four brand new hours are before me. I vow to live fully in each moment and to look at all beings with eyes of compassion[23]." In my own life, the practice of becoming present has enabled me to slow things down, feel more spacious, and access greater clarity. Through mindfulness I became aware that moments are strung together in minutes and hours, but often they evaporate quickly amidst the hectic nature and mindless pursuits of my day. Now, even when my days are busy, I can connect to my breath and stay present to all that is before me.

The phrase "present moment, wonderful moment" holds immense wisdom even in its simplicity. We can literally create anxiety and stress in the body when the majority of our thoughts exist in either the past or the future. This doesn't mean we should gloss over our lives and ignore incidents from the past or desires for the future; rather, it means we can employ conscious exploration and willful manifestation to guide and co-create our reality. In essence, the past and future both exist in the present moment, as what has happened in the past affects us now, and our actions now will indeed contribute to the moments of our future. Our past is valuable because it is akin to having a wise ancestor by our side, our future exists as a powerful vision for our aspirations, and the present moment is like having a dear friend reminding us we are not alone and that we are supported from all directions[24]. When I split up with my partner, my present-moment experience was constantly hijacked by thoughts of the past, which only served to perpetuate the same patterns in the present. The voices within kept asking, "What went wrong? What could I have done to make it work? Why is the universe doing this to me?" I had entered a vicious cycle. At first, my approach was to ignore these thoughts and make them wrong. I later realized, however, that because these emotions had found their way into the present, they were my "present moment, wonderful moment." I was alive, conflicted, feeling, and—although the subject matter belonged to the past—it was still very much alive in my everyday decisions and interactions. When I stopped resisting and allowed the thoughts to simply exist, there was a softening that eventually allowed them to dissipate and enabled me to integrate their imprints and move on.

Thich Nhat Hanh orders the words "present moment, wonderful moment" this way intentionally; the saying isn't "wonderful moment, present moment" for a reason. This is because those moments we traditionally think of as wonderful (*noticing a flower, listening to birds sing, making love*), are natural doorways to being fully absorbed in the present. But Thich Nhat Hanh reminds us through his careful wording that we must also open to the idea that being present with each experience—whether mundane, dark, or bitter—will allow us to encounter the wonderful, even if we only sense it days, weeks, or years later. Jack Kornfield writes: "Boredom comes from lack of attention…We get bored because we don't like what is happening and so don't pay attention. But if we stay with it, a whole new level of understanding and contentment can grow…Note it, feel its texture, its energy and the pains and tensions in it, the resistances to it[25]."

Inquiries

On the Mat: Use the breath to anchor each pose, and notice whether it provides you the space to relax, feel, watch, and allow. Explore the quiet power in returning to the centering and stabilizing nature of each inhalation and exhalation. As thoughts arise, identify them, thank them for their insights, skip the process of evaluating them as good or bad, and return your attention to breath and body. Investigate how slowly you can move your body through your chosen sequence of postures, constantly revisiting the power of the breath.

Off the Mat: Pick one task usually labeled as mundane as a vehicle for cultivating mindfulness. It might be brushing your teeth, washing the dishes, folding laundry, changing a diaper, or driving to work.

Practices

I celebrate the present

I find the value inherent in each moment

Supportive Words
present: *current, immediate, now*
moment: *instant, juncture, point, time*

Visualization
Taking in the color and smell of a single flower in bloom.

Complementary Breath
natural
Spend time becoming aware of the quality of your breath from one moment to the next.

Closing Ritual
walking meditation
Instead of a traditional seated centering, use a walking meditation to transition into the practice of mindful breath and movement.

I acknowledge how both my past and future are embedded in the now

With the intention to live wholeheartedly

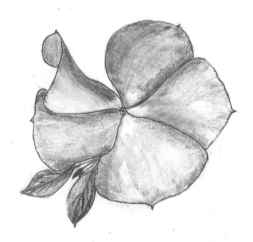

Armor & Softness: {*inspired by Yoganand Michael Carroll*}

Moving around has been a significant part of my life's journey; from Israel to Los Angeles, back to Israel, then to London, a few years in Florida followed by a few in Denver, then to Los Angeles again, Boston after that, then Vermont, and finally to the Berkshires of Western Massachusetts. My initial move from Israel to Los Angeles was the hardest one, as I felt like I had been ripped from my natural habitat. When I arrived in California, I didn't know any English. I was teased in school, and all of a sudden I was dependent on a car to get everywhere as opposed to the freedom of movement I had known as a child in Israel. Needless to say, the more threatened I felt, the more armor I donned, and I eventually retreated to life in my internal world, trusting only my family and my imaginary friends. As I continued to move around and engaged in more interactions and relationships with others, I started noticing a pattern. Each time I would get angry, find myself in conflict, or be on the verge of another move, I would use the tactic of withdrawal and retreat to the safe space I had created inside. It was easier to barricade myself and shut people out of my life than to try to work things out or simply be present with what I was feeling. The unacknowledged anger and pain brewed inside, compounding the distance I felt from others. When I began to practice yoga, though, both my physical and subtle bodies began to open up. The knots inside began to unravel, and I glimpsed the simple beauty and benevolence life has to offer. I learned that a protective casing is not inherently negative; there are effective ways to use it to set clear boundaries and stand in one's truth. Increasing my capacity for savoring life more fully, however, involved learning how to let my guard down.

In the first months and years of our lives, we thrive as a result of being nurtured by caregivers with food, constant eye contact, loving touch, and gentle words. This consistent love enables us to meet the world with curiosity and heart. Life is joyful because our boundaries are soft, and we marvel at the simplest objects and events we encounter, sensing that they are all manifestations of an essence that also lives in us. As we age, we realize that a certain amount of sheilding is necessary to establish safe and appropriate boundaries. As a result of extreme experiences in youth, many of us are compelled to overprotect ourselves, and we end up closing ourselves off from our truest nature and likewise from those around us. These extraneous layers of armor are often the product of severe physical pain, emotional neglect, religious dogma, situational conflict, degrading verbal violence, and other types of trauma. They show up in the body as symptoms such as physical knots in the muscle tissue, tightness in the shoulders and hips, contraction of facial muscles, and shallow breathing among others. Over time, we become more and more guarded, and our life experience begins to feel increasingly unsafe as we glean the message that the world is out to get us. Sadly, our beliefs, feelings, and thoughts act like magnets; as we focus on what isn't going well, we attract more troubling experiences that affirm our stance of vulnerability. If we are able to recognize this vicious cycle as it recurs, however, we can begin to witness it and extract lessons from it. By immersing ourselves in communities and experiences that counter this notion of life as unsafe, we can reclaim the sense of openness we knew as children. Through taking the time to cultivate uplifting moments in our lives, we can return to a more optimal balance of protective covering and openness. The key is to maintain the power to adjust our defenses in accordance with the various obstacles we encounter instead of always walking around overly protected.

Haven Trevino graciously writes:

Firmness is incomplete
Without softness to receive it.
Embrace these two,
and a child is formed,
Perfect, innocent, and free.

Give to the day
Receive from the night;
Honor these two,
Become the ritual of life.

Live your highest aspirations
In an unassuming way:
Cupped hands at the crystal spring.

Be the lump of clay
And the sculptor too:
A universe of unlimited potential[26].

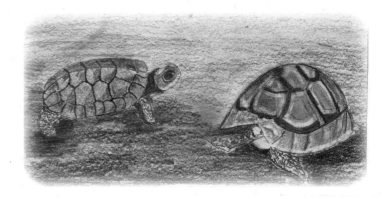

Inquiries

On the Mat: Sense whether you heavily armored in your physical or emotional body. If this is the case, use this practice session to work on deepening your breath, softening the skin and muscles, and becoming more skillful at recognizing when and where to let your guard down. If you are in an overly receptive state and unable to skillfully shield, practice asserting yourself. Set clear boundaries with your poses and root into your personal strength. In either case, remain curious about aspects of your being that might thrive with lowered defenses while identifying other areas that could benefit from added protection. Study the symbiosis of these two energies, as intentional strengthening in one area allows us to release in another. Dedicate the first half of your sadhana to exploring more vigorous movements and utilizing armor to your benefit. As you begin to wind down, shift gears by invoking heightened receptivity through forward bends and twists. Investigate sun salutation, standing forward fold, down dog, standing wide-angle forward bend, head to knee, cow face, tortoise, and reclined tortoise.

Off the Mat: Identify one specific area of your life in which additional armor might help you preserve your sacred space. Identify another in which you might be best served by softening.

I recognize the optimal place between armor & softness in this moment. I actively channel breath to areas of my being that feel constricted. I open to a sense of receptivity within, trusting that my outer frame will sustain my inner suppleness.

Supportive Words
armor: *casing, protective covering, shield, shell*
softness: *openness, pliability, suppleness*

Visualization
The turtle carrying its exquisite shell maintains its softness on the inside, which provides the strength necessary to uphold its external armor. It knows when to move inside for protection and when to extend outward in order to encounter the world.

Complementary Breath
ujjayi
Focus on the softness it creates.
kapalabhati
Focus on the strength it engenders.

Closing Ritual
self/partner massage
Offer yourself a squeeze or two of shoulders, hands, and feet. Better yet, find a friend to do this for you.

Same, Same, but Different: {*inspired by Mihal Arguetty & Douglas Brooks*}

When my sister traveled to India for the first time, I was still in college, and the thought of journeying to this foreign land was the furthest one from my mind. As I listened to the stories of her adventures and watched her video footage of this colorful, festive country, I was intrigued by the differences I witnessed, but my curiosity ended there. During one of our conversations, my sister mentioned that one of the sayings she often heard uttered in India was that of "same, same, but different." I liked the way the words rolled off my tongue, but I never gave them much thought beyond that. Studying philosophy with Douglas Brooks years later, however, I was sparked by words that reminded me of what my sister had shared. This motivated me to contemplate the idea anew, and I began to recognize its profound message.

The first statement of "same" communicates the idea that we are all fundamentally comprised of the same stardust as the cosmos. As we delve beyond the physical and cultural planes of our existence to examine life at the microscopic level, we find the intrinsic threads connecting us all. In fact, more than 99% of our DNA is identical to that of our fellow humans (*and even some animals*), which means that only a single percent is responsible for the existing diversity[27]. These strands of connectivity entwine the lives of all humans. Moreover, they link us to all creatures on Earth, to the planet herself, and to everything that exists as the known universe. Acknowledging this sameness enables us to feel greater understanding and concern for the people and species around us, as we are inspired to honor our commonalities even in light of our differences. Even the person who challenges and provokes us most is made up of this same substance that comprises all that is.

The middle concept of "same" acknowledges the idea that in spite of being unique individuals, we do share certain traits and characteristics. Humans have the same basic facial structure, possess fingerprints, consume food and drink for nourishment, partake in cultural rituals, and interact with the natural environment. It is these similarities that allow us to access empathy and compassion when disaster strikes on the other side of the planet, lend a helping hand to a neighbor, or relate to a friend experiencing heartbreak. This sense of kinship encourages us to step into the shoes of another in order to feel his experience and contemplate the steps we would take if faced with the same joys, dilemmas, or life challenges.

The idea that we are "different" relates to the fact that all human beings are unique individuals, with distinct facial features, one-of-a-kind fingerprints, diverse nutritional needs, and a multitude of cultural rituals, professions, and ways to share and interact with the world. These differences enable us to create abundant richness as we journey through embodied life. Imagine if there were only one profession to choose from or only one meal you could eat day after day. Thankfully, through both our diverse collective cultures and our individual desires to pursue varied interests, we weave a multicolored tapestry that amplifies our own joy while creating gifts for those around us.

A more tangible example of these concepts can be found by examining the foods of different cultures. In many places throughout the globe, flour, water, and salt are combined to create a staple food. Indians mix these ingredients to make a flatbread known as chapati or roti. People of the Middle East combine them to form pita bread, and the same items are mixed to make pizza crust in many Western cultures. Even within these different traditions, each of these breads has a unique taste depending on the intention, the cook, the origin of the wheat, and the method used for baking. In essence, this is the same phenomenon we experience when dining out at an ethnic restaurant or at a friend's house. These settings offer us the chance to enjoy unfamiliar dishes as well as the subtle differences of familiar dishes made by others. The power of living our lives rooted in this recognition of both similarity and diversity is that we can navigate easily between these territories based on the situation at hand, equally affirming areas of stark difference, those of essential likeness, and finally the currents of deep, integrated connection underlying all. Some yoga traditions encourage us to strive towards the first idea of sameness and thus encourage us to eradicate our differences. Tantra, however, teaches us that while it is vital to recognize our interconnected nature, it is equally important to assert our preferences and honor our distinctive offerings. "Same, same, but different"; these are indeed wise words that honor our uniqueness as individuals while also acknowledging our shared identity as brushstrokes comprising the masterpiece of life. As Zen Master Dogen writes:

Everywhere in each tree, rock, bird, and beast, I meet myself. It is at once me, and I am not it[28].

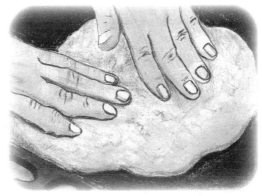

Inquiries

On the Mat: Apply this inquiry to a class. In yoga, we experience the three levels of "same, same, but different" every time we practice. During a class, each person practices at his or her own level of ability and embodies a given asana in a completely unique way. At the same time, there is a blanket of shared experience among the participants as they all proceed through the specific sequence of postures offered by the teacher. Finally, through their explorations on the mat, students cultivate awareness of the subtle thread linking them to their greater surroundings. Explore these three distinct expressions of "same, same, but different" all at once. Take time to appreciate the ways in which your individual practice is unique, and then notice your resonance with others around you. Finally, tune into the greater connection you share with your classmates and your environment on the subtle, cosmic level.

Off the Mat: Make time to invite two or three friends into a conversation about a meaningful topic. Some ideas include spirituality, eco-friendly living, personal health, or a current issue in your community. As you talk, take note of the various points of commonality, empathy, and difference.

Practices

Supportive Words
same: *alike, comparable, related, similar*
different: *dissimilar, distinct, diverse, unique*

Visualization
Water, flour, and salt combined to make pita bread in the Middle East, chapati or roti in India, and pizza crust in the West. These breads are simultaneously not alike, extremely similar, and essentially made out of the exact same ingredients.

Complementary Breath
dirgha, ujjayi, kapalabhati
same, same, but different

Closing Ritual
Chant five rounds of continuous "aum", and notice the similarities and differences present in each unique sound.

Teacher's Note
Lead a fishbowl-style exercise in which four students volunteer to come into the middle of the room to do a specified symmetrical pose. Ask other students to gather around and assume the role of conscious observers. Once you guide the volunteers into the pose, focus first on the uniqueness of each person's posture. Invite the observers to comment on some of the distinctions they see. The second time, ask them to expand their vision to notice the similarities. Finally, invite everyone into the posture to highlight the invisible thread of shared experience.

I embrace the elements of my life that are wholly personal to me. I acknowledge the similarities I share with those around me. I honor the points of connection between me and all of creation.

Sitting in the Fire of the Heart: {*dedicated to Leonie Arguetty*}

My little sister Leonie was a true embodiment of heart energy and universal love. Her light radiated from deep within, and simply being around her opened people's minds and hearts to greater beauty. In February of 2001, Leonie was involved in a skiing accident and passed on; although she is no longer here in the physical form, I still feel her presence, guidance, and love. At the time of her passing, though, I was overwhelmed with grief. Once the reality of her death sank in, I felt like I had been thrown into a pressure cooker that was about to explode. More than anything else, I wanted to run away and hide from the world in attempt to put out the fire raging inside. In my prolonged struggle to answer the question of why this tragedy had occurred, I eventually came to a crossroads. My choices were to give up and shrivel into nothingness, or to remain in the cooker and be with everything that was showing up. Although my life became incredibly hazy for the next six months, I worked to remain present and witness my feelings. The stew of my experience fluctuated between pangs of bitterness, moments of intense spice, and—after some time—small glimmers of sweetness. Sitting in the fire of my heart was the only way to cope with the pain and weather the pure, raw emotions that bubbled up. I wasn't sure when things would change, but I trusted that if I held myself there long enough, I would someday emerge on the other side. Eventually, I found my way out of the encompassing haze, and I was motivated to restructure my life in ways that reflect deeper appreciation for the gifts of this embodied form.

While taking care not to dwell in them for too long, it is important to recognize the inherent potential of periods of extreme darkness for bequeathing us some of the most precious lessons and heart-opening experiences of life. Giving ourselves permission to be present with uncomfortable and intense sensations, though often difficult in the moment, is ultimately of tremendous value. Through connecting with breath and nature, sourcing genuine self-compassion, and welcoming the support and love of others, we can begin to rebuild and move back into life with enhanced perspective and a renewed desire to savor the gift of human existence. To revisit an earlier metaphor, our raw emotions are just like the raw ingredients of a soup. Through the forces of heat, pressure, and careful tending, what is raw softens, cooks, and eventually combines to form a satisfying meal. The key is to give the ingredients ample time to blend, resulting in a wholly new substance abundant with fresh textures, smells, and flavors. In the very same way, we can allow challenging experiences to settle, soften, and morph into something of greater value and complexity. As Rumi eloquently writes:

A chickpea leaps almost over the rim of the pot
where it's being boiled.

'Why are you doing this to me?'

The cook knocks him down with the ladle.

'Don't you try to jump out.
You think I'm torturing you.
I'm giving you flavor,
so you can mix with spices and rice
and be the lovely vitality of a human being.

'Remember when you drank rain in the garden.

That was for this.'

Grace first. Sexual pleasure,
then a boiling new life begins,
and the Friend has something good to eat.

Eventually the chickpea
will say to the cook,

> *'Boil me some more.*

Hit me with the skimming spoon.
I can't do this by myself.'

'I'm like an elephant that dreams of gardens
back in Hindustan and doesn't pay attention
to his driver. You're my cook, my driver,
my way into existence. I love your cooking.'

The cook says,

> *'I was once like you,*
fresh from the ground. Then I boiled in time,
and boiled in the body, two fierce boilings.

My animal soul grew powerful.
I controlled it with practices,
and boiled some more, and boiled
once beyond that,

> *and became your teacher*[29].

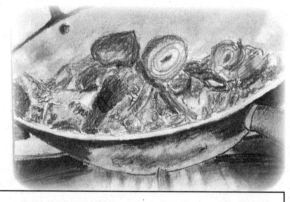

Inquiries

On the Mat: Utilize longer holdings of your postures to generate the stamina to sit in the fire of the heart and illuminate the nature of your inner conversations. As you linger with the sensations of a particular pose, allow your inner dialogue to simmer and soften. Rest in your inner knowing that integration is occurring on both the cellular and emotional levels as the flavors of your practice stew and blend. Sequence your sadhana so that you build to a peak pose of longer holding (*about eight to twelve long, rich breaths*) followed by a few moments of integration and journaling about the experience. Utilize chair pose as the first pinnacle pose, followed by a two-minute rest in corpse pose. Before continuing, take a few moments to write about an intense situation currently manifesting in your life. Use warrior three as the second peak posture, followed by a two-minute integration in child pose. This time, write a few thoughts about how you find balance and nourishment in the midst of intensity. Investigate twisting triangle as the last long holding, followed by two minutes of the channel-clearing breath. Recall one experience in your life in which sitting in the fire brought about profound learning and transformation, and make note of this, as well.

Off the Mat: Purposefully place yourself in a situation that is likely to invoke vivid sensation, strong emotions, or intense heat. Choose to remain in the fire of this experience longer than you normally would. Journal about what transpires.

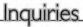

Practices

Supportive Words
abide, hang in, linger, pause, remain, stay put

Visualization
The raw ingredients of a soup slowly cooking and melding into a new substance over the course of a few hours.

Complementary Breath
ujjayi

Closing Ritual
ritual of lighting a candle, candle meditation

Teacher's Note
Utilizing the sequence above, encourage students to observe the unique alchemy of each posture and to notice what occurs after lingering for several rounds of breath in a given pose. At the end of the practice, leave time for students to share in groups of three. Allow time for each person to share one insight with the group.

Playing the Edge {inspired by Yoganand Michael Carroll}

Hatha yoga is a physical practice that has been around for a couple thousand years and was traditionally practiced on a variety of surfaces. The sticky mats of today are comfortable and can be a valuable tool in support of our practice, but they always lead me to wonder, "How did the yogis do it hundreds of years ago?" In my first yoga teacher training at Kripalu, my teacher Yoganand pointed out that the early practitioners of Kripalu Yoga practiced on carpet. As such, he challenged us to explore our practice without a sticky mat to see what might change. I followed his advice and found that my asana practice was extremely different on a carpeted surface. Muscle groups that had never been activated in my practice before sprang to life and began to communicate with the rest of my body. Continually using the mat had habituated me to one way of doing things, and as a result some of the most vital muscles in my body were being left out of my postures. Practicing on a rug brought me to uncharted edges of asana experience, provided new information, and enabled me to access previously unexplored realms of both body and mind.

In much the same way, it can be easy to get comfortable and settle into habitual behaviors and life-detracting patterns. If we become accustomed to avoiding difficult conversations, putting off tough decisions, or dwelling in feelings of unworthiness, we will likely continue to do so just out of habit. When we play the edge, though, we shake things up. At first this may feel decidedly uncomfortable, as there is often resistance holding us back and amplifying our fear of looking over the perceived cliff. In intimate relationships, for example, there are many moments when we simply want to withdraw and throw in the towel. Often, this response is triggered when a partner pushes us into a place that feels edgy, or when a corner we have occupied contentedly for decades is suddenly thrust into the spotlight. Eckhart Tolle surmises in *The Power of Now* that relationships exist not only to make us fulfilled or happy but also to make us more conscious[30]. In the same way, we can become more fully conscious and awaken to our potential when we confront our internal boundaries. Venturing out to this edge takes courage and steadfast intent, and it is vital to remember that there is no one right way to approach a given situation. It is also helpful to remember this undertaking needn't be laden with seriousness and struggle. What is required is acknowledging our resistance, softening the heart, and becoming more humble as we explore how far we want to go. Ultimately, challenging a perceived limit empowers us to become more awake, engaged, and present to life. As Hafiz shares:

Fire has a love for itself –
It wants to keep burning.

It is like a woman
Who is at last making love
To the person she most desires.

Find a Master who is like the Sun.

Go to His house
In the middle of the night.

Smash a window.
Act like a great burglar –
Jump in.

Now,
Gather all your courage –
Throw yourself into His bed!

He will probably kill you.

Fantastic –
That's the whole idea![31]

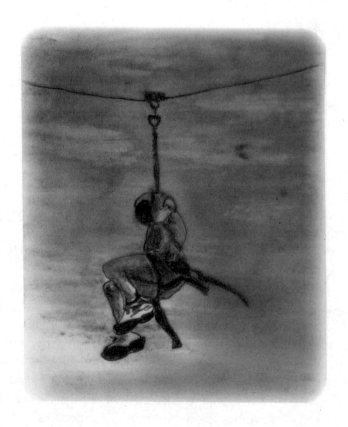

Inquiries

On the Mat: Assess whether you have fallen into any habitual routines in your practice of yoga. Bear in mind that the brain literally thrives on stimulation, which can come in the form of new poses, more advanced variations, or longer holdings. As you explore a new or demanding pose, make room for what feels uncomfortable or impossible at first, and know that this feeling is a clear indication of voyaging to the edge. The skill of playing here involves finding the place where you are challenged but still supported by the structure and stability of the asana. Erich Schiffmann writes, "The body's edge in yoga is the place just before pain, but not pain itself. Pain tells you where the limits of your physical conditioning lie. Edges are marked by pain and define your limits. How far you can fold forward, for example, is limited by your flexibility edge; to go any further hurts and is actually counterproductive. The length of your stay in a pose is determined by your endurance edge. Your interest in a pose is a function of your attention edge[32]." As you identify these various edges, proceed mindfully and approach them with astute awareness. Notice any resistance that surfaces in the process or any desire to retreat to the habitual corners of your practice as you move into deeper asanas. Likewise, take time to acknowledge when you have probed an edge effectively. Explore arm balances, standing splits, standing yoga mudra, humble warrior, L at the wall, and handstand at the wall.

Off the Mat: Identify an edge that impacts your daily life. Make one mindful yet courageous move to challenge yourself in this specific area. Share the results of this experiment with a friend or loved one.

Practices

I utilize my breath to safely explore my edge   I notice the

feelings that arise

places in my practice that

Supportive Words
boundary, brink, extremity, fringe, limit, outskirt, periphery, rim, threshold, verge

Complementary Breath
alternate-nostril kapalabhati

Visualization
A zip line; exploring the edge of the platform before stepping into mid-air.

Closing Ritual
journal contemplation
What is a specific posture that brings you to your edge? Why and how does this relate to your life?

I explore new ground with a sense of curiosity, honoring any   seem habitual or stagnant

The Ripples of Inspiration: {*inspired by Yoga Teachers in Training*}

Every once in a while, the thought, "Does anything I do really matter?" creeps into my mind. At other times, I notice myself being inspired by the smallest, simplest actions of those around me. In these moments, I fully comprehend the impact of even seemingly insignificant actions. An acquaintance shares his intention to take a yoga class, and the next moment I am motivated to go to my own mat and practice. Another friend shares her experience of compassion and understanding for her family during Easter dinner, and I am inspired to accept my own family more fully. A deep learning takes hold as I watch another friend wash the dishes. Instead of letting the water run the whole time, she fills a container with water and soap, washes the dishes, and then rinses them with clean water. My life is forever impacted by the simple act of observing another person's routine, as I realize how little water is actually needed to complete this task. What fascinates me most about these examples is that none of them was a message targeted directly towards me. Rather, I was stirred by the ripples that naturally emerged from each of these occurrences.

Moving through life with an awareness of these ripples of inspiration can enable us to retreat from the habit of devaluing our offerings and instead recognize how our seemingly trivial actions have deep significance for the world around us. Sometimes, we might ignite an awakening for another person right in the moment of a particular act. In other instances, what we share with others through our words, actions, or thoughts may not resonate until they are faced with a similar situation later on. We may never personally witness how we have affected someone, but it is vital to remember that everything we say and do has the potential to influence another. More difficult to imagine but perhaps even more important is how the wake of our behavior radiates outward in all directions, carrying the potential to touch and transform thousands of people. For this reason, dwelling in our truth and living our lives from a place of heart is absolutely essential. There are countless examples throughout history of people simply being themselves with the result of deeply impacting cultural and societal norms. During the 2008 United States Presidential elections, a wise soul said, "Rosa sat so Martin could walk…Martin walked so Obama could run…Obama is running so our children can fly!" As with the undulation created when a pebble lands in water, the wake eventually disappears from view, but the vibration continues long after the visible signs have vanished.

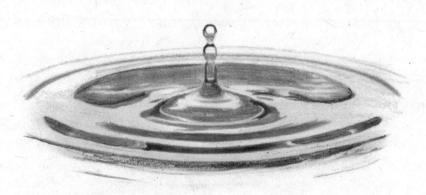

Inquiries

On the Mat: In this practice, invite a friend to join you. When we practice in community, we can be moved physically, energetically, and vibrationally as experience is shared and transferred. Seeing another in a posture we find challenging or intimidating might allow us to recognize the possibility of the asana becoming accessible to us, as well. As we receive the gifts others offer, we ride the wake of their intentions, drawing inspiration that can sometimes last for months. These ripples of energy and inspiration we absorb become integrated into our own essence, and we, in turn, inspire others. In this way, the original vibration grows and expands. When we approach the mat, our primary dedication is to our own practice. Still, yoga is a co-creative experience whether we are alone or in a class setting. We explore our inner landscape through the acts of trying to kick up into a demanding inversion, embodying our poses with brightness and vigor, or simply showing up to practice. As with the metaphor of the pebble, this process results in a ripple effect that can indeed alter the fabric of existence. Move through a practice blending various types of postures, including standing forward fold, parsvotanasana, bound angle, reverse table, cobra, head-to-knee, down dog, locust and purvottanasana with hands clasped.

Off the Mat: While simply being who we are gives rise to ripples of inspiration, we can utilize our actions to intentionally generate them, as well. Pick one or two ways to initiate such a ripple. Whether this takes the form of paying a toll for another car, leaving an unexpected gift for a loved one, or buying a farm animal for a family in Africa, choose a specific action and trust the ripples to emerge.

Practices

I hold true to myself and affirm how my unique way of being

Supportive Words
ripples, undulations, wake, waves

Visualization
As a pebble is dropped into a body of water, the waves flow outward, creating a ripple effect felt far beyond the point of contact.

Complementary Breath
kapalabhati
Notice the power of this breath to leave ripples of vital energy coursing in the body for hours after practice.

Closing Ritual
Rub your palms together rapidly for a few moments to create heat and friction, and then separate the palms slightly. Notice the energy flowing between your hands and extending out in all directions. If you are practicing with a friend, repeat the process, this time mirroring your palms to one another.

Teacher's Note
When you reach the peak posture of your sequence, pause and ask students to partner up. Have them observe one another in a meditative, supportive way as they take turns exploring this pose without words. Afterwards, ask them to share with one another their experiences by describing any vibrations they felt while witnessing the posture.

ripples of inspiration all around me

affects others

I open to the possibility

With a sense of reverence, I embrace the

that my life has the power to inspire others

Honoring the Endings: {*inspired by Todd Norian*}

When my teacher training with Todd Norian was coming to an end, I felt a sense of sadness and a desire to numb myself as this five-month journey drew to completion. As part of our closing ritual, Todd led us in a series of heart-centered exercises that involved sharing, chanting, and staring into the reflection of ourselves as children. Within minutes, the room erupted in tears, but they were tears of triumph, authenticity, and joy. It was truly a gift to devote so many hours to bringing our training to an end with deep integration, celebrating the closure and savoring it wholeheartedly. Endings tend to have a bittersweet quality and can leave us feeling melancholy even in spite of excitement for the next chapter. When an ending is near, we might experience discomfort, annoyance, sadness, or avoidance as we prepare for changes in our world. In the marrow of each conclusion in our lives, though, lies a unique opportunity for ritual, celebration, pause, and contemplation. Moreover, the way we complete one event or stage of life often sets the stage for how the next chapter will manifest.

Endings are a natural part of life. The darkness envelops the last glimmer of light as the sun sets, a goodbye culminates with a warm embrace and a gentle tear, and the last bite of a lovingly prepared meal is savored with a long pause. Indeed, the way we approach these moments can determine how our experience of each one will be imprinted. During a funeral, a profound sense of sadness is undoubtedly present in the wake of losing a loved one. Yet beneath this lives the possibility of shifting into a state of appreciation as we acknowledge and remember all this person shared and offered. This practice of recognizing the value of endings manifests in many other instances in life, including times of work transition, the conclusion of a relationship, or the celebration of a fully lived day. In the Tantric world view, we are eternal beings, so even our death—which might be considered the most frightening ending of all—is in fact just the closure of another episode leading to a new beginning. By taking time to pause in ritual acknowledgement as we encounter endings on our path, we enable healthy integration of the impending transition and turn what might be culturally perceived as a

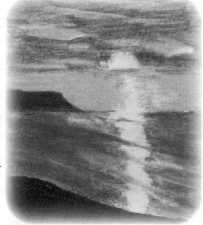

negative event into a beautiful, rich experience of the fullness of life. One of the best ways to become more fluent with endings is to start acknowledging them more consciously in daily life. Some closing rituals include: gathering in a circle and holding hands, verbalizing feeling words at the end of an experience, offering a warm embrace when saying goodbye, writing about a particular event or learning, and burning or burying an object that is related to a passing time. In addition to the above, we can also gather around a bonfire, chant "aum", bow in acknowledgement of another, rest in corpse pose, celebrate the end of a long workday by eating a delicious piece of chocolate, or go on retreat to honor an ending that has occurred. Charlie Mehrhoff writes:

the sun
she
is setting
in the tall grass
beneath the pine

where the heart
beats
one with the land

where the mule deer
approach
their antlers raised

where with palms
upturned
we pray[33]

Inquiries

On the Mat: Take note of what shifts when you fully savor the final moments of each asana. Sense whether you tend to rush ahead to the next posture in your sequence, which leaves less time for mindful closure of the pose at hand. Explore following through completely with each asana, and take two complete breaths to fully acknowledge the end of each experience and absorb its imprint. As you rest in savasana *(corpse pose)*, affirm this posture's incredible capacity to facilitate integration of endings, and remember that even from this asana associated with death, we transition into a fetal position, rise up, and begin anew.

Off the Mat: When you hug a friend or loved one before parting, hold the embrace for three full, rich breaths. Notice how your experience of this moment is impacted as you remain wholly present to saying goodbye.

Practices

Supportive Words
closing, closure, completion, conclusion, culmination, finish

Visualization
Savoring every moment of a beautiful sunset, the array of colors merging in celebration of the day.

Complementary Breath
viloma *(exhale)*
Focus on the final moments of each phase of the breath.

Closing Ritual
Practice by candlelight, and honor the ending of the session by blowing out the flame as you chant the closing "aum".

Teacher's Note
closing circle
Holding hands, invite students to open their eyes, look around the circle, and absorb the beauty and sweetness of closure. Then guide them to close their eyes and turn inward, chanting "aum" to complete the class.

I embrace the endings that emerge along my path

closure in everyday life

I carve out

I treasure the moments of

space for creating closing rituals to help me integrate and thrive

the wisdom
of yoga

"As one goes through life, one learns that if you don't paddle your own canoe, you don't move."

-Katherine Hepburn

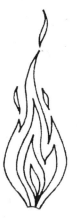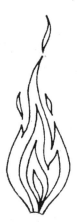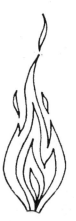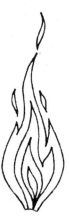

One of the most potent elements of the teachings of yoga is the structure they provide for helping us understand how the world, and consequently our lives, function. The philosophy of yoga is vast, and it has expanded and evolved through the pre-classical, classical, and post-classical eras. As a branch of this greater body, Tantra encompasses many diverse concepts and beliefs. Douglas Brooks writes, "Speaking of the 'Tantras' as if they represent a homogeneous body of thought can be extremely misleading[1]." The schools that comprise Tantra yoga philosophy range from the more orthodox examples constituting the tradition's mainstream to those with a reputation of dark magic, unruly sexual activity, and immoral behavior. The word "Tantra" translates as "loom" and reflects the metaphor that knowledge, intention, and practice can be interwoven to create enhanced empowerment on the human path. Many streams of Tantra embrace the teachings of the Vedas and Classical Yoga as valid tools for deeper understanding, synthesizing and refining fundamental ideas of each of these earlier schools of thought. At the same time, it is vital to understand that there are clear distinctions between the Tantric approach and the schools that preceded it.

Douglas Brooks writes, "While classical yoga maintains that yoga is the way human beings realize that the immortal is not to be confused with the mortal, the unconditioned with the conditioned, and the eternal with the temporal, the Rajanaka seeks to understand how one is actually the other. Yoga then is not merely how we would go about deriving our own perfectly lucid self-realization. Yoga in the Tantric mind is precisely how the Divine itself goes about expressing, choosing, and coming into its own infinite possibilities." In this way, we are invited into a voyage of discovering how to see the Divine reflected in the common world through objects, relationships, thoughts, feelings, and experience. Brooks continues, "In short, the Rajanaka believes everything is the Divine, which is ever-becoming more of itself, not simply a singular core from which all things originate and to which all things return, but an infinitely expanding reality[2]." This last point is a key distinction, as even some Tantric models are based on a theory rooted in the unification of polar opposites, like Siva and Shakti or dark and light. In these systems of thought, yoga is used to mitigate the opposing forces by striving towards a singular core. Rajanaka, however, welcomes a constant unfolding that nurtures both opposites and the vibrant paradox they create; the endeavor is not to cancel them out by finding their mean but rather to appreciate the unique conduit of exploration offered by each.

What follows in this section are contemplations and insights inspired by the philosophical tenets of yoga. Although many of these ideas are rooted in the pre-classical or classical time periods of the tradition, I have personally experienced them through the Tantric lens and therefore comment on them accordingly. The potency of the Tantric world view is that it does not reject ideas that precede it but instead chooses to update and build upon fundamental principles, especially when they serve the greater endeavors of expansion and inquiry. As Doug Keller beautifully communicates, "We actively create the world—not just in our own minds, but in reality, because reality is made of Consciousness, just as we ourselves are nothing but Consciousness…Tantra calls us to participate in the world (rather than only seek liberation from it) because the world is us—and we are free to make it better or worse by the very way in which we see—and thus co-create—it[3]."

Perfect Fullness: {inspired by Bella Arguetty}

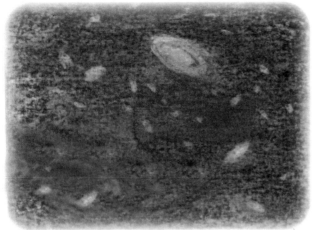

My mom has been an artist her whole life, crafting her magic in the realms of sculpture, set design, oil painting, and photography. At the age of fifty-six, she decided to return to art school for a second time in order to reenergize her skills. When she submitted her application, she was rejected because the school felt she had too much experience. Eventually, though, after talks with the headmaster, she was allowed to enroll. When I asked her why she was going back to school to study what she had already learned, she said she wanted to stretch herself further and remarked that there is always room to develop one's knowledge. Her comments inspired me to approach more areas of my life with an ongoing desire to expand my vision while continuing to honor exactly where I am in the moment.

In the Tantric world view, we are born from perfection into perfection, and we are whole even in the very first moments of our lives. Purnatva, or purna, is the Sanskrit word translated as fullness, riches, or perfection[4] used to signify this state of wholeness and abundance. We are complete because we embody and carry the energy of the entirety of creation. Life would be uninteresting and unproductive, though, if we simply basked in our divine beauty upon recognizing this fullness. Intuitively, we begin to stretch out from our already perfect state to seek even more fulfillment. We expand outward in new directions for the joy and radiance that come from filling up with the delights of the world. Babies are an inspiring example of this phenomenon. They freely channel the energy of the divine and yet they are not satisfied with an idle existence; contrarily, they eagerly explore their environment to enhance an already precious state.

This innate tendency we possess as babies follows us through the rest of our lives, mirroring the same dynamic in the universe at large. The cosmos is already quite full, with seventy sextillion known stars *(7 followed by 22 zeros, or 10 times the amount of grains of sand on all the world's beaches and deserts)*[5]. Even with this many stars, though, the universe continues to expand by birthing new celestial bodies every day. Why does the universe continue to reproduce in this way? Tantra maintains that the motivation is merely the delight of experiencing itself in as many forms as possible. Likewise, each new form offers us another distinctive conduit for seeing, feeling, and sensing the masterpiece all around us. There is an important distinction, though, between this idea of fullness and the act of simply stuffing ourselves with items, events, or thoughts that do not serve us. In a state of purnatva, the fullness we experience is spacious, aligned, and bright. We might tap into this sense of fulfillment through the celebration of a rare ten-course meal, or it might arrive in the pleasure of a single small dish created with intention. While it is easy to succumb instead to thoughts of what we are lacking, we can counter this by acknowledging we are doing our best in any given moment and recognizing our efforts as whole and complete. From this vantage point, we open to the possibility of stretching even more fully into the intentions of our lives. As Lisa Masé elegantly writes:

I invited a guest
to sup with me last night
and left the door ajar
to make passage easy as evening's breeze.
While onion crescents simmered to sweetness,
I chopped carrot tops with ease.
Stirring the stew in delight, I knew
it was time to eat the most delicious dish
I had ever tasted. I offered my heart
and asked for nothing,
yet the ecstatic guest arrived
and fed me the finest divine satisfaction
I have ever known. To taste each bite
beyond ingredients is bliss enough
to fill every living creature
and cover the Earth in love pudding[5.5].

Inquiries

On the Mat: Take time to methodically deepen each inhalation and establish the foundation of the breath. Notice how the tissues of the lungs literally loosen up after a few rounds of breath, inviting even more oxygen into the body. The wonder of the breath is its ability to constantly expand as we assimilate the life-giving force it so graciously offers. As you flow through your asana sequence, remember that each posture has a capacity for experience that is always beyond what you may have encountered before. Affirm the perfection of each pose regardless of its outward appearance, and at the same time feel the excitement of extending yourself more fully into the delights of your sadhana. After every two or three asanas, pause your movement and affirm the energy of purna by stating silently or aloud: "I am perfect in my imperfections. I am full yet open to expansion. I am at once all-knowing and constantly evolving." Explore knee-down lunge, hands inside foot in knee-down lunge, quad stretch in knee-down lunge, high lunge, cobra, locust, down dog, bound angle, cow face, baby dancer, and pigeon.

Off the Mat: Identify one area in your life in which you feel perfect, whole, and complete at present. Spend the next week observing whether this is a fixed state or whether there is an element of changeability even with regard to this particular facet of your being. Consider how your sense of fullness in this realm might be continuing to grow and expand.

Practices

Supportive Words
abundant, bursting, complete, entirety, fullness, wholeness, expanse

Visualization
The living, thriving universe, already complete and whole, yet continually unfolding expanding into more.

Complementary Breath
dirgha

Feel the way the breath continually expands.

Closing Ritual
chant or play

Aum purnam-adah purnam-idam; Purnaat purnam-udachyate; Purnasya purnam-aadaaya; Purnam-eva-avashishyate.

This is perfect. That is perfect. From the perfect springs the perfect. Take the perfect from the perfect and only the perfect remains.

Mindful Witness: {inspired by Kripalu's Spiritual Lifestyle Program}

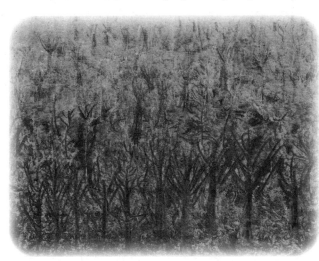

During my time volunteering at Kripalu, I decided to limit myself to having desserts only on Saturdays. My sweet tooth was challenged, but I wanted to experiment with exercising this kind of self-discipline. I will never forget sitting with a few friends at the Kripalu Cafe on a particular weekday afternoon. One of them bought an assortment of high-quality organic chocolate bars and generously laid them out on the table for all to share. The fragrant scent of orange-infused 70% dark chocolate reached my nose, and my thoughts began their dance. In a split second, my composure dissolved as my mind raced with the impulse to grab as many cubes as I could. Witnessing this, I began to deepen my breath and watch my thoughts as the sensations of needing and wanting the chocolate made their way through my skin, muscles, and bones. After a few breaths, my mind relaxed and the temptation dissipated as a deep sense of calm slowly enveloped my being. In this moment, I understood what aware observation was all about. When we can be both inside and outside of an experience at the same time while fully participating, life begins to slow down, and we are no longer enslaved by unconscious reactions.

Unusual circumstances, agitating people, and unexpected events are guaranteed to manifest in our daily lives. When a wave of emotion hits, we often get swept into a reactive state. We go around blaming everyone else for our problems, and we are unable to recognize the triggers and negative mindset framing our life. Yoga invites us to slow down and engage our own thoughts, external circumstances, and other people with greater skillfulness. When we can willfully take the seat of the watchful seer, we can empower ourselves by deepening our capacity to respond rather than react to the various facets of life. Through this ability to respond, we are in essence affirming the freedom embedded in the very fabric of our being. Even amidst the most horrible circumstances, there are tales of those who manage to hold on to the essence of this inborn individual liberty by responding to life. Viktor Frankl, an Austrian neurologist and psychiatrist, survived the Holocaust and authored the celebrated book *Man's Search for Meaning*. In this work he writes, "We who lived in concentration camps can remember the men who walked through the huts comforting others, giving away their last piece of bread. They may have been few in number, but they offer sufficient proof that everything can be taken from a man but one thing: the last of the human freedoms—to choose one's attitude in any given set of circumstances, to choose one's own way[6]."

A true, complete response involves connecting to the breath, feeling emotions, watching the experience as it unfolds, and allowing it to integrate and move through us. Attuning to the big picture in this way, we can choose how to navigate situations with more intelligence and grace. The key awareness with regard to mindful observation is that there is never a good or bad choice in any given situation. There is simply the distinction of whether we choose a given behavior (*i.e. a friend makes you angry, you feel your emotions, and you choose to have a piece of chocolate*), or whether it is merely an unconscious reaction (*i.e. a friend makes you angry, and seconds later, the chocolate is in your mouth*). The tool of witnessing is literally like a muscle we develop and strengthen as we step into relationship with the many areas of our lives including eating habits, interpersonal relationships, and self-discovery. In some schools of thought, the concept of aware observation is described in terms of separation, implying that being in this state is superior and wholly independent from our usual mode of operation. In this view, the goal shifts to first identifying and then transcending an illusory world of names and forms that block our way, or in other words, eradicating the different aspects of inner self (*the neurotic, joyful, angry, or excited*) to arrive at a supreme, steady oneness. In the Tantric perspective, attentive seeing is instead the capacity to see and be present with all of these facets in their incredible diversity. The aim here is ultimately to be able to recognize the multiple ways in which the divine is present in ourselves and in the world. As we delve more deeply into our own experience, we become more astute at identifying how these varied expressions actually enable access to deeper levels of relationship with both our inner and outer realms. As Henry David Thoreau writes in Walden:

> Only that day dawns to which we are awake. Jon Kabat-Zinn comments: "If we are to grasp the reality of our life while we have it, we will need to wake up to our moments. Otherwise, whole days, even a whole life, could slip past unnoticed[7].

Inquiries

On the Mat: Utilize this practice to strengthen the muscle of mindful observation as you hold your postures and focus on your breath. As you come into an extended holding of a pose, your mind might be inclined to trigger a hasty release. Usually, the mind reacts this way because the posture is raising heat and ushering emotions to the surface. Our animal brain is instinctually designed to avoid pain and seek pleasure, but there is a vast and rich field of experience between mere discomfort and potentially injurious pain. As you settle more deeply into a given posture, notice when you arrive at a definitive edge that is the fine line between true pain and uncomfortable but ripe sensation. Allow your thoughts and any physical messages to merge, and notice new insights that arise in your body or as intellectual reflections. Focus on standing poses with mountain, warrior one, warrior two, lateral angle, chair, goddess, plank, tree, and eagle.

Off the Mat: Food is a wonderful arena for strengthening the muscle of witnessing. Dedicate a week to exploring your relationship with one of your favorite foods. Once a day, take at least five minutes to engage it solely through the senses of sight, smell, and touch. Simply be with the breath as you explore what comes up, and feel free to journal about your emotions. On the seventh day, make time to mindfully savor this particular food, and notice what results.

Practices

I observe my experience with focus and dedication. I choose to watch and feel the insights revealed in each breath. I slow down and savor the moments of my practice.

Supportive Words
attentive, aware, conscious, observant, tuned in, watchful

Visualization
Trekking through a forest too dense to allow a clear view, and then gaining altitude and looking down to plainly see the area from an expanded perspective.

Complementary Breath
anulom vilom
With each subsequent retention of the breath, be present to what shifts and arises anew.

Closing Ritual
seated meditation
Breath, relax, feel, watch and allow.

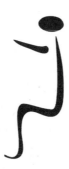

Skillfulness in Action: {*inspired by Douglas Brooks & Dinabandhu Garrett Sarley*}

When I assist yoga teacher trainings at Kripalu, I am always amazed by the stories students share of what it took for them to make space for 200 hours of training. Some students share their struggles to take time away as busy working mothers, while others comment on how many years it took to save the funds for tuition. Some for whom English is a second language speak of their trepidation regarding studying outside their native land. I am continually inspired by witnessing what people can accomplish when they align with their highest intentions, move towards that which is unknown or uncomfortable, and ride the waves of experience with deep knowledge that whatever surfaces is of benefit.

The word yoga refers to a path that encompasses more than just the physical asanas so familiar in the West. The poses are the portal through which many students begin their journey of yoga, and they indeed serve as a launch pad for practitioners' exploration of the other realms that comprise this time-honored tradition. As teachers and students, it is at once heart-opening, inspiring, and startling to awaken one morning to realize the practice of yoga has expanded far beyond the boundaries of the mat and that all of life is, in fact, an experience of this divine pulsation. As yoga invites us into deeper contemplation of the ways in which we lead our lives, it asks us to consider how we can traverse our path in the most effective and skillful ways. Through endeavoring towards this refined way of being, we begin to shift our values and generate more vitality both for ourselves and for the world we inhabit. In chapter two of the Bhagavad Gita, yoga is defined simply as "skillfulness in action." The first step in this endeavor towards being adept at the way we live our lives is identifying what it is we most desire for our own sense of well-being and for the well-being of the world. In some yoga traditions, desires are considered "unspiritual" and are to be avoided. In the Tantric world view, however, these personal wishes are embraced because they provide us with important information and give us direction. Having wants is an intricate part of human nature that can ultimately be a doorway to fulfillment and happiness in our lives when approached mindfully. Although many people share similar desires, our ability to isolate the specific elements we seek or that differentiate our particular lens inevitably points us in our own unique direction. According to Dinabandhu Garrett Sarley, it is up to us to align our words, thoughts, feelings, and actions with this desire once a direction becomes clear. In this way, we begin to craft an environment of support for what we are attempting to accomplish.

Through the inquiry of our thoughts and feelings, we can reflect on how much we value each desire that arises in our lives. Establishing a hierarchy of importance for all of our many wants is essential for determining where to first direct our energies. When I graduated from college, I had many desires, including finding a graphic design job, locating housing in Los Angeles, exploring intimacy, and making new friends. Each of these wants had to be prioritized with respect to the others. Upon reflection, I determined my primary goal was finding a place to live, followed by steady work, then social connections, and finally an intimate relationship. The dynamic nature of desires, though, means that this hierarchy needn't be locked in place, as their level of priority can change in accordance with our shifting circumstances and inner awakenings.

The final component of lining up with skillfulness involves the specific actions we take. One of my friends is studying to be a doctor, and I have been privileged to witness his journey. I am constantly amazed at the gut-wrenching decisions he has had to make time and time again to stay the course. When we have clarity regarding the nature of our most urgent desire, we can begin to formulate concrete steps and clear intentions that move us toward our goal. This final aspect of skillfulness also asks us to consider whether this most conspicuous desire is truly authentic. When we get real about what is required to fulfill a particular aspiration, we can attain clear perspective and open to the idea of shifting our hierarchy of value if need be. For example, at one point in my life I was flirting with the idea of becoming a commercial pilot. When I began contemplate whether I was truly prepared to take the steps necessary to fly planes, however, I soon realized my heart and dedication were not fully attuned to this endeavor.

In the course of our lives, we encounter instances that feel deeply right and moments when what we say, feel, think, and do fully echo our intention. When we can move into life with more skillfulness in our actions, we gain greater access to stores of inherent fullness. Doors open up that may have otherwise remained shut, and we summon deep belief in ourselves and trust in the support of outside forces to bolster us in our journey. The endeavor of skillfulness in action is not an easy one, as often our words, feelings, and thoughts are not fully in line with one another. It might be that we feel and communicate what we want, but are afraid to initiate the actions needed to accomplish our goal. Alternatively, it could be that we are striving in the direction of our innermost calling, only to have our internal dialogue constantly berating and contradicting our external efforts. As Goethe states:

> *Until One is committed, there is hesitancy, the chance to draw back, always ineffectiveness. Concerning all acts of initiative there is one elementary truth, the ignorance of which kills countless ideas and endless plans: That the moment one definitely commits oneself, then providence moves, too. All sorts of things occur to help one that would never otherwise have occurred. A whole stream of events issues from the decision, raising in one's favor all manner of unforeseen incidents and meetings and material assistance which no man could have dreamed would come his way. Whatever you can do or dream you can, begin it! Boldness has genius, power, and magic in it.*

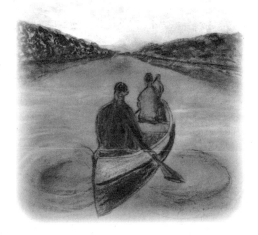

Inquiries

On the Mat: As you start your practice, first identify what it is you desire most from this time on the mat. Do you want to build strength, flexibility, and mental clarity? Do you likewise feel drawn towards a vigorous workout? Are you also in need of deep relaxation? Recognize that to accomplish all of these at once, you would have to do yoga for the rest of the day, so instead prioritize. As you determine what aspect of practice to focus on in this particular practice, start to align your thoughts and feelings accordingly. Note whether your tendency is to be clear in your desires but then become overwhelmed by your thoughts. Do you want to explore new poses but never allow yourself to step onto the mat in the spirit of play? Do you make time for yoga but then become mired in an internal dialogue of unworthiness or lack of knowledge? Once you become aware of your thoughts and actions, utilize your skillfulness to inform your decisions. As you become more skillful at aligning your desires, words, thoughts, and actions, you will become more adept at recognizing your limitations, easily determining when it is of value to push and when it will better serve you to back off. Explore a balancing sequence with standing half moon, lateral angle, warrior three, standing crane, tree, eagle, balancing half moon, and revolved balancing half moon.

Off the Mat: Reflect on a decision you need to make in your life, applying the principles of skillfulness in action to explore whether all parts of you are unified to support this choice. Take time to inquire into any resistance, and notice whether your alignment shifts in one direction or the other after this spell of mindful consideration.

Practices

With intention and courage, I align my words, feelings, thoughts, and actions

Supportive Words
ability, aptitude, dexterity, experience, proficiency, technique

Visualization
Paddling a canoe in harmony with the currents of the river; steering and staying on course with a sense of certitude.

Complementary Breath
ujjayi
Focus on the skillfulness of this breath and its ability to simultaneously energize and soothe.

Closing Ritual
journal contemplation
What is one way in which skillfulness in action is manifesting in your life at present?

heart, and speak my truth

I awaken my mind, feel my

turn into the waves of doubt and willfully pursue my dreams

The Practice of Yoga: {inspired by Douglas Brooks}

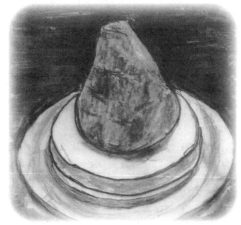

One of the first concepts that struck me regarding the practice of yoga was the emphasis on the word "practice." This teaching of being complete in my offering without concrete notions of success or failure became even clearer in my role as a yoga teacher. When I teach, there are times when a class that starts well suddenly morphs into a whirlwind of reaction and disappointment. Sometimes a mere awkward look from a student *(who is likely simply in the depths of her practice)* throws me into a tailspin of misconception. I instantly stamp my performance with a letter grade, and yet there is an inner voice of composure if I choose to listen. Even if my students do pick up on the mistakes that inevitably pepper my classes, they are usually grateful for the imperfection and realness they represent. As a teacher, I can model how to embrace the unrefined aspects on both the internal and external planes. On a personal level, this kind of openness deepens my capacity for meeting others, as well as myself, as being in the process of a practice.

Being in an ongoing sadhana *(forms of practice[8])* fuels further inquiry, allows us to build a more stable knowledge base, and invites us into the delight and joy of simply being in process. What if we let go of perfection and allow our efforts to be good enough as they are? How can we embrace the questions and unfinished parts of ourselves and know that just like the universe, we, too, are unfinished masterpieces gradually but constantly being revealed? The idea of being in progress—unfinished, asymmetrical, and rough—can be challenging to embrace because there are so many signs pointing us towards predetermined notions of perfection. Whether it is the right body type, the best grade, or the most desirable and newest gizmo, there is often an underlying message that arriving at some preordained destination will bring us true happiness. Luckily, many people discover that these landmarks are also just part of the journey and by no means guarantee a permanent, blissful state of being. Life is almost never about finished products or perfect packages because the very nature of the universe is one of evolution and flow. By expanding into this awareness and softening into its implications, we can access a richer, more fulfilled way of being. Rainer Maria Rilke writes:

> *Be patient toward all that is unsolved in your heart and try to love the questions themselves like locked rooms and like books that are written in a very foreign tongue. Do not now seek the answers, which cannot be given to you because you would not be able to live them. And the point is, to live everything. Live in the questions now. Perhaps you will then gradually, without noticing it, live along some distant day into the answer[9].*

Inquiries

On the Mat: Yoga itself is a work in progress, and it invites us to revel in the novelty and richness of the incomplete each time we engage in asana practice. Welcome the process of practice as you grow more comfortable with the ever-shifting elements of yoga and honor the physical idiosyncrasies that make certain poses awkward. Approach the mat with this awareness, and discover areas in which you place a demand on yourself to be finished and whole. Explore the unrefined and messy elements of each posture while admiring the beauty in the roughness. Allow intention and effort to be the focus, as these carry the weight of our sadhana and resonate more deeply with our spirit than preconceived notions of success or failure. Explore back extensions with standing forward fold, standing yoga mudra, lateral angle, warrior two, reverse warrior two, humble warrior, pigeon, quad stretch in pigeon, parsvotanasana, twisting chair, revolved tree, cobra, locust, crocodile, half frog, bow, and camel.

Off the Mat: Dedicate a half hour for three consecutive days to creating a collage. Although you might wish to finish it on the first day, purposefully stretch out the process, and witness what surfaces. On the third day, whether you feel it is "finished" or not, share your collage with others.

Practices

I embrace the unrefined parts of myself

Supportive Words
evolution, practice, process, unfolding

Visualization
A rough, wet lump of clay, with infinite possibilities of form.

Complementary Breath
dirgha

Closing Ritual
Draw your hands to heart center, silently bow, and flow quietly into the next experience of your day.

I honor the questions

I explore my preconceived notions of

and expand beyond my known ways of being

success and failure

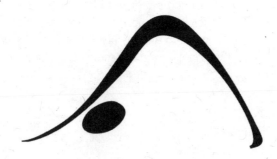

The Blessed Glow of Sun & Moon: {inspired by Deb Neubauer}

Hatha yoga is the common name used for the physical asana practice of yoga. In Sanskrit, one definition for ha is sun, while one interpretation of ta is moon. Together, they are translated as violence or force, alluding to the early history of the yoga tradition. At the time when hatha yoga was first developed, there was a pointed focus on "purifying" the physical body by beating it into submission. Later on, Jnaneshwar, a poet-saint, strived to create more balance to reflect and honor the composite roots of the tradition. Doug Keller writes, "His Jnaneshwari is a profound effort to unite the teachings of the hata yogis and of the philosophies of the yoga tradition with the way of the heart taught by Krishna from the time of the Bhagavad Gita…Jnaneshwar wished to redress the balance between practice and devotion, between effort and grace, [and] between mastery and surrender[10]." As a result of this new perspective, hatha yoga evolved into the inquiry of how we can best align ourselves with these two supreme energies influencing our daily existence.

The sun is a potent energy source that both illuminates our world and nourishes myriad forms of life. Without its resplendent light and energy, little on our planet could exist or function. The word "solar" is associated with daytime, bright light, heat, and power. This greatest of stars is a symbol of abundance, and it exudes masculine characteristics. In us, these solar qualities are associated with the active, masculine, and passionate aspects of ourselves, and they reside in the right hemisphere of the body. Here, breath that enters through the right nostril activates the pingala nadi, which is the subtle energy conduit that begins and ends on the right side of the central channel. When the pingala is activated through intentional breath practices, we can experience increased heat, stimulation, and vitality. The solar aspects of ourselves illuminate our unique gifts and offerings as individuals. These fuel our passions and will and empower us to engage fully in the world as we maneuver through life.

The moon is a more subtle power source, and yet it is an influential player in the dance of life on the planet. The moon's magnetic relationship to the Earth is readily apparent, as it literally tugs the ocean waters towards itself. Instead of giving off its own light, the moon reflects the sun's glow once we rotate out of its direct range. Like the coals that continue to glow even after the fire has been extinguished, the moon is a reminder that light is never truly absent. As such, the moon symbolizes the abundant, ever-present light of universal consciousness that is ours so long as we acknowledge it even in its subtlest forms. Lunar energy corresponds to qualities of night, reflection, coolness, and calm. It is associated with the feminine, more receptive aspects of our personalities. Indeed, the moon serves as an apt metaphor for the parts of our multidimensional selves that are not apparent in the light of day yet always present. Although we cannot possibly see all facets of ourselves all the time, we can explore these latent realms through the subtler, indirect means of reflection. Just as the right hemisphere of the body gives us access to our solar power, the left correlates to lunar energy and is home to the ida nadi, which is the subtle energy conduit that begins and ends on the left side of the central channel. When the ida nadi is activated by focused breathing, we can experience increased comfort, calm, and coolness. The lunar aspects of ourselves illuminate our eternal connection to all that is, which—like the moonlight—is always present but not always visible. These qualities which encourage us to soften, trust, and receive grace allow us to recognize that we do not have to stand alone in the face of life's tasks.

Nature requires that we be soulful and therefore requires a dimension within us where darkness and light may meet and know each other. Mornings and evenings somewhere inside, with similar qualities to the mornings and evenings of the earth. Qualities of gradual but vast change; of stillness and tender transference, fading and emerging, foreboding and revelation[11].

Inquiries

On the Mat: Many yoga classes incorporate both heating and cooling movements to access the unique energies inherent to each of these celestial bodies. The key is to have equal, ready access to both our passionate, individual self as well as our subtler, reflective side. Feel and explore the solar and lunar as they surface through various facets of your practice. Notice how different postures and categories of poses embody the complementary energetic signatures of sun and moon. Become acquainted with your own solar and lunar qualities, honing your connection to both. Take time to develop a deeper relationship with these distinctive realms of your being, and sense whether you can utilize them more skillfully to maximize your intelligence and vitality in life situations. Use sun salutes to draw forth the heat and individual power of surya, and then flow into moon salutes and forward folds to invoke cooling, softness, and awareness of overshadowed parts of the body. If possible, increase the level of light in your practice space during the sun salutes, keep your eyes open, and utilize a stronger ujjayi breath to engage sun energy. Once you begin to cool with moon flow and forward folds, turn the lights down, soften your gaze, and shift your focus to the introspective nature of ujjayi. Explore sun salutations *(any variation depending on your energy level, taking time to pause in plank or low push-up)*, moon salute *(mountain, standing crescent, goddess squat, five-pointed star, triangle, intense stretch, runner's stretch, extended leg squat, full squat)*, and forward folds.

Off the Mat: Next time the moon is full or nearly so, spend a few hours in the sun before nightfall, and then sit in the light of the moon once it has risen. Meditate, contemplate, and dialogue with others on your direct experience of these primal energies that form the backdrop of our lives.

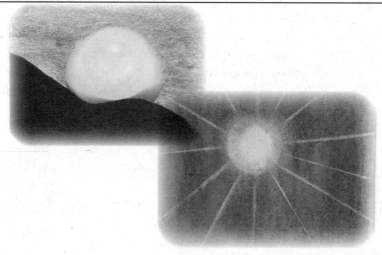

Supportive Words

solar: *heated, life-giving, masculine, potent, powerful*

lunar: *cool, feminine, reflective, stabilizing, subtle*

Visualization

The brilliant, life-giving radiance of the sun; the sweet, reflective glow of a full moon

Complementary Breath

surya bhedana

Activates solar energies, at the beginning of practice. *(With the left nostril closed off, breathe in and out of the right.)*

chandra bhedana

Activates lunar energies, at the end of practice. *(With the right nostril closed off, breathe in and out of the left.)*

Closing Ritual

When you return to a seated position after relaxation, place one hand at heart center and the other on the lower back, simultaneously sensing both the solar and lunar planes of your being.

life to reflect the intention of my spirit

of darkness, I sense the omnipresence

Like the moon reflecting the light of the sun, I allow the situations of my

of subtle lunar light

The Gift of Community: {inspired by Wild Geese}

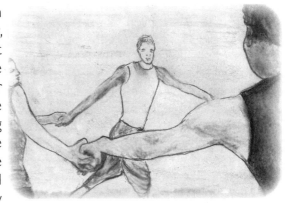

When geese fly together, they essentially form a traveling community. As one goose tires of leading, it maneuvers its way to the rear of the flock where it finds support from the draft of those ahead. The same phenomenon occurs when we as individuals lead our lives in the context of community. Just like the geese, we uplift one another to shine more brightly. By opening to our own inner light in tandem with others who are doing the same, we generate a potent wake that can have tremendous influence on the world around us. When I guide meditations at Kripalu, guests often remark how much easier it is for them to sit and center in the presence of a group. Yoga offers us the tools not only to engage in personal inquiry through dedicated action of body and mind but also to deepen this through mindful interaction with those around us.

There are numerous examples in life in which singular entities gather together to function as a collective. Animals travel in herds, our cells gather in community to form larger systems in the body, and an infinite number of celestial bodies comprise the known universe. In these examples, the singular elements that constitute the greater whole are indeed numerous and diverse, but they are never separate from all of existence. There exists a mutually dependent relationship; without the parts, the collective wouldn't function as a whole, and without the whole, the parts wouldn't have purpose. Among animals, our bodies, and the larger universe, fluctuations arise when there is separation, as stray animals, afflicted cells, and disconnected components no longer function in harmony with the larger whole. This same phenomenon occurs when people become isolated physically or energetically from family, friends, and networks of support; struggles with depression and other physical maladies are oftentimes manifestations of this distance. In truth, we can never totally disconnect from one another as we are always in relationship on some level, but we can "mis"connect with the life that is before us through our conscious and unconscious choices.

In the Tantric world view of yoga, we are reminded that engagement with community is vital, as we enhance our own capacity for growth by supporting the skillfulness, awareness, and heart of those around us. In a sense, the ever-evolving, collectively rooted enlightenment described by this tradition invites us to acknowledge the intimate relationship between our journey as individuals and the spiritual health of our greater community. As we step into our various life roles and offer our personal gifts to each particular tribe (such as those of family, colleagues, nature, social networks, or hobby groups), we can recognize and utilize the gifts of others, as well. This model, therefore, does not require us to do everything ourselves. Instead, it holds that calling upon the expertise of others honors them while simultaneously allowing us to focus our energies on our true passions. As Mary Oliver describes so elequently in *Wild Geese* no matter who we are and how lonely we may be, the world is there full of its imagination. The harsh moments and the exciting times call out, over and over, announcing our place in the family of things[12].

Inquiries

On the Mat: Even though you may be practicing alone, explore the concept that you are not truly isolated in your experience, as the invisible thread that binds us all is ever-present. As you dive into practice, invoke the support of the various tribes of your physical body as well as the literal families that sustain you. Alternatively, take this inquiry into the classroom and contemplate how your yoga community nourishes both your practice and life. Explore a back extension practice with knee-down lunge, cobra pulsation, warriors one and two, humble warrior, knee-down lunge with quad stretch, sky gazer, locust, reclined hero, and camel variations.

Off the Mat: Call to mind something you have always tried to do alone but know deep down you need more help to accomplish. Reach out to your community to ask for assistance. As you become more comfortable enlisting supporters on your path, notice whether you encounter more opportunities for sharing your own unique light through extending help to others.

I step into each moment wholly

Supportive Words
community, tribe, family, clan

Visualization
A group of people holding hands in a circle.

Complementary Breath
ujjayi

Closing Ritual
three rounds of "aum"
Dedicate the first round to yourself, chant the second for the loved ones who comprise your family at present, and sound the last one for all the beings who form your larger community.

Teacher's Note
Begin class by inviting students to find a partner who is the same size and asking them to arrange their mats in concentric circles facing one another. Set up your mat in the center, but make sure there is enough space for you to walk through and around. Start class with students sitting back to back in pairs. As they feel their own breath as well as their partner's, guide their awareness to the connection that binds us all. Encourage students to notice how the presence of others contributes to the overall experience of practice. Repeatedly bring the group back together by guiding synchronization of the breath and allowing pauses for students to sense the collective energy. Use plenty of partner poses to connect them to one another physically. In addition, lead the class in a few full group experiences. Guide utthita hasta padangusthasana *(extended hand to foot)*, lining students up so they are side by side with an arm's distance between them *(you might have to organize this in rows depending on the constraints of your space, but attempt a single line if possible)*. As you guide them to take their leg *(or bent knee for the modification)* out the side, request that neighbors support one another by gently holding the ankle of the extended leg in front of them, reminding students to communicate whether they need additional support or added stretch. Next, line students up shoulder to shoulder as in the previous posture, and guide warrior three. With arms extended like wings, invite students to take hold of their neighbors' hands or shoulders.

assured of my eternal connection

the unique gifts I contribute to my community

I acknowledge

of community to expand my horizons

I utilize the power

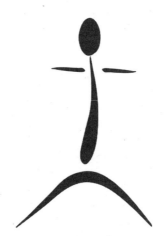

I am that I am: {*inspired by Dinabandhu Garrett Sarley*}

During my college years, I experienced intense confusion and inner turmoil in my struggle to come to terms with my sexual orientation. Initially, I was unable to tolerate the consequences of being who I truly was because I had so many fears. I thought being gay would mean not having a family, contracting a life-threatening disease, and being isolated as a result of my unfamiliarity with gay culture. When I finally began to accept myself, though, I rediscovered a sense of profound connection to my authentic nature. I approached my life with renewed confidence, excited to explore this new dimension of myself. Rooted in this radical affirmation for every facet of my being, I was able to move on with my life and more freely share my gifts with others.

In the Tantric world view, our inherent splendor is comprised of both darkness and light, and therefore enduring courage is needed to shift the embedded misperceptions of our inherent value. Dinabandhu Garrett Sarley describes one aspect of yoga as the ability to tolerate the consequences of being ourselves. Acknowledging and affirming all parts is something many people find extremely challenging. The process of recognizing why we are not able to tolerate being who we are equates to finding the layers and obstacles hindering our ability to affirm our own beauty. As young children, we are deeply connected to the source of our inherent self-worth. Over time, though, certain life experiences communicate to us in one way or another that we are not of value. Slowly, our inner belief system shifts, and we begin to live our lives from this devalued state of being. This deflated identity becomes apparent in the words we choose to describe ourselves, the physical posture we adopt, and in our interactions with those around us.

To work with accepting the consequences of who we are, we must employ an ample dose of love and compassion, step into our power, and trust wholeheartedly that we are enough. It can be so easy to fall victim to the stories we accumulate or to become entangled in the harsh, derogative voices within. When we find ourselves in this space of diminished self-worth, we can pause to connect to the breath, build upon trust in the greater web of energy, or seek guidance and support from others. One of the journals I keep by my bed helps me tolerate myself even in the most challenging of moments. Whenever I have an uplifting experience in my life, like a student offering an affirmation of my teaching or a moment of feeling proud of the way I handled a particular situation, I write it down. If I suddenly find myself bombarded by my inner critic, I read my journal and remind myself of these other voices in my life. Once we begin to embrace the power of self-affirmation, life responds by co-participating in our healing. The world reciprocates the affirmation we muster within, and we begin to find ourselves in more situations that bolster our feelings of inner value. Patterns of self-criticism are seductive and create a deep, internal divide between the parts of the self we promote and those that we lock up and hide away. Embracing all aspects of who we are, though, can allow us to rediscover that there is more than just one way to live a worthy life. Marianne Williamson reminds us:

> *Our deepest fear is not that we are inadequate. Our deepest fear is that we are powerful beyond measure. It is our light, not our darkness, that most frightens us. We ask ourselves, who am I to be brilliant, gorgeous, talented, fabulous? Actually, who are you not to be? There is nothing enlightened about shrinking so that other people won't feel insecure around you. As we let our own light shine, we unconsciously give other people permission to do the same. As we are liberated from our own fear, our presence automatically liberates others[13].*

Inquiries

On the Mat: Yoga can serve as an effective vehicle for moving into the layers separating us from our own inherent brilliance. In this practice, endeavor to locate the underlying, unresolved issues at the root of any intolerance you feel towards yourself. Sit with the postures that challenge you, connect to your breath, and attempt a pose you never thought possible. Regardless of the outcome, the inner self is bolstered by our willingness to attempt something different and new. Initiate an internal dialogue with the question, "How can I be loving towards myself in my practice today, both internally and out in the world?" In every pose, silently repeat the affirmation, "I tolerate the consequences of being who I am." During the cool-down phase of your practice, use some restorative postures to fully honor who you are. In restorative yoga, lingering in passive poses for longer periods of time allows the body to fully reap the benefits of these positions. Each restorative asana is a literal gesture of being present to both our physical and energetic bodies. Investigate a potpourri practice incorporating both active and restorative postures, including: chair, high lunge, knee-down lunge, hands inside foot in knee-down lunge, lateral angle, warrior two, pigeon, easy pose twist, easy pose forward fold, bound angle, child over bolster, twist over bolster, legs up the wall, and reclining bound angle over bolster.

Off the Mat: Upon waking, write down one positive affirmation about yourself, stand in front of the mirror, and say it aloud three times. Continue this exercise each day for a full week, adding a new affirmation each morning and repeating the previous ones, as well. When the week is complete, take some time to reflect on the effects of having started your days with this positive vibration.

Practices

I affirm the limitless possibilities that dwell within me

Supportive Words
appreciation, esteem, merit, tolerance, value, worth

Visualization
A mother hugging her child with love and acceptance; envision offering that same kind of love to yourself.

Complementary Breath
natural
Focus on the breath as being enough as it is in the present moment.

Closing Ritual
mantra meditation
"I am enough." Or chant So Hum, So Hum; So Hum, Shivo Hum; I am that I am

part of human life

I stand firm in my actions

I make room for the inevitable mistakes that are

and embrace the outcome

The Depth of Participation: {inspired by Douglas Brooks}

When I graduated from college, I thought having a degree would provide me with direction and security. Little did I know that confusion would ensue over the next several years as I began to wander and explore what mattered to me most. Today, I have an entire computer file entitled "ideas" that serves as a reminder of all that I would love to do in my life. When I distill my passions, they boil down to interests in yoga, nutrition, and care for the environment. It is through this clarity of knowing what it is I value most that I can participate in my life with deep passion and determination.

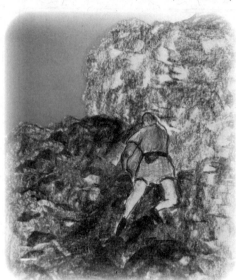

Some spiritual traditions subscribe to the belief that the events of our lives are predetermined such that we simply ride the various waves that emerge. In the Tantric world view, however, we are made up of the same elemental substance that is the universe, and as a result we have the ability to align with this greater energy and steer our own path. We honor the power of the universal source, but at the same time we acknowledge that we have been invited to co-participate in our experience. In this view, we are not merely observers on the sidelines watching as the universe enfolds and unfolds; we are instead part of what moves the layers of existence in a particular direction. Some yoga schools encourage us to disassociate from the worldly plane and seek transcendence of the embodied experience, but even this endeavor to disengage is a kind of subtle engagement. Tantra invites us to contemplate what we actively choose to engage with in life. In other words, what is of such high value that we choose to give it our wholehearted participation? It might be the quest to heal the environment, couples counseling to overcome challenges in a relationship, or the commitment to being a professional dancer. In each instance, we channel our energy and move in a direction that fosters expansiveness and growth. We recognize the circumstances appearing en route while actively participating in fulfilling our heart's intentions. The reality of being in the world is that things are going to get messy; this is the nature of life. There are diverse opinions, a multitude of motivations, and an infinite number of layers comprising the many views on a single issue. The key, therefore, is to embrace what we have chosen while preserving space for others to be just as they are. As we hold fast to what we value most and simultaneously maintain a sense of openness, we can engage with the flow of existence as we creatively sculpt a life of active participation while honoring diversity. As Douglas Brooks writes:

> Immanence is Transcendence. The real world of decision-making, law, real estate, human choice, and the blessings and tragedies of embodied life is the place where the ultimate meaning of life is to be created, sustained, and finally decided...We are not living to get to heaven after death...but rather deciding how we might experience more fully the divine while we are living[14].

Inquiries

On the Mat: Choose to participate in asana with greater enthusiasm, and sense the different parts of your internal and external being that awaken as a result. Note that even the tiniest effort will yield huge results. As you take a single step towards aligning with the intelligent matrix that is the universe, you will feel the winds of change start to blow. First, examine your relationship with the breath. It is common for practitioners to either over-control or under-engage with regard to deep breathing. Experiment with breath awareness that is active but respectful of the natural flow. As you transition to asana, engage muscle groups you might not normally use. Awaken your hand and forearm muscles and explore the toes and shins as ways to participate fully in your sadhana. Revel in the gifts of participation, and sense the power and depth of skillful engagement. Explore high-energy postures like dolphin, L at wall, down dog, plank, high lunge, knee-down lunge, upward boat & core strengtheners, standing splits, and handstand at the wall.

Off the Mat: Choose a time frame that works for you *(it might be weekly or monthly)*. Journal about one aspect of your life with which you aspire to be more involved. List five action steps to take over the course of the next week or month to create more engagement.

Practices

I cherish the moments that beckon a deeper involvement in life

Supportive Words
engage, involve, partake, take part in

Visualization
A rock climber, engaged with his entire being to support the steep, upward climb.

Complementary Breath
ujjayi

Closing Ritual
journal contemplation
What is one area of your life in which you want to participate more fully? What is one action you can take towards that deeper engagement?

I participate in the world

I choose to

I honor the ways in which

engage wholeheartedly as I sculpt the life I most want to live

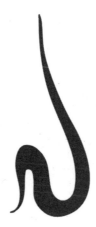

The Creative Nature of Shakti: {inspired by Bella Arguetty}

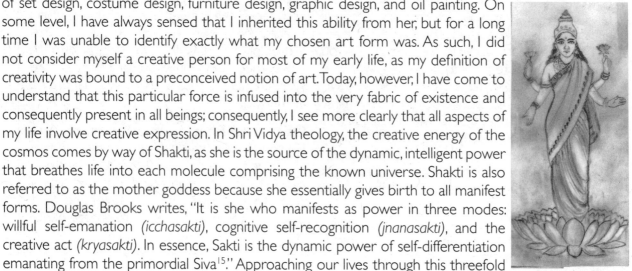

My mom is an amazing artist who has expressed her creative talent through the varied media of set design, costume design, furniture design, graphic design, and oil painting. On some level, I have always sensed that I inherited this ability from her, but for a long time I was unable to identify exactly what my chosen art form was. As such, I did not consider myself a creative person for most of my early life, as my definition of creativity was bound to a preconceived notion of art. Today, however, I have come to understand that this particular force is infused into the very fabric of existence and consequently present in all beings; consequently, I see more clearly that all aspects of my life involve creative expression. In Shri Vidya theology, the creative energy of the cosmos comes by way of Shakti, as she is the source of the dynamic, intelligent power that breathes life into each molecule comprising the known universe. Shakti is also referred to as the mother goddess because she essentially gives birth to all manifest forms. Douglas Brooks writes, "It is she who manifests as power in three modes: willful self-emanation (icchasakti), cognitive self-recognition (jnanasakti), and the creative act (kryasakti). In essence, Sakti is the dynamic power of self-differentiation emanating from the primordial Siva[15]." Approaching our lives through this threefold lens of creativity, we can utilize action to step into our desires, employ knowledge to get the ball rolling with skillfulness, and make use of our innate creative essence to make an offering.

The creative nature of shakti is in us and all around us, but just like any other force in the universe, it circulates, reseeds, and then grows. There are days when we might witness this energy manifesting in our lives as generative ideas, unbounded inspiration, or pure physical stamina to support our endeavors. At other times, we might find it challenging to access the inner well of imagination. Through embracing this particular dance with its moments of activity and pause, we become artists of life, sharing our deepest intentions in manifest form. The idea of art here is much more expansive than the traditional understanding of the word, as our creativity can manifest in unique and unexpected ways. If the universe herself is in essence creative life force, we indeed possess the innate ability to craft any feature of our path with imagination and vigor. It is thus through shakti that our intentions and knowledge can assume form and enrich our lives and the lives of others as tangible energetic offerings. As Symeon the New Theologian (English version by Ivan M. Granger) shares in the Fire Rises in Me.

The fire rises in me,
    and lights up my heart.
Like the sun!
Like the golden disk!
Opening, expanding, radiant—
    Yes!
    —a flame!

I say again:
    I don't know

what to say!

I'd fall silent
—If only I could—
but this marvel
> *makes my heart leap,*
it leaves me open mouthed
> *like a fool,*

urging me
> *to summon words*
> *from my silence*[16].

Inquiries

On the Mat: Think of your practice as an opportunity to activate the creative power that resides within your being. Set an intention to honor your desires for this practice, and acknowledge your accumulated understanding of asana. Combine these with the enlivening force of shakti to engage your postures anew and dance with your breath. Enjoy a fluid practice, literally creating art in each moment. Remember to utilize the rich palette of your asana practice to cultivate, nurture, and share the breadth of your generative potential. Explore a spontaneous flow of a variety of postures.

Off the Mat: Identify one area of your life that you consider lacking in creativity. Spend one week in the inquiry of infusing imagination into this part of your life utilizing your intention and your knowledge as raw materials. At the end of the week, write in your journal about anything that shifted.

Practices

I use my breath to fuel the animating power of shakti residing within my being. I move

Supportive Words
imagination, ingenuity, vision, innovative, inspired

Visualization
A glowing goddess rooted firmly in intention while offering up her spirited, creative nature through gesture, sound, and color.

Complementary Breath
ujjayi

Closing Ritual
At the end of your practice, use crayons or markers to illustrate whatever may be present for you in the moment. Soften around any criticisms of your drawing if they arise, and instead honor it as the embodiment of shakti.

Teacher's Note
For this class, call upon your ability to generate a flow based on the moment-to-moment experience. Forgo planning and tap into both your inner and outer awareness, and lead the class utilizing the creative stream of shakti.

and flow of creative life force

I honor the natural ebb and flow of creative life force towards my personal vision, sculpting the life I want to live

Aum: {inspired by the Teachings of Yoga}

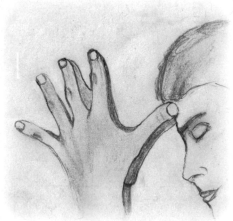

The sacred sound that has become commonplace in yoga classes throughout the world holds uncommonly profound meaning. Aum is said to be the universal sound or the sound of all sounds, and it is referred to as the Maha Mantra *(great mantra)* in Sanskrit. Aum is first mentioned indirectly in the Yajur Veda, where it is described as pranava *(the mystical or sacred syllable)*. In a later text, the Maitri Upanishad, it is written that "aum" is the primordial throb of the universe and is the sound of Atma, or consciousness. Chaitanya Kabir writes, "The whole universe comes out of a single vibration…whether we call it the 'Big Bang Theory' or we call it 'AUM,' it's the same thing. There is a single vibration that went forth from pure consciousness and elaborated itself so much that, eventually, it created the impression that there are solid things here, physical things here. But even physics will tell us that almost all of the physical space of an atom or solid material is emptiness. There's just a tiny bit of matter there, and that is just waves meeting. It's waves giving the pretense of matter[17]."

The actual pronunciation of "aum" is comprised of four parts: the "ahhh," the "oooo," the "mmmm," and silence to end. The "a" sound is the first letter of the Sanskrit alphabet and represents creation, birth, and new beginnings. The "u" is the first vowel in the alphabet and indicates sustenance of that which has been created. The "m" is the last letter in the Sanskrit alphabet and stands for dissolution as creations return to their place of origin. Finally, the silence is symbolic of the eternal nature of all of existence and reminds us that these three natural cycles pulse infinitely in our surroundings[18]. The sound of all sounds encapsulates the essence of our lives, as we, too, experience creation, sustenance, dissolution, and reabsorption on so many levels of our existence. The breath enters the body, pauses, makes its way out, and is then reabsorbed into the air around us. The seasons also follow suit, each coming into the fullness of its respective qualities, lingering for a spell, then dissolving into the advent of the next cycle. In this way, the universal sound of "aum" mirrors our own participation in this natural progression. When we are able to flow with this cyclical vibration as it manifests in our lives, we can live in a more awakened state. Dullness results when we resist new beginnings, refuse to pause with what is, or attempt to defy an ending that occurs as part of the natural course of things. Indeed the sound of "aum" has immense power, as it is a vibration that affects us on the psychological level as well as the physical. Robert Gass writes that: "Contemporary medical research has shown that chanting and other forms of vocalization actually oxygenate the cells, lower blood pressure and heart rate, increase lymphatic circulation, increase levels of melatonin, reduce stress-related hormones, [and] release endorphins[19]." By chanting this great mantra, we can better align ourselves with the energy of the heart; as with a finely tuned instrument, we can then offer ourselves more fully from a place of clarity and connection.

Inquiries

On the Mat: Use the intelligent structure of your practice to identify and explore the potency of this sacred sound. Begin in savasana *(to represent your eternal nature)*, and then slowly awaken movement using warm-ups *(occasionally chanting the first sound of "aum", "ahh")*. Next, move into standing postures and heating poses to sustain your practice *(sporadically chanting the middle sound "ooo")*, and then wind down with cooling forward folds and twists *(intermittently chanting the final sound "mmm")*. To close, return to savasana to symbolize this idea of reabsorption into our eternal, universal nature. In addition to emulating the cycle in this way, focus your awareness on other manifestations of this vibration throughout the course of your sadhana, such as breath, individual postures and movements, and thoughts that emerge and dissolve in your mind.

Off the Mat: Choose one day when you will make note of any cycles—at any level of awareness—that you notice throughout the course of your various activities and interactions. On this day, spend a few minutes chanting "aum" in the morning, afternoon, and evening.

Practices

I attune to the natural cycles of life, both internally and externally

Supportive Words
cycles, loops, phases, rhythms, rounds

Visualization
The vibrating sound of "aum" echoing off the vast sandstone walls of a desert canyon.

Complementary Breath
dirgha & aum pranayama
pausing at the third eye

Closing Ritual
Chant seven rounds of continuous "aum".

Teacher's Note
Guide a continuous "aum" in a circle, with students taking turns in the middle to receive the power of the sound.

The Divine Within You: {*inspired by Anjali Budreski*}

Namaste is the gesture used to acknowledge the completion of a yoga practice and is commonly used in India for greetings and partings. The word and accompanying gesture combine to convey a respectful acknowledgment of one another's embodied divinity. Ways of translating "namaste" include: "I bow to the divine light in you," "I salute the light of God in you," and "I honor that place where you and I recognize our interconnectedness." Ram Dass translated namaste in a poetic and beautiful way, and when we add a Tantric spin to his original words, the meaning of namaste becomes, "I honor that place in you where the entire universe resides, where lies your light and your shadow, your love and your truth, your uniqueness and your peace. When you are in that place in you and I am in that place in me, our light as individuals expands to enhance the luminosity of the greater, shared tapestry of all life." The offering of namaste is rooted in anjali mudra, the sacred gesture known as the lotus of the heart. As we enact this seal, we awaken to the light in ourselves despite our many flaws. We focus actively on our many blessings and gifts, recognizing that these will develop further over time. The motion of drawing the palms together in front of heart center is significant as an outward expression of this empowered inner state. From this reflective seat of the lotus, we can then unfurl our own petals in acknowledgment of the inherent divinity that radiates from others.

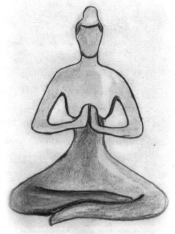

At the end of a yoga practice, there is an atmosphere of sweetness wherein we affirm ourselves and honor our fellow practitioners. The true potency of namaste, however, lies in its capacity for shaping our interactions with those around us in daily life. As we connect more fully to ourselves through dedicated mindfulness practice and self-compassion, we can further recognize our shared humanity with those we encounter. When we take namaste to the streets, so to speak, we actively acknowledge the light in all who surround us. Even when we meet people who are not aligned with our own way of life, we can honor them as embodied spirit. We can recognize that they might be rooted in fear, stress, or genuine lack of awareness, and we can choose to either offer support and skillfully engage or walk away respectfully in lieu of blaming them. Remember that when we say and practice "namaste" both at the end of a sadhana and in life, not only are we bowing to the universal energy that is us, but we are also reminding ourselves and one another of our true nature through this tangible acknowledgement of our interconnection. As Albert Einstein writes:

> *The most beautiful emotion we can experience is the mystical. It is the power of all true art and science... To know that what is impenetrable to us really exists, manifesting itself as the highest wisdom and the most radiant beauty...this knowledge, this feeling, is at the center of true religiousness. In this sense, and in this sense only, I belong to the rank of devoutly religious men.*

Inquiries

On the Mat: In yoga, we can explore this idea of rooting into ourselves through the use of breath, asana, and mudra while at the same time offering our blessing to those practicing around us. Experiment with bringing anjali mudra into your postures, and notice the potency of this sacred gesture. Take time to allow an outer expression of your inner intention to take form in each asana. As you hold poses with hands at heart center, silently connect to the reverent nature of namaste. Sense both the deep connection to self and the more expansive feeling of interconnectedness

invoked even if you are alone on your mat. Explore hands in anjali mudra or reverse in: warrior one, warrior two, lateral angle, chair, twisting chair, twisting warrior, fish, back extension in mountain, tree, wide-angle standing forward fold, and parsvotanasana.

Off the Mat: For the span of one day, silently offer namaste to people around you regardless of whether you know them or not. If possible, draw your hands into anjali mudra as you offer your blessing.

Practices

Supportive Words
celestial, divine, eternal, omnipresent, sacred

Visualization
Hands in anjali mudra, offering the blessing of namaste.

Complementary Breath
ujjayi

Closing Ritual
aum pranayama
Take three seated sun breaths. Following the last round, transition into three rounds of

aum pranayama, drawing the palms together overhead and slowly bringing the hands towards heart center as you chant "aum".

Teacher's Note
Have students sit facing one another in pairs. Invite them to draw their hands into anjali mudra, close their eyes, and spend a few moments retreating within. After a few breaths, have students open their eyes and simultaneously bow to one another while saying namaste; they can then bow to a few others nearby.

Sacred Gestures of Light: {inspired by Kripalu's Houshold Staff}

Kripalu is one of the major yoga centers in the United States. As a result, every week and weekend there are program rooms in use, yoga classes in session, and guests arriving and departing. Each morning after a yoga class ends, our household staff comes in to clean before the program assigned to the space begins the day's sessions. One day as I lingered after class to do my personal practice, two of our veteran household staff, Jose and Rosa, came in to organize and clean the room. I had seen them many times before, but on this day I happened to notice how much grace and care they brought to seemingly simple tasks like folding blankets, vacuuming, and organizing props. I was reminded of the idea that each and every one of us leaves an energetic imprint everywhere we go throughout the day. When I enter the room to teach, I don't often think about how it is that the blankets are so neatly folded or the cushions so tidily stacked, and yet the energy created by this order and attention to detail supports me in my teaching. This particular encounter seeded a desire in me to be more conscious of all the actions I take in my day-to-day life. Simply interacting with a grocery store clerk, wiping the sink clean, or leaving a secret note for a friend could make a subtle but vast difference. Every action we initiate throughout the day leaves a mark that has the power to uplift and support others.

Science defines light as energy, or as the way in which nature transfers energy through space. What usually comes to mind when we think of the word "light" is the manifestation we can see; however, it actually encompasses a much broader meaning. In physics, the terms "luminous energy" or "radiant energy" are used to describe the electromagnetic radiation to which our organs of sight react. The light we see with our eyes is only a tiny portion of a vast range called the electromagnetic spectrum. This spectrum includes gamma, ultraviolet, infrared, X-rays, and also microwaves and radio waves, all of which are part of the same wave with no divisions or boundaries. You might think of them as the parts that would show up if we were dissecting a strand of light. The main point to understand here is that light is typically depicted as a wave because it carries a vibration. In other words, "Light is vibration and vibration is light. The universe is vibrationally based, and you—as physical extensions of this nonphysical energy that has created all of this—are vibrational beings, too. Everything vibrates, and everything is communicating and reacting, responding and integrating with other things that are vibrating[20]." As such, if we are vibrational beings and light is the means by which we transfer our energy through space, our "fingerprints" of light are left everywhere we go.

In our practice of asana, each posture in effect becomes an energetic imprint of light that conveys experience and sensation from one moment to the next. The Sanskrit word "mudra" is usually defined as "seal" or "sacred gesture." As such, asanas are essentially forms of mudra. When we position our bodies in an asana, we are in fact embodying a sacred gesture that facilitates deeper absorption with consciousness and moves us towards greater awakening from the inside out. Just like the wax seals that protect the contents of confidential letters, our postures form energetic seals that provide us the space to explore the characteristics and workings of our inner landscape. The process of mudra is a two-way street, as sometimes a posture will effect a shift in our inner realm (*i.e. a forward bend creating a sense of calm*), while at other times our inner experience will dictate what sort of seal the body assumes (*i.e. intuition moving us into a heart-opening backbend*). As we begin to tune into the feeling state each posture offers, we are no longer simply utilizing asana merely as a means of movement. Instead, we intentionally engage an ancient and time-honored practice that holds tremendous possibility for impacting the whole of our life experience. B.K.S Iyengar says, "The body is my temple and asanas are my prayers[21]." When we express our own unique mudras, we pay homage to the light of our inner spirit, acknowledging our divinity and our connection to the universal. Doug Keller adds, "Just as in a temple, hatha yoga is practiced with an attention to our inner state no less than our outer body. It's a tool for working not only with the body, but also with our emotional being, uplifting and transforming our everyday feelings into qualities of the heart far greater than anything we ever thought we had within ourselves[22]." David Whyte so eloquently elaborates in *Working Together*:

We shape our self
to fit this world

and by the world
are shaped again.

The visible
and the invisible

working together
in common cause,

to produce
the miraculous.

I am thinking of the way
the intangible air

traveled at speed
round a shaped wing

easily
holds our weight.

So may we, in this life
trust

to those elements
we have yet to see

or imagine,
and look for the true

shape of our own self,
by forming it well

to the great
intangibles about us[23].

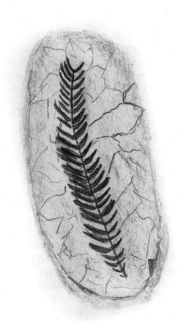

Inquiries

On the Mat: Pay attention to the imprint of the various poses and recognize the qualities unique to each seal. Notice how your internal state manifests outwardly in certain postures and how the outer placement of the body likewise influences the internal landscape. As you transition from posture to posture, contemplate what kind of imprint you are leaving behind. Finally, explore utilizing each pose to literally emboss certain qualities *(such as the balance, stability, and courage of warrior one)* into the fabric of your life through your creative and dedicated engagement on the mat. Explore a potpourri practice with standing yoga mudra, seated yoga mudra, head to knee, baby cradle, high lunge, knee-down lunge, hands inside foot in knee-down lunge, pigeon, warrior one, lateral angle, triangle, reverse warrior two, goddess, chair, dolphin dog, and humble warrior.

Off the Mat: Take one full day to explore the imprints of your physical body on both your own energy and the energy of those around you. Work in front of your computer in slumpasana and take note of your inner state, and then reverse the inquiry by assuming a more supportive posture as you continue to work. In addition to this exploration at the personal level, investigate how your interactions with others are impacted by a more closed physical posture as opposed to a more open expression.

Practices

I acknowledge the sacred gesture I create through the physical embodiment

Supportive Words
embed, etch, inscribe, instill, mark, stamp

Visualization
The ancient imprint of a fossilized leaf in stone.

Complementary Breath
nadi shodana
Focus on Vishnu mudra.

Closing Ritual
Sit in a comfortable way and place your hands in chin mudra *(thumb and index finger touch to make a small circle, palms down, on knees/ thighs)*. Take a few moments to imprint your practice by simply being.

mark on the tablet of life

of each pose   I humbly

enter the temple of my heart   I use each moment of life as an opportunity to inscribe my

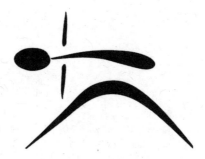

The True Teacher: {inspired by all who teach}

Who has been your greatest teacher? When I consider this question, I am always stumped. Indeed I wonder if there has been any person, incident, or conversation that did not have a lesson tucked inside. Yet the most profound effect of all of the teachings that have graced my life has been their enrichment of the guide residing within. In Sanskrit, "sat" means "true," and "guru" is translated as teacher, as well as "that which is valuable, precious, or heavy." In the Upanishads, it is written, "In the presence of the satguru; Knowledge flourishes (Gyana raksha); Sorrow diminishes (Dukha kshaya); Joy wells up without any reason (Sukha aavirbhava); Abundance dawns (Samriddhi); and all talents manifest (Sarva samvardhan)[24]"

Reflecting on times when I have felt all of these criteria at once, I remember my first meditation retreat in Malibu, California, the first time I ate a conscious meal, a week spent in the magical desert of my homeland of Israel, a study retreat with my teacher, and a lasting intimate connection. What ties all of these experiences and many others like them together is that they contributed to my practice of savoring the richness of life. For me, this has manifested as a sense of inherent fullness and the small voice within becoming more lucid and brave. Through connecting to the satguru, our self-trust is fortified, and suddenly we are able to grasp the concept that the answers to all we have been seeking indeed reside within. Even after we establish this relationship with satguru, though, it—like any relationship—requires nourishment and maintenance. By employing mindfulness, cultivating witness consciousness, doing yoga, sitting for meditation, and being in the presence of a teacher, among other things, we can strengthen this guide who dwells in the heart.

Although there are many experiences that can bolster our internal compass, history clearly demonstrates a strong emphasis on student-teacher relationships, apprenticeships, and dedicated learning with an experienced guide. When I first heard the term "guru," my preconceived notion that this word signified a pledge of allegiance to only one teacher and one set of teachings brought up uncomfortable associations of dependency and restriction. What I soon came to understand through my relationships with teachers is that what I had previously interpreted as mindless worship was instead a natural manifestation of loving devotion and gratitude for all that these guides had awakened inside of me. Furthermore, I realized that a true mentor is not interested in dependency; instead, she seeks to enlighten and empower her students so they can function as self-reliant individuals exercising their own voices.

An authentic teacher entertains the difficult questions, doesn't pretend to know it all, and is more interested in an ongoing conversation than a final destination. The true measure of a guide lies in his or her ability to support us in cultivating the seeds we have always possessed inside. The Rig Veda states, "The one who does not know the way asks of him who knows it: taught by that knowing guide, one travels forward. Truly, this is the splendid blessing of instruction: one finds the path that leads onward[25]." In asana practice, we seek guidance from an experienced mentor who offers both presence and instruction. When we step onto the mat in a class, we extend a measure of trust, signaling our intention to follow the lead of the teacher with consciousness. Through this practice, we discover our own unique expression of the asanas, ultimately sculpting an authentic inner guide. The range of experiences we meet in the practice awakens something inside, leading to greater trust of the satguru. As the class progresses, we might encounter blissfulness, the challenge of a difficult pose, the distraction of low self-worth, or the recognition of our limits. All of these come together to enable us to know ourselves more fully. Through these internal and external relationships, we can absorb teachings, wisdom, and guidance, and yet we are always the ones who must ultimately make decisions and act in accordance with our own hearts. In essence, "we are all sufficient unto our own enlightenment[26]," meaning that although others can support us on our path, we already possess the innate ability to fulfill our deepest calling.

There are two kinds of intelligence: One acquired,
as a child in school memorizes facts and concepts
from books and from what the teacher says,
collecting information from the traditional sciences
as well as from the new sciences.

With such intelligence you rise in the world.
You get ranked ahead or behind others
in regard to your competence in retaining
information. You stroll with this intelligence
in and out of fields of knowledge, getting always more
marks on your preserving tablets.

There is another kind of tablet, one
already completed and preserved inside you.
A spring overflowing its springbox. A freshness
in the center of the chest. This other intelligence
does not turn yellow or stagnate. It's fluid,
and it doesn't move from outside to inside
through the conduits of plumbing-learning.

This second knowing is a fountainhead
from within you, moving out[27].

Inquiries

On the Mat: Take this inquiry into a class and notice the play between the outer teacher and your own inner teacher. When do you need to listen more to your own voice? In what ways are you supported by the wisdom of another?

Off the Mat: Spend three days carefully observing your internal teacher. Make note of instances in which you discount this personal wisdom. Use the three days that follow to actively cultivate the strength of sourcing decisions from this place of deep inner knowing.

Practices

Supportive Words

guide, guru, mentor, teacher

Visualization

Think about someone who has been an influential teacher for you, and envision this person residing inside your heart, seated in a position of strength, dignity, and grace.

Complementary Breath

ujjayi

Closing Ritual

journal contemplation
What qualities of your external teacher do you most admire? What qualities of your inner teacher do you most value? How are they similar? How are they different?

Teacher's Note

Pick three poses from each of the main planning categories (*standing, inversions, arm balances, hip openers, backbends, forward bends and twists, relaxation*). During the class, create space for students to choose one posture from each group in which they feel they could use support, and have them work with a partner. Remind students that this support from the outer teacher (*the partner*) helps reinforce the inner teacher, or the satguru.

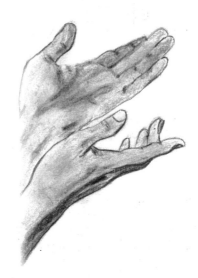

The Yamas & Niyamas: {*inspired by Todd Norian & Kripalu's Spiritual Lifestyle Program*}

During my time as a volunteer at Kripalu, I engaged in practices that generated a tremendous amount of energy. Raising energy through asana and breath in this way, I experienced shifts that provoked new feelings and sensations inside. My vitality was increased, and the conduits of my body were literally rushing with increased life force. One of the metaphors used to teach us how to interact with this heightened level of energy was that of gradually strengthening a container to prepare it to sustain increased volume. In this way, I built a strong foundation to ensure that I was able to consciously utilize heightened levels of energy on the physical, emotional, and intellectual levels. Still, there were a few times when a jolt of life force caught me unprepared with the result that I ended up betraying my original intentions by indulging in large quantities of unsupportive food, handling sexual desires in an imbalanced way, or mismanaging day-to-day tasks. As a strategy for becoming more skillful with regard to the heightened levels of prana in order to avoid outcomes such as these, we can embark upon an inquiry of the yamas and niyamas.

The yamas and niyamas are part of Patanjali's eight-limbed path of yoga. In classical thought, the system is structured like a ladder; one must progress sequentially through each limb in order to arrive at the pinnacle of liberation. Patanjali introduces the yamas and niyamas as the first two limbs of his eight-fold path, with the implication that study and practice of these concepts should precede engagement with any of the other limbs. According to the Tantric reinterpretation of Patanjali's path, though, the system is less linear. A seeker can start with asana, concentration, or meditation and later learn about the yamas and niyamas to further enrich his yoga practice. In the West, many yoga students have not been introduced to these concepts, as the third limb of asana (*the seat or physical posture*) is the most frequently emphasized. That said, there are potent benefits to studying these guidelines before or in conjunction with the practices of asana and meditation. The yamas are a set of externally-oriented strategies that support us in navigating our relationships with other people and our interactions with the outside world. The niyamas are more personally oriented ones for sustaining us in the exploration of our inner landscape and embodiment of spirit. Essentially, these first two limbs comprise a foundation of contemplations with direct application to life both on and off the mat in support of our deeper physical and energetic practices.

The potency of the yamas and niyamas is their role as conversation starters to stimulate meaningful practical inquiry and an enlightening internal dialogue through questions like: How does nonviolence apply to this situation? What would happen if I utilized more softness in this incident? Can I manage my energy more effectively this week? Through engaging in dialogue with these ideas, we can learn how to fully embrace each experience even if it is ripe with discomfort. The benefit of this particular approach to these principles is that they become our own guidelines as opposed to rules etched in stone or regulations imposed by someone else. There are many possible interpretations for each yama and niyama, and this enhances their value. All of the yamas and niyamas provide us food for thought in this regard; they challenge us to mindfully tailor our interpretations based on our individual lives and the situations we encounter. This is indeed the true grandeur of these principles; they serve as our tools in the workshop of life as we ask the explorative questions that move us closer to what feels most authentic in each passing moment.

Ahimsa:

As human beings, we naturally encounter moments that tempt us to diminish one or several parts of our being. This tendency might manifest in the desire to have a body part look differently, a repetitive cycle of thoughts and feelings of unworthiness, or actual physical violence resulting from deep inner frustration with ourselves or with the world at large. Ahimsa, or the yama of peace making, offers a useful lens through which to explore our inner landscape. It sets the challenge of walking our path with the intention of harming neither ourselves nor those around us. Although it can be tempting to assign a clear-cut definition of ahimsa, in reality this must be skillfully adjusted based on the situation at hand. How could there be just one way to look at nonviolence? One could argue that nonharming means being a vegetarian and not killing animals. Another could argue that by not eating some food from animal sources, she is being violent to herself because she has discovered that her body does not function well without a certain amount of animal protein. As with this example, the fundamental question becomes whether there is a way to be conscious and have our needs met at the same time.

Furthermore, what might seem like a practice limited exclusively to the physical realm actually applies to all facets of life. A true exploration of ahimsa, for example, extends even to the realm of habitual communication, as words don't simply say things but in fact create our experience of reality. Many people move through their days leading peaceful lives externally, but internally they are beating themselves up, judging every action and living in turmoil. In addition, the violent thoughts and words we direct towards others have an energetic imprint of their own. The tone, volume, and pitch of our voice can convey significant emotional information, and our nonverbal expressions are also powerful indicators of what is happening inside. In a sense, the endeavor to lead lives of nonviolence encourages us to become more attentive to, and conscious of, the full spectrum of our interactions with the world. Simply plowing through daily experiences, challenges, and confrontations is a common mode of operation. With ahimsa guiding us, though, we can contemplate how to most skillfully engage with each situation that arises and actively choose the most nonviolent action while still acknowledging our boundaries. As Judyth Hill writes:

Wage peace with your breath.

Breathe in firemen and rubble,
breathe out whole buildings and flocks of redwing
blackbirds.

Breathe in terrorists
and breathe out sleeping children and freshly mown fields.

Breathe in confusion, and breathe out maple trees.

Breathe in the fallen and breathe out lifelong friendships intact.

Wage peace with your listening: hearing sirens, pray loud.

Remember your tools: flower seeds, clothespins, clean rivers.

Make soup.

Play music. Memorize the words for "thank you" in three

languages.

Learn to knit, and make a hat.

Think of chaos as dancing raspberries.
Imagine grief
as the out breath of beauty
or the gesture of fish.

Swim for the other side.

Wage peace.

Never has the world seemed so fresh and precious.

Have a cup of tea, and rejoice.

Act as if armistice has already arrived.
Celebrate today[28].

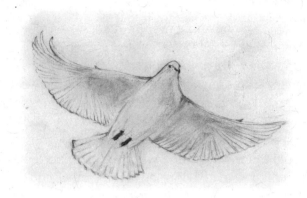

Inquiries

On the Mat: In yoga, our tendencies can be illuminated by simply noticing the level of violence we are enacting in each posture and asking ourselves, "Am I finding my edge, or am I straining to prove something to myself or the world?" Take note whether the adage, "No pain no gain!" has trapped you into believing that the harder you work, the greater benefit you will receive. In this practice, explore modifications *(easier versions of postures)* and variations *(more difficult versions of postures)*, while taking the responsibility to find your own expression of nonviolence in each passing moment. Move beyond the notion of ahimsa on the physical plane, and excavate the concept more deeply, identifying the subtle ways in which you assail yourself through repetitive unsupportive thoughts, words, and habits. Explore a potpourri session with mountain, standing half moon, tree, standing forward fold, runner's stretch, twisting high lunge, warrior one, twisting warrior, down dog, three-legged dog, leg twist in down dog, lateral angle, intense stretch, baby cradle, reclined hand to big toe, and revolved reclined hand to big toe.

Off the Mat: Take one week to investigate both the subtle and obvious ways in which you are violent to yourself and those around you.

Practices

Today I stand in mindful exploration of nonharming

words with others

I choose to observe

Supportive Words
consideration, empathy, non-harming,
nonviolence, soft-heartedness, tenderness.

Complementary Breath
digha

Visualization
A white dove spreading wings wide and
soaring high with gentleness and strength.

my relationship with myself as well as the ways in which I utilize the power of actions, thoughts, and

Satya:

The concept of truth is one of the most enigmatic topics in life. Standing in certainty and letting our light shine fully can feel more intimidating than climbing Mount Everest. If we make a habit of choosing to act and speak from our deepest sense of integrity, we will inevitably be required to do so in situations that will challenge our limits. By declaring, "I am an artist, and this is my passion!" we indeed open ourselves to tests of our resolve. Aligning with this authenticity, it is up to us to manifest our best, most authentic embodiment of this affirmation. As per this example, truthfulness within is indeed the groundwork of satya. Only from the foundation of honesty with ourselves can we authentically interact with the world. Sometimes we create truths geared towards pleasing others, but in reality these are often masks to hide our authenticity, which can be frightening or overwhelming. Rumi writes "the heart is comforted by true words just as a thirsty man is comforted by water[28.5]." With this knowledge, can we open to recognizing our innermost certainty, no matter how scary it might be? When I began to realize I was attracted to men, I was extremely afraid. I wanted to hide this fact because I knew doing so would be easier than the alternative. Ultimately, though, the energy of that fear was exactly what I needed to propel me forward, as it allowed me to shed the inhibiting layers and step into alignment with my heart.

Some schools of thought maintain that there is one essential, unchanging truth with which we must align as we quell the distractions of our creative mind. In the Tantric reinterpretation of this yama, though, the fact that everything in life shifts and changes is recognized even with respect to satya. Our deepest certainty today might differ from that of a year ago. The nature and identity of our certainty might shift because we have acted with integrity and thus unearthed a new knowing, or, contrarily, because we have retreated due to fear. Both are equally valid catalysts, and the manifested truth should be held with admiration and respect. After several years together, a friend's partner decided he wanted to be in a more open relationship. That was his genuine stance at the time, and he was not able to budge, for doing so would have meant disregarding this internal knowing. She felt extremely challenged because her conviction was one of monogamy, but she also loved him dearly. Herein lies the simultaneous beauty and tyranny of truth. In this instance, my friend's partner was not bad, nor was she good; they were simply in different places. When we encounter a situation like this in which we are merely rooted in a different vision than another, we can recognize that it is time to agree to disagree with open hearts, acceptance, and respect for the other's position. In this way, the practice of satya carves out space for ownership of our feelings, practice of conscious communication, and embodiment of integrity, honesty, and authenticity. As Danna Faulds writes:

> "There are as many paths
> to truth as there are
> heartbeats, leaves, fireflies
> in summer twilight[29]."

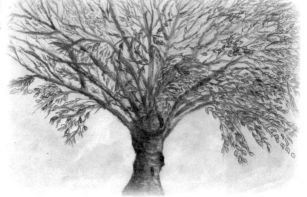

Inquiries

On the Mat: We can reflect upon whether we are standing in our truth with regard to the practice level we are choosing and our approach to the postures. As a pointed inquiry, return to warrior two often in your sequence, and tune into your personal integrity in the moment as you hold the posture longer with each repetition. Deepen the front thighbone each time you explore the pose, and notice how the reality of what nurtures you shifts and changes. Explore a strong standing pose practice with standing forward fold, mountain, flying warrior one, chair, standing half moon, goddess, tree, standing marychiasana, down dog, leg twist in down dog, reverse warrior two, and warrior two with eagle arms.

Off the Mat: Take a few days to clearly identify the central ideas comprising your certainty at present. How have these changed over time? Is the truth you are rooted in now the same as that of months or years ago? Compare your notions of authenticity with those of someone else in your life. How are your visions similar, and how do they differ?

Practices

Today I take comfort in the light of my truth

Supportive Words
authenticity, certainty, honesty, genuineness, integrity, truthfulness

Complementary Breath
bhastrika

Visualization
An oak tree rooted strongly in earth, yet responsive to the changing winds of nature.

ways that nourish and strengthen my spirit. I stand in my authentic certainty even in the midst of

I honor myself fully in

challenge

Asteya:

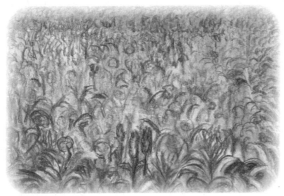

Asteya translates as "non-stealing" or "non-devaluing" and invites us to contemplate how our words, thoughts, and actions towards others and ourselves affect our life's vibration. As we move through our days, we can be easily swept into a whirlwind of drama, gossip, and nitpicking others' faults. When we find ourselves in a rampage of unfounded criticism without the ability to examine what is being triggered inside of us, we are in a sense stealing the right of another to exist in his or her uniqueness. While asteya can sometimes be interpreted as a moratorium on all evaluative judgment, the Tantric mindset maintains that there is value in having conscious discernment with regard to people, events, and life choices. The refinement of this practice is understood as the ability to critically assess and also hold space for a diverse view. Instead of diminishing the other vantage point, we are invited to acknowledge our disagreement but also open to understanding that this alternate perspective indeed has value, even if only for the other person. Non-stealing can also be understood more literally as not taking things that do not belong to us whether they are someone's material possessions, creative ideas, or time in the spotlight. Finally, the principles of asteya are equally as useful in our relationship with self. Our internal self-talk as well as our conversations with others can reveal the unconscious ways in which we devalue ourselves every single day. This can manifest as unintentional yet consistent use of disempowering language that simply fills empty space and lacks an empowered quality. Regular use of the word "sorry" after each statement or overuse of adverbs like "maybe," "perhaps," and "kind of" signal the subtle ways in which we steal our own inherent potential. As Hafitz writes:

> What
> We speak
> Becomes the house we live in.
>
> Who will want to sleep in your bed
> If the roof leaks
> Right above
> It?
>
> Look what happens when the tongue
> Cannot say to kindness,
>
> "I will be your slave."
>
> The moon
> Covers her face with both hands
>
> And can't bear
> To look[30].

Inquiries

On the Mat: Take this inquiry into the studio, and notice whether you easily slip into a mindset of looking at others and identifying their inadequacies. Do you have a constant, running critique of the teacher or the form of other students' postures or bodies? Investigate the moments when you feel the desire to steal another's masterful expression of an asana, even though you are not ready or able to come into the same pose. Gauge whether you spend precious practice time scrutinizing the ways in which you yourself are not measuring up to a preconceived ideal of perfection and thus subverting your own meaningful intention. Each of these is an example of stealing, as we rob ourselves of the potential for deeper connection with the current experience by engaging in these thoughts or practices. Instead of giving full attention to that which yields growth and expansion, we devalue the moment and create barriers to the energy of possibility. Use the practice of coordinated breath and movement to aid you in pinpointing awareness of the obvious and subtle ways in which you debase your own experience. As we become more conscious of the recurring patterns that detract from our practice, we can begin to choose a different path and honor ourselves as we are.

Off the Mat: For a period of two weeks, maintain an asteya log. Cultivate heightened awareness of how much time and energy you spend focusing on others faults, gossiping, and creating drama. When you notice these behaviors, make note of them in your log. Briefly describe each incident, and take a few moments to formulate a hypothesis of what deeper issues may be at the root.

Practices

Today I value the unique offerings of others I allow them to move through

Supportive Words
cheapen, debase, devalue, diminish, non-stealing, talk down, write off

Visualization
A meadow of wildflowers, each shining in its own way; because of the diversity, the overall beauty is amplified.

Complementary Breath
natural

life at their own pace honoring their light

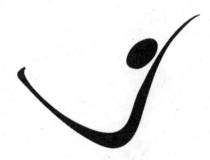

Brahmacharya:

Brahmacharya translates to "walking like or towards Brahma, the deity of creation," and has traditionally been used as a term to describe a life of strict practices, dedicated learning, and deep introspection. In classical thought, celibacy was one of the primary criteria of this yama, as sexual energy was viewed as an obstacle to true enlightenment and happiness. The practice of repressing and disciplining the source of these disturbances was thought to allow practitioners to move closer to the energy of the divine. As yoga philosophy evolved and changed, however, other interpretations emerged to contend that true embodiment of consciousness comes through embracing our whole selves. These models encourage mindful exploration of sexuality and other desires, recognizing that the resulting energies can serve as remarkable opportunities for learning by virtue of their intensity. Entering this realm of more pervasive exploration, we must still bear in mind that anything in excess can cause distress and lack of focus. The remedy, however, is not repression, but rather a watchful and moderate engagement. As a result of these shifting interpretations, Brahmacharya has come to be defined as energy management, conscious self-restraint, or conscious moderation with regard to various forms of stimuli including food, intimacy, thought, and action.

Dinabandhu Garrett Sarley offers the perspective that yoga is that which creates the most vitality in our lives. In other words, whatever generates a charge, increases life force, and enhances energy is the practice of yoga. In this interpretation, any experience such as one of art, intimacy, asana, meditation, music, friends, or nature can be labeled yoga when approached with mindfulness and clear intention. We can utilize the practice of energy management in any of these realms to engage in the inquiry of prioritizing vitality. Many individuals turn to the practice of yoga after reaching an extreme in their lives that spurs a desire to live a more authentic life. Typically, we are bombarded with constant stimulation from television, advertising, work, family, shopping, and other demands on our time. People get burned-out as a result of overcommitted schedules, addictions to unhealthy foods, and lack of self-nourishment. If we open to the idea that everything in the physical world breaks down into a vibrational frequency, which in turn has profound effects on our energy, we can better choose those elements of life that renew us and enable us to function optimally. What would happen if we could pause before every action to contemplate whether it would augment or deplete our life force? Work can be a conduit to increased energy and vitality if we have a professional passion. It can also be a complete drain. A relationship can be an expansive channel for heightened life force, or it can be an immense weight dragging us down. How would things shift if we infused more conscious choices into all areas of our lives?

The first step in working with energy is becoming aware of how our choices impact our daily lives, either uplifting or depleting our vitality. The second phase of the process involves recognizing times when we have become mired in a depleting pattern, acknowledging the contrast and taking steps toward a more life-enhancing way of being. The third skill necessary for walking the path of moderation is flexibility, adjusting our energy management based on each individual situation we encounter. As we engage these steps to temper a habitual behavior that is depleting our life force, we are likely to feel more centered and vital. At some point, we may retreat into a choice that depletes our life force. The key here is simply to recognize the learning available to us in these moments as we stay the course of developing a more conscious relationship to our management of time, our food choices, and the company we keep. The power of yoga is that it helps us develop fluency in this practice. As Dinabandhu states, "A yogi doesn't stop making mistakes; he just doesn't make the same mistake twice." If we make a choice that does not reverberate with the positive charge of amplified energy, we simply recognize that we would choose another avenue the next time around.

Inquiries

On the Mat: As our sadhana progresses, we seek to harness and distribute our energy in even and supportive ways. Explore your relationship to energy management through your approach to asana. Do you dive straight into vigorous postures, tire quickly, and then find yourself unable to sustain the rest of the experience? Or do you take too long to start up and feel your energy fizzle in the absence of sufficient stimulation? In addition to its applications to the whole of your practice, investigate energy distribution at the level of each posture. In standing poses, what shifts when you distribute the breath more fully to the lower part of the body? Likewise, note whether your experience of arm-balancing asanas differs if you allocate more energy to the upper body. In addition to these inquiries, notice any shifts in energy with respect to the time of day you do your sadhana. In a morning practice, you might start slower but conclude with less emphasis on cooling postures so you are alert and ready for your day. In an afternoon or evening class, most of the day's activity is already done, so ending with more forward folds, hip openers, and twists can support deeper relaxation and preparation for rest. Observing your thoughts and the energy they produce is another avenue for gauging how you choose to generate and allocate life force. Explore a varied practice with standing half moon, standing crane, tree, warrior one, high lunge, knee-down lunge, hands inside foot in knee-down lunge, quad stretch in knee-down lunge, arms at side in warrior three, balancing half moon, eagle, eagle back extension, cobra, boat, and bow.

Off the Mat: For one week, track both the sources of your energy and your expenditures. Take note of specifics. If you go for a hike, do you feel a peak in vitality? What happens when you watch TV for several hours? How are your food choices affecting your energy levels? Who contributes to your energy, and who drains your life force? At the end of the week, write about the effects of this inquiry and consider what changes you might make to help balance your life force.

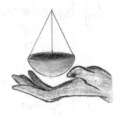
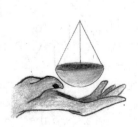

Practices

Supportive Words
*balance, center, midline, middle place,
moderation, skillful restraint*

Visualization
Your own hands as scales, with palms facing up,
weighing what will keep you vital.

Complementary Breath
nadi shodana
Focus on the ability of this breath to create a
sense of ease and moderation from within.

Aparigraha:

One of my own personal encounters with letting go surfaced in the process of moving from Los Angeles to Boston. Knowing where I wanted to live in Boston but not wanting to make the trip cross-country to look for an apartment, I searched online and found a studio apartment that seemed spacious and nice. A friend who was living in Boston offered to check the place out on my behalf and reported that it was pleasant, so I decided to take it. When I arrived at my new abode, I was shocked to discover that the entire studio was the size of my bathroom in Los Angeles! I was in mid-breakdown when I realized I had no option but to soften into the reality of the moment, as the lease had already been signed. My ill-proportioned belongings arrived from the West, and somehow I managed to construct a livable space. Before long, I was quite comfortable in my new, albeit tight, quarters. Months later, I came to appreciate having had the experience of living in such a small room. It encouraged me to consider more carefully what things I truly needed to feel a sense of abundance. When I traveled to India later that year and saw the sizes of homes that sometimes housed entire families, I was humbled further.

Non-attachment is the practice of letting go of those elements of our lives that continually cycle through draining our vital life force. By clinging to people who have passed, places we have left, unresolved feelings, or circumstances beyond our control, we can potentially brew tremendous discomfort and suffering for ourselves and others. Living in a state of attachment not only stifles the possibilities of the present moment, but also diminishes our ability to create an optimal future. Our most significant encounters with non-attachment usually occur at times of change such as the loss of a job or the death of a family member. When we cling to any aspect of our existence with anger, frustration, desperation, or anxiety, we end up thrusting ourselves against the proverbial brick wall, with only pain and bruises to show for our efforts. In addition to intense moments of life transition, attachment can surface in the day-to-day as we interact with partners, friends, work, and material possessions. When we develop strong attachments to any of these, we naturally feel compelled to guard against their loss with an attitude of desperation. As a result, our focus shifts from abundance to lack, and this defensive stance roots our actions in fear and worry as opposed to trust. In the Tantric world view, the invitation to non-attachment does not require disengaging from our surroundings or disconnecting emotionally from our relationships and lives. Instead, it encourages us to recognize letting go as a normal part of life that has the potential to create space and possibility. Our emotional states naturally follow the contour of a wave, with peaks and valleys that cycle continuously. Any emotion we experience is likely to linger for a while, float away, and eventually return. Instead of holding on to extreme joy or pushing away extreme grief, we can step into the dance of maneuvering this natural flux with skillful non-attachment. As Danna Faulds writes:

The first of this year's
leaves lets go and drifts,
no breeze to bear it.
With lazy grace the leaf
unwinds its growing
season in a dancing
downward spiral, lands
in silence, making of
itself a perfect offering
to the altar of the earth[31].

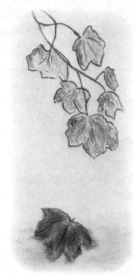

Inquiries

On the Mat: In yoga, it is important to have a certain amount of attachment to the way we engage our practice. Yet there are times when we cling so strongly to one way of being that our sadhana starts to lose its luster. Notice if there are moments when you become so fixated and inflexible regarding the outward manifestation of your yoga that you become disconnected from your true essence. Attachment appears on the mat as the belief that we must do a particular sequence of asanas even if it isn't fully serving us, as irritation when presented with an unfamiliar posture, or as clinging to a single, rigid idea of a particular pose. Experiment with letting go of attachment to notions of "right" postures or ways of practice. Approach your experience with beginner's mind, and hone your awareness of moments when frustration arises. Stretch your capacity to hold diverse feelings, sensing how letting go augments your life force even though it may initially bring about discomfort. Set an intention at the beginning of practice to investigate areas of your life in which you are unnerved by your own grasping tendencies. In savasana, use a complete body scan to encourage ease and letting go as you transition into relaxation. Explore forward folds like standing forward fold, humble warrior, hands inside foot in knee-down lunge, child, down dog, head to knee, cow face, and wide-angle forward fold.

Off the Mat: Go to a closet or storage area in your house, and find an item you have kept for years but never use. Notice what thoughts or feelings come up when you consider giving this object away. Intentionally choose to let go of this item, and note the effects of this action.

Supportive Words
letting go, release, unconstrained, unwind, clutching, non-attachment, non-clinging, non-possessiveness.

Visualization
A brilliant yellow maple leaf in autumn, gently floating towards the earth.

Complementary Breath
dirgha
Focus on every exhalation.

in each moment

my attachment to any

people, possessions, and thoughts that are blocking my way. I affirm that I am doing the best I can.

Saucha:

The first niyama aids us in establishing order in our lives on all the various planes of existence to serve our deepest intentions and desires. Leading a conscious life is no small task; it requires ardent dedication, acute awareness, and ready compassion. In the context of a conscious life, saucha is often interpreted simply as devotion to physical cleanliness or a preconceived notion of purity. While bodily hygiene is indeed important, this principle encompasses much more. Saucha encourages us to ask deeper questions regarding the structure and ordering of our lives, such as, "What do I need to clear out of the way so that I can focus on what I came here to do?" This niyama helps us identify what blocks, both external and internal, we must remove to make progress and follow our objectives. At times, we are extremely clear regarding our purpose, but practical realities or internal emotional knots impede the path that leads there. Through a practice of saucha, though, we can begin to refocus and reorganize our lives so that our external circumstances and surroundings facilitate our internal process. When we clean, arrange, and let go of items that are no longer of use, we stimulate renewed flow of energy and access previously unknown channels of creativity. During the process of writing this book, daily attention to saucha was vitally important; doing regular asana practice, paying the bills, prepping food, and keeping my living space tidy all influenced my ability to nestle in and write. When these tasks remain undone and start to accumulate, I feel increasingly overwhelmed, and my ability to focus is compromised. Through implementing the skillful guidance of saucha to smooth everyday functioning, we can find support in honoring the commitments of our path and do what is necessary in order to further our goals. Ways to cultivate this practice include: daily rituals to cleanse the body *(pranyama, internal flushing with water, belly pumping, skin exfoliation, tongue scraping)*, to-do lists to support organization, and mindful arrangement of living space and work environment. As the Mother beautifully writes:

> *You carry with you, around you, in you, the atmosphere created by your actions, and if what you do is beautiful, good, and harmonious your atmosphere is beautiful, good, and harmonious*[32].

Inquiries

On the Mat: Notice how yoga enables you to connect more fully to your body and breath, which in turn allows you to step into your decision-making process with greater clarity and ease. In the mat practice itself, cultivate saucha by focusing on postures and sequences that aid in clearing your physical body of any internal or external obstructions. Sense the resulting increase in vitality as breath reaches further into your extremities and the brain is literally rebalanced. Use your asanas to focus on revitalizing and aligning the body in a more refined, conscious way. Note whether this intention supports you in better organizing your life to serve your calling when you step off the mat. To highlight the qualities of saucha, focus on deep, cleansing pranayamas, energizing standing postures, and refreshing twists. Identify any obstacles crowding your path, and position your body with precision to align the physical and energetic planes of each pose. Utilize the cleansing effects of twisting postures and pranayama to advantage to clear out internal clutter and make room for that which will most deeply nurture your body, mind, and spirit. Explore twisting postures with high lunge, knee-down lunge, warrior one, standing marichyasana, twisting warrior, lateral angle, bound angle, easy pose twist, half lord of the fishes, head to knee, Marichyasana one, and revolved head to knee.

Off the Mat: Choose to reorganize your altar, a shelf, or an entire room. Change the location of sacred items, rearranging them in the spirit of saucha to invoke renewed energy and clarity.

Practices

Supportive Words
organization, lucidity, hygiene, exactitude

Visualization
An organized living space nurturing clarity and openness.

Complementary Breath
kapalabhati

Today I use saucha as a reminder that my

Focus on the cleansing properties of the breath.

Teacher's Note
Invite your students to arrange their mats in a new pattern that will serve the inquiry of saucha.

of energy in my life

outer environment serves

my inner intention, I mindfully clear away any physical or emotional obstacles constricting the flow

Santosha:

One of the gifts of living in a region with a long winter is the contrast offered by the arrival of spring. By late spring, I typically feel the veils of winter lifting and enter a spell of enthusiasm, passion, and joy as the climate shifts in earnest. One spring, after several days of feeling blissful, I awoke with a different sentiment in my heart. I paused to contemplate how to label what I was experiencing. It didn't feel like eagerness, happiness, or even hopefulness; it was merely contentment. With the contrast of delight suddenly absent, there was a distinct quality of sweetness to the sense of equanimity that remained in its wake. I wasn't overwhelmed or underwhelmed, ecstatic or sad; I simply felt present and full of peace. Santosha is the practice of cultivating this state of contentment, which resides in the space between uplifting emotions (*eagerness, enthusiasm, love*) and more subdued ones (*boredom, pessimism, frustration*). It relates to the quality of being wholeheartedly present and not worrying about the past or anticipating the future for a period of time. Contentment can sometimes manifest as a moment of simply sitting still or an ordinary yet mindful task repeated in a soothing and constant rhythm. This sense of equanimity is characterized by the practice of living with the elements of life that are already before us instead of wanting or seeking more. In our modern day culture, this can be an incredibly challenging practice; moments of santosha can become rare as we rollercoaster between the extreme highs and uncomfortable lows triggered by external stimuli. In fact, because many people spend their lives constantly amped up by television, caffeine, consumerism, entertainment, and the like, what might actually be a moment of contentment is often mislabeled as mundane. Instead of pausing to savor a space before us, we race to fill it with the next distraction and thus miss out on the richness embedded in simply being. To practice contentment is to say, "This is enough, this moment is enough, this person is enough, this meal is enough right here and now." As Gary Snyder writes:

> It is as hard to get the children herded into the car pool and down the road to the bus as it is to chant sutras in the Buddha-hall on a cold morning. One move is not better than the other, each can be quite boring, and they both have the virtuous quality of repetition. Repetition and ritual and their good results come in many forms. Changing the filter, wiping noses, going to meetings, picking up around the house, washing dishes, checking the dipstick—don't let yourself think these are distracting you from your more serious pursuits. Such a round of chores is not a set of difficulties we hope to escape from so that we may do our "practice" which will put us on a "path"—it is our path[33].

Inquiries

On the Mat: Yoga is a practice that targets the nervous system directly and can help bring us back into balance if we have grown accustomed to oscillating between extremes of being overwhelmed and underwhelmed. Yoga can support us in building the internal muscle to savor moments of contentment through focus of breath and presence of body. In this practice, focus on moving the body in a steady way that is not overly fast or overly slow. Choose one posture that typically infuses you with high energy, and practice it in a modified way. For example, instead of half lotus in tree, practice the posture with the foot on the inner shin. Can you tap into a sense of tranquility without the immediate high? Next, choose a posture that had been frustrating you recently because of its challenging nature. Use as many props and supports necessary to engage the pose and remain present for five to ten cycles of breath. Even amidst the slight discomfort, can you locate an experience of santosha? Explore easy pose twist, bound angle, head to knee, standing yoga mudra, hands inside foot in knee-down lunge, parsvotanasana, twisting warrior, wide-angle seated forward bend, and revolved wide-angle seated forward bend.

Off the Mat: For the duration of one week, pause once each day to acknowledge and record something with which you are wholly and simply content.

Practices

Supportive Words
contentment, tranquility, relaxing into life, self-trust, peace

Visualization
Swinging in a hammock on the first day of spring, bathed by sun and air that is just warm enough.

Complementary Breath
ujjayi

Today I deepen my relationship to equanimity. I honor both the ups and downs of life and bathe in the contentment available at present.

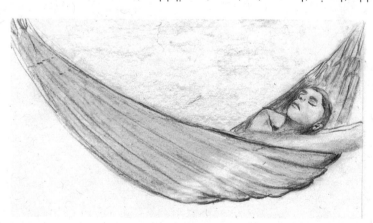

Tapas:

Real intensity is not something many people seek out on a daily basis, yet the practice of tapas beckons us into its fires to experience deep transformation. As we organize our lives and gain clarity with regard to our path through saucha, we can begin to explore practices that challenge limits and build dedication through the transformative heat of tapas. Encounters with intensity are true tests of how much we value what we are moving towards in life. By approaching these moments with curiosity instead of recoiling from them, we can build energy and begin to peel away the layers masking our inner brilliance. Once these have eroded, we can experience deeper expansion and live our lives more authentically. Engaging the intelligent discipline of tapas

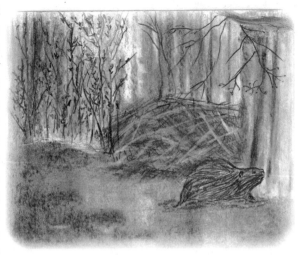

involves imposing a limitation on a particular aspect of our experience. This restriction serves as the foundation of our practice, and ultimately it is friction with this boundary that generates the ensuing sensation and fire. Initially, the constraint might seem like a suffocating mandate, but it almost reveals itself to be a gift in disguise. Through intentionally adopting various limitations, we ultimately find our way to enhanced freedom. For example, limiting unsupportive foods often leads to more vitality, and creating clear boundaries around social interactions and media consumption typically makes more space for time in nature or self-reflection. In nature, beavers build intricate dams that harness flowing waters to create lush wetlands. These wetlands attract more fish, ducks, frogs, and other wildlife while providing the beavers a safe haven from natural predators. It is thus through their implementation of a firm boundary that they engender more possibility for themselves as well as the surrounding environment[34].

The practice of tapas can be daunting at first because the entity *(physical, behavioral, or energetic)* we choose to limit is often one to which we are very attached. Although we may recognize that a particular vice is detracting from our life force in the long run, taking the step of limiting ourselves is the hardest part of the process. The key to the practice of tapas is choosing self-imposed limits not as a form of punishment but rather one of inquiry. These restrictions spawn intensity and heat that provide us with contemplations and rich life lessons, which serve as gateways to savoring more of life. The practice of tapas invites us to stray from the path of our habitual behaviors into the fertile territory of challenge in order to discover new features of our ever-changing internal landscape.

Inquiries

On the Mat: Our yoga practice is the perfect laboratory for working with the niyama of tapas. The first application is in the basic discipline of showing up on the mat, whether in class or at home. By setting a firm commitment to your practice time, you create a boundary that supports your overall schedule as well as your dedication to having a regular yoga sadhana. By imposing limits on a particular area of the body through the technical details of our postures, we can experience openings in another. In cobra pose, try rooting your legs and tops of the feet firmly against the earth, and sense whether more freedom becomes available in your torso as you rise up and expand into the pose. In pincha mayurasana, utilize a strap to impose constraints. Bind the forearms, and note what happens to your ability to maintain the pose. As you deepen the breath in your centering, place your hands at the sides of your rib cage, feeling how the internal limit of the ribs channels the flow of prana into the rest of the body. Move through a sequence to open the hamstrings utilizing isometric resistance for deeper expansion. Explore high lunge, knee-down lunge, down dog, warrior one and two, runner's stretch, triangle, lateral angle, hamstring stretch in standing forward fold, one foot behind the other in down dog, and reclined hand to big toe pose with a strap.

Off the Mat: Call to mind some habits that are currently not serving you, such as lack of physical activity, overconsumption of caffeine or sugar, or addiction to doing. For a period of three days, try placing a limit on one of these habits. At the end of each day, journal about what has transpired for you physically, mentally, and emotionally.

Practices

Supportive Words
heat, dedication, commitment, intelligent limits

Visualization
A beaver dam, sturdy and strong as a boundary, yet engendering more possibility.

Complementary Breath
alternate-nostril kapalabhati
Focus on how limiting and closing one nostril creates more openness and energy on the opposite side.

Today I choose healthy limits that support my overall well-being and life's purpose

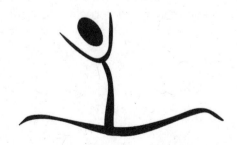

Svadyaya:

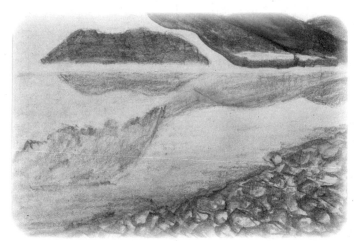

Self-study is one of the most beneficial practices of the yoga experience, as it is the primary seed for deepened and awakened consciousness. In the light of intentional contemplation, we begin to see previously obscured features and details of our actions, thoughts, and words. When we inventory the many qualities and patterns comprising our being, which in turn deeply influence our interactions with others and the world, we access a more conscious locus from which to make decisions. Through self-study, we get to know ourselves better, becoming acquainted with our likes and dislikes as well as our deeply-held values and beliefs thereby gaining clarity with regard to our priorities in life. This is often extremely challenging given that we are not typically attuned to the deeper implications of our actions on others and, likewise, on ourselves. To be sure, self-exploration promises to be a lifelong journey, as there is an ever-emerging stream of new catalysts for awakening and a vast array of situations and experiences in the works, each of which is a unique lens through which to study our inner workings. May Sarton writes: "One does not 'find oneself' by pursuing one's self, but on the contrary by pursuing something else and learning through some discipline or routine *(even the routine of making beds)* who one is and wants to be." During my time as a volunteer at Kripalu, I worked in our household department making beds, cleaning toilets, and mopping floors. When I was first assigned to this department, my initial reaction was, "You expect me to do what?" By the end of my stay, though, I was surprised at how much I had learned, shifted, and grown on the inside. One of my greatest lessons involved the ability to recognize that any type activity can be a catalyst for deep self-reflection when approached with an intention for learning.

The concept of svadyaya also encourages study of scripture, which can be interpreted as anything that has the power to inspire and motivate, from ancient texts to contemporary writing in the form of poetry, novels, plays, and film. Certainly, sacred texts have been designated as such because they have the power to spark internal revelation. In the same way, insightful stories and conscious contemporary media can allow us to glimpse a reflection of our own humanity through the eyes of another. As William James states:

> *Man is made or unmade by himself. In the armory of thought he forges the weapons by which he destroys himself. He also fashions the tools with which he builds for himself heavenly mansions of joy and strength and peace.*

Inquiries

On the Mat: Yoga offers us a safe space for exploring the ways we relate to the world. Everything that surfaces during asana is a reflection of how we are behaving in life, and thus yoga provides a means of developing a more intimate relationship with the various aspects that comprise our being. Explore what shows up when you hold a posture for a longer period of time, when your transitions are slowed, or when you step into a more vigorous practice. Choose a specific technique like flowing through the postures at a different pace, using pranayama to raise energy, experimenting with a longer meditation, or exploring mantra to foster an atmosphere of self-study. Acknowledge the awarenesses that emerge through each of these gateways.

Notice sensation in the physical body, the effects of each technique on your mental state, and the influence of a given practice on your breath, emotions, and internal dialogue. Explore inversions with standing forward fold, standing yoga mudra, warrior two, plank, humble warrior, triangle, lateral angle, goddess, down dog, dolphin dog, standing wide-angle forward fold, and tripod headstand.

Off the Mat: Once a week for four weeks, choose a favorite book or favorite reading to study. After reading, spend ten minutes in silent meditation to contemplate this wisdom. Following your meditation, write about how it might support your life.

Practices

Today

I choose to mindfully

Supportive Words
self-observation, contemplation, self-study, mindfulness, self-exploration

Complementary Breath
natural

Visualization
A clear lake reflecting and holding all of the beauty below, above, and around

study and learn from my thoughts, words, and actions

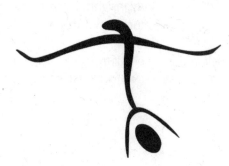

Ishvara Pranidhana:

The concept of surrender is one that spans many spiritual and religious traditions. In the early days of yoga, surrender was perceived as the act of setting aside the oars to float down the river of life, wholly subject to the will of a greater external being. Although the tradition encouraged building a tool bag of skills for maneuvering around obstacles with greater effect, all was subject to the decisive will of something greater. As yoga evolved, Tantra revamped the idea of surrender to include our co-creative power as embodiments of the same consciousness that makes up the cosmos. Even though active participation is one of the central philosophies of the Tantric path, the ability to soften our boundaries in order to receive is highlighted as another extremely valuable skill. Still, the process of choosing to open to what is before us can at times be enormously challenging.

Through my own engagement with the practices of yoga, I began to notice that one of the most predominant aspects of my constitution is that of air, referred to as vata nature in Ayurveda. I found that I would start one thing, then quickly get interested in another, and move right away to the next. Although this fluidity of focus was actually serving me, I constantly fought it and labeled myself as overly ungrounded. I berated myself for not sticking to one particular interest, even though I genuinely knew that I would never be satisfied with just one. Even today, I find the various facets of my life drawing me in many diverse directions. In my yoga practice, I have delved deeply into three different styles and utilize them all to create my own flow. In my work life, I teach yoga, offer nutritional consultations, and express myself through graphic design. One day, I finally realized that instead of fighting my variable nature I had the option to embrace it, acknowledge it as a gift, and open to the diverse possibilities it offers. Instead of standing in my own way, I now choose to soften any resistance that surfaces and give more of myself—in all of my fluidity—to what is before me.

The process of softening as an active intention requires that we choose receptivity in order to fully absorb the gifts we encounter. This is quite distinct from the notion of releasing as giving up and simply hoping for the best; we instead engage by consciously choosing to receive, even when what is before us does not conform to our desired ideal. In the course of daily life, we might engage this by radically opening to a passion we have been ignoring for years, receiving a gift graciously without any sense of obligation to reciprocate, or actively embracing the natural timing of a particular process, the consequences of our actions, or the various roles we play. As David Whyte eloquently writes in his poem, *Enough*:

> *Enough. These few words are enough.*
> *If not these words, this breath.*
> *If not this breath, this sitting here.*
>
> *This opening to the life*
> *we have refused*
> *again and again*
> *until now.*
>
> *Until now*[35].

Inquiries

On the Mat: Exploring the areas of the back body where our gaze cannot reach is one of the most powerful ways to develop our ability to open. In this practice, soften your gaze and observe your felt sense of the entire posterior plane. Focus your practice on back extensions, working with postures such as bridge, bow, camel, upward bow, and standing drop backs (*at the wall for less intensity*). Experiment with your ability to remain anchored while softening into the receptive space of each asana. Throughout your sequence, find moments to pause in stillness (*such as supine mountain, reclined bound angle, or fetal position*) and fully receive the vibration of the pose. In addition to these inquiries, identify any areas of your practice in which you are overly controlling and unable to welcome new experience. Use the breath to soften these areas and invite flow in accordance with the natural rhythm of life.

Off the Mat: Choose one facet of your life currently in process to which you have dedicated much effort and will. Instead of focusing on the outcome, redirect your energy towards simply being in the process and trusting its intelligence. Invoke the inherent lessons and riches of this approach and soften into the act of receiving the full wave of experience.

Practices

Supportive Words
mindful opening, love, receiving life, softening, trust

Visualization
A gentle flower bud curled tightly against the cold slowly opening to receive the warmth, light, and moisture of the day.

Complementary Breath
ujjayi

Teacher's Note
To help students embody the concept of surrender while fully supported, lead upward facing bow drop back in groups of three. Alternatively, lead a trust circle, with one person at the center falling into waiting hands that gently lift and redirect them around the circle.

Today, I soften to the flow of life. I open to receiving the many precious gifts that appear along my path

The Layers of Being: {inspired by Todd Norian}

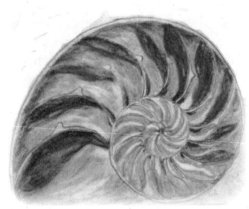

In yoga philosophy, our singular body is actually three: the physical body, the subtle body, and the causal body. These three bodies are composed of five distinct but not separate sheaths known as the koshas. Anamaya is the food sheath and is contained in the physical body. Pranamaya is the life- force sheath, manamaya is the mental and emotional layer, and vijnanamaya is the discriminative mind; together these three comprise the subtle body. Anandamaya kosha is the bliss sheath, and it is located in the causal body. In some yoga systems, the koshas are seen as coverings that veil the light of the true self, and so the intention of life's journey is to transcend the first four to arrive at bliss. In Tantric philosophy, however, everything is contained in everything, so this journey takes a different form. For Tantrikas, the goal is to awaken to the presence of ananda (bliss) in each one of these layers. In lieu of a systematic journey wherein the mission is to travel through each kosha in turn to find joy only in the last, we engage in an ongoing dynamic dance that unearths the ecstasy embedded in each sheath.

One summer morning, I was riding my bike to work while the day was still cloaked in darkness. As I coasted downhill with visibility low and wind blowing in all directions around me, my whole being suddenly resonated with insight. For the first time, I felt the various layers of my being illuminated all at once. My physical body was engaged, with all senses active; my breath sheath was pulsing; my mental and emotional body was spacious yet present; my intuitive layer was awake, navigating my course from within; and in the midst of all that was transpiring, I felt like I was floating on a bed of clouds in sheer happiness. Prior to my immersion in the study and practices of yoga, I don't think this moment could have occurred; I spent the majority of my time engaged only on the physical plane, with the others largely dormant or unnoticed. Today, I feel like I am able to see, feel, and interact with the various layers of my being in order to thrive more fully in life. As I learned from my experience on the bike, the layers of being are interwoven, each one supporting our exploration of the others. For example, when we ingest high-quality food, more prana is available to the cells of the body. With the organs and systems of the body bolstered both physically and energetically, our mental/emotional realm becomes increasingly clearer, which leads us to make more conscious decisions that leave us feeling more aligned overall. A potent image for visualizing the arrangement of the five sheaths is that of a nautilus shell. These radiant shells have a fluidly interwoven structure, with an inner matrix that has no real beginning or end. The shell is built layer upon layer, with each compartment connecting downward towards the infinite spiral center.

Sensing the World:

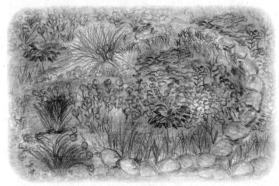

Yoga is a path that encompasses altered energetic states, which usually begin with physical experiences that ignite the senses. Anamaya Kosha, or the food sheath, corresponds directly with the sustenance we ingest to provide energy and life force for the body. The body is the sacred container for the radiant energy infusing our being, so there is tremendous value in keeping both the external form and internal functions healthy through careful decisions regarding this sustenance. Additionally, anamaya kosha encompasses what we absorb through the full spectrum of our senses, including smell, sound, sight, and touch in addition to taste. Swami Niranjanananda Saraswati writes, "Although, scientifically, we look at the physical body as different systems which control the bodily functions, yoga says that these functions are nothing but manifestations of the interaction between energy and consciousness[36]." According to this perspective, everything we encounter in life has a vibrational effect on the external and internal health of the physical body. This view thus encourages us to make wise choices regarding the media we absorb, the colors that decorate our living space, the kinds of food we eat, and the fabrics we put against our skin. The experiences we ingest through our various senses have a profound effect not only on the framework of the physical and subtle bodies, but also on the level of joy and well-being we experience on a daily basis. As we become more conscious of what we bring into our lives, we can make intentional decisions that honor the unique nature of our physical gifts. Once we recognize how discernment at the level of the senses increases our vitality and opens the doorway to inherent bliss, we can more easily see and experience the divine in the material realm. As Thich Nhat Hanh shares in *Transformation and Healing*:

> Our eyes, ears, hearts, half-half smiles, and breathing are wonderful phenomena. We only ned to open our eyes and we can see the blue sky, the white clouds, the rose, the clear river, the golden fields of wheat, the shining eyes of a child. We only have to attune our ears to hear the whisphering pines and the waves washing up on the shore...In us and around us, there are so many wondrous phenomena in nature which can refresh and heal us[36.5].

Inquiries

On the Mat: In yoga, asana practice aids us in reconnecting to the body, specifically to the treasure trove of sensory experience available to us in the human form. Use this practice to know your senses more fully and become more skillful at utilizing each one. Note whether retreating from overwhelming and life-detracting sensory experiences by way of your practice serves to revitalize your senses. Think of your sadhana as an opportunity to relearn how to use them in a more present and mindful way. Some things to consider include: the color of your practice space or yoga studio, the effects of different types of music or silence, the smells that surround you, the texture of your clothes and props, and the food and drink you consume before and after practice. As you flow into the various forms of the practice including postures, breath, meditation, and mindfulness, distinguish which sense is most activated by each one and take note of the information it provides at the level of the body as a whole. Practice with your eyes open. Draw your attention to the tactile sensations of the postures, especially the points of contact on the feet and hands. Listen to the sounds of your body, and invite sounds to arise from within. Take time for an extended savasana, and guide yourself through a detailed relaxation allowing each body part to soften in turn. Finally, try using a soothing essential oil during relaxation. Explore a potpourri practice with standing yoga mudra, plank, down dog, three-legged dog, three-legged dog twist, high lunge, knee-down lunge, hands inside foot in knee-down lunge, and side plank.

Off the Mat: Go for a walk in nature or in a nearby park if you live in the city, and be sure to leave your cell phone at home. Bring special awareness to softening and opening your senses. Take time during your walk to experience the surrounding environment through each of the five senses in turn. Afterwards, journal about what you saw, heard, smelled, touched, and tasted.

Practices

I reflect upon how I choose to feed my body

Supportive Words
consume, ingest, imbibe, surrond, take in

Visualization
Being in a luscious, colorful garden, all the senses delightfully stimulated and alive.

Complementary Breath
ujjayi

Closing Ritual
Try a sweet treat meditation using dark chocolate or dried fruit. Be fully present, and take your time to savor all the senses that awaken.

of being in the world

With my eyes open

I connect to the vital sensory experiences

I relish the beauty of my physical sheath

Breath Body:

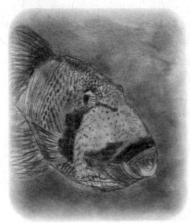

One of the most powerful therapies I have experienced is rebirthing breath. Through this practice, the body is flooded with an enormous amount of oxygen. One of the most significant revelations I had as a result of this practice was grasping the ability of the breath to circulate through the whole body as opposed to only being limited to the space of the lungs. The breath layer stores and carries the life force continually being channeled to the physical and subtle parts of our being. On the physical plane, oxygen nourishes the blood, organs, cells, and various systems of the body. Breath and oxygen provide us with constant fuel, allowing the millions of physical mechanisms, chemical exchanges, and neural communications to do their work and provide us with energy as we move through the activities of each day. The more air we consume, the more potential we cultivate for increased liveliness and seamless, stress-free functioning. In addition to supporting the internal processes of the body, taking deeper breaths aids the outer form in staying supple, firm, and fit.

As babies, our breath is extremely uninhibited and it blends effortlessly with the external environment. As we grow older, though, the breath can become stagnant and less fluid. With less oxygen circulating throughout the breath body, energy is lowered, cells are starved for vital nutrition, and muscles begin to tighten. In addition to its effects on our internal organs and outer form, yoga invites us into a contemplation of how the flow of prana affects our subtle energetic architecture. The nadis, which are defined as conduits or veins, are the carriers of energetic life force permeating every part of the body. Conveyed by these conduits, the life force generated by the breath activates and charges various energy centers known as the chakras. As these energy centers open up, we can begin to access repressed emotions, stored traumas, and accumulated life patterns. If the flow of breath, and thus prana, through both our gross and subtle realms is hindered or decreased, we ultimately spend more time in a contracted state of being. This physical and energetic shift, which often results from a learned pattern of holding, can eventually lead to a profound sense of isolation and separateness. Conversely, the more we nurture the breath body, the more sensitive we become to our internal and external worlds; from this space of attunement, we are better equipped to make conscious, empowered decisions in life as pranamaya kosha also serves as a bridge between our physical body and our mental/emotional body. Doug Keller writes:

> I experience the prana as an intelligent force, an energy that permeates the atmosphere, binding all things of life through the process of breathing. It's neither my personal possession nor something entirely separate from me; it's both 'mine' and more than 'mine'[37].

Inquiries

On the Mat: Yoga postures are the outer forms of inner energetic activity, but without prana, they lose their luster. As the physical body opens up more fully, our capacity for receiving breath expands. In this practice, focus on your breath and its ability to nourish you on both the physical and subtle levels. Take time to center, and spend a few moments noticing the way your whole body breathes before actively engaging pranamaya. Center yourself lying on your back as you focus on building the breath in this relaxed position. Place a cushion on your belly to increase your perception of the expansion and contraction resulting from full breath. Note whether you experience reluctance in letting go or if there is a constant desire to pull, hurry, or control the breath. From this basis of skillful alignment with prana, partner with the dance of the breath, and begin to integrate breathing exercises in order to explore the diverse energetic and physical effects of each breath on pranamaya kosha. Focus your awareness on any physical sensations or subtle shifts of the internal flow of prana as you experience the unique imprint of each exercise. In addition to specific breathing techniques, allow the asana portion of your practice to take the form of a meditative dance with the entire breath body serving as an intelligent guide supported by the senses. To highlight the power of breath, include deep backbends in your sequence, as they open more space in the legs, lungs, and spine for the breath to flow.

Explore the following breaths in your practice. *Centering:* natural breath, dirgha, ujjayi; *warm-ups:* coordinate ujjayi breath with movement; *standing poses:* kapalabhati, alternate-nostril kapalabhati, bhastrika, pigeon, head to knee, easy pose twist, bound angle, bramari, fish, block at sacrum in bridge, seated forward fold, half lord of the fishes, anulom vilom; *savasana:* long blanket roll from shoulder blades to low back, focus on the return to the natural breath

Off the Mat: For four days of a given week, commit to doing a ten-minute breath practice upon waking. Note the effects on your pranamaya kosha.

Practices

I connect to the animating power of prana

Supportive Words
breath, life, life force, vitality

Visualization
A fish with its whole body immersed in the water, breathing through its gills.

Complementary Breath
Follow sequence in inquiries.

Closing Ritual
A guided meditation moving progressively inwards through the layers of the body *(from skin to muscle to bone, then to veins and organs, then to subtle conduits and energy channels, and finally to prana as breath).*

entire surface of my body

In each moment I allow

I breathe through the

the breath to craft the form of my pose from the inside out

Potent Mind:

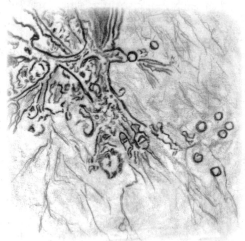

The mental layer, or manamaya kosha, is comprised of our thoughts, emotions, and psychological presence. What we ingest through the five senses is processed and assimilated here, directly affecting the central nervous system and our emotional states. This sheath also encompasses the mental dimension of linear and sequential thinking, as well as memory and observation. Technically speaking, manamaya is linked to the functioning of the body through its processes of digesting sensory input and directing oxygen and blood through the physical systems of the body. Just like pranamaya kosha, manamaya is interspersed throughout the entire body, including our organs, muscles, and cells. Yoga teacher Shiva Rea calls this sheath the body of awareness, alluding to the idea that thought and emotion imbue every part of our being. As such, we can envision every part of the body as having its own mental/emotional capacity and thought pattern even though the brain is the central processor of information. This layer is truly a marvel of our existence, as it is responsible for the autonomous behaviors of the body. Specifically, it governs the basic drives common to all humans, including survival instinct, fight-or-flight response, and reproduction among others. Developing a conscious relationship to the mental/emotional layer opens the door to an inquiry of the effects of our thoughts through the feelings, stored traumas, and unsupportive behaviors that stem from them.

It is in this sheath where many of us find ourselves stuck in grooves of habitual action. Like a scratch on a compact disc, these grooves go unnoticed in the course of our everyday experience and quickly become deeply ingrained and difficult to escape. There may be times when we experience deep resistance because this programming is not in-line with our highest purpose, and yet we are prone to overlook these habits as the origin of the disturbance. When we are born, our minds are a fairly smooth slate free of deep conditioning, but through life experiences we develop grooves that can stop us in our tracks. These ruts might result from trauma in childhood or adulthood, growing up in a challenging environment, or being around people who degrade our individuality and confidence. Jack Kornfield writes: "When any experience of body, heart, or mind keeps repeating in consciousness, it is a signal that this visitor is asking for a deeper and fuller attention[38]." The deeper the impression, the harder it is to change the pattern and return to a ground of equanimity. Yet our deepest grooves can also help us become experts in a given area, and once we awaken to a new way of being, we can aid others who are stuck in a similar predicament.

In order to empower ourselves in relationship to the stagnant patterns of the mind, we must first slow down, become more introspective, and attune to the many rhythms at work in the body. As we focus on the breath, heartbeat, and undulating dance of thought and emotion, we can enjoy the spaces comprised of the brief moments between waves of experience. We can utilize these spaces to become more conscious of the chronic blocks littering our internal matrix and empower ourselves to move towards change as a result of this awareness. Daniel Odier writes regarding the mind, "Everything can arise, everything can be reabsorbed, all states become passages, crossings. And when we leave behind the perception of a fixed state we are now necessarily in continual movement. Emotions can circulate freely, and we realize that, when we allow things to circulate, they become immediately tuned to the rapid functioning of the mind[39]." In these ways, manamaya kosha invites us into conscious exploration of our functioning on the mental and emotional levels and aids us in illuminating the deeper realms of our psyche. In some yoga traditions, the mission is to fully cleanse manamaya kosha in order to attain ultimate liberation. Tantric thought, however, maintains that our deepest patterns will inevitably reemerge from time to time regardless of how much we succeed in bringing awareness to them. When they do, though, the key distinction is that our newfound positioning will empower us to meet these familiar patterns with the skill and grace of a dancer, clear and attentive while also responsive to what we encounter. As Katherine Mansfield shares:

> The mind I love must have wild places, a tangled orchard where dark damsons drop in the heavy grass, an overgrown little wood, the chance of a snake or two, a pool that nobody's fathomed the depth of, and paths threaded with flowers.

Inquiries

On the Mat: Utilize this practice to hone the skills that lead to more fluency in the language of the mental layer. First, simply note the wonder and power of the mental sheath and its vital role in our lives. Sense how mental patterns create vibrations that translate into emotional states. Acknowledge the role mental function plays in breathing, movement, tissue repair, immune support, and digestion. In asana, connect more fully to your body and your breath. As you become more astute and more relaxed through the physical practice, take note of any fresh insights that arise in this influential dimension, and start to notice the places where routine functioning or mental impressions are no longer serving you. Take time to move through your practice in deep meditation. Through repeatedly meandering to and from one place of focus (*usually the breath works well*), cultivate a sense of spaciousness to bring ease to manamaya kosha. Explore inverted poses in order to stimulate the mental layer in its full scope. Step into the inquiry of inversions with mountain, eagle arm rotations, standing yoga mudra, bridge, down dog, dolphin dog, L at wall, head on block in standing wide-angle forward fold, headstand, and shoulder stand.

Off the Mat: Dedicate three days to locating the sources of unsupportive repetitive thoughts in your life and make note of them. Include both the roots of these thoughts as well as the behaviors and choices that result from them. Use the three days that follow to journal about the ways in which the repetitive functions of the body and mind are an asset to your life.

I affirm the wonder of the mind and acknowledge the thousands of repeated
actions it implements seamlessly in each moment
king, and I notice how they are holding me back
I identify my ingrained ways of thin
I am learning about my inner habitual functioning
I am open to learning about

Supportive Words

emotions, imprints, mind, grooves, thoughts

Visualization

The cells in all of our organs and tissues as intelligent, pulsating components of life.

Complementary Breath

viloma *(inhale & exhale)*

Feel the space between each segment of the breath, and notice the cyclical nature of the mind and emotions.

Closing Ritual

trataka, or candle flame mediation

Provides a single constant stimulus for our attention while freeing up space for us to attune more fully to the intelligent functioning of manamaya kosha.

Teacher's Note

Pair students up, and instruct them to talk at their partner at the same time without listening, by completing the statement, "My life sucks because…" for thirty seconds. Laughter is common here. Tell students that this exercise demonstrates what happens when we become overwhelmed by the turbulent grooves marking our consciousness. For the second round, invite them to share what they are grateful for right now for thirty seconds each while the other student holds the space and actively listens. Switch, and then invite them to share their insights about this exercise. Tell students that this second part symbolizes our ability to hold space for ourselves as we become more aware and skillful in maneuvering the realm of unsupportive thoughts.

Inner Wisdom:

The previous layer of manamaya kosha supports us in moving into the realm of automatic functioning to illuminate fixed and constricted aspects of our inner workings. Once aware of what is holding us back, we can tap into the discriminating power of vijnanamaya kosha. This space of concentrated wisdom is connected to intuition, insight, and internal reflection. In this sheath, we encounter our deepest knowing and our ability to discriminate between what will be life-enhancing and what will detract from our vital energy. This sheath is what sets humans apart from animals by empowering us to make choices based in value judgments and analytical thinking. To build our connection to this layer of being, we must become more sensitive and exercise trust in our deepest intuition. In daily life, we utilize the visual sense as a primary way of interacting and moving about the world. By simply pausing to close our eyes, we can dive more fully into the space of vijnanamaya kosha. As the body demonstrates through the wonder of proprioception *(the unconscious perception of movement and spatial orientation arising from stimuli within the body itself [40])*, there is deep insight aiding us in staying centered even when vision is obscured. As we hone this internal sense bolstered by the previous sheaths, we can begin to feel and experience a unique radiance in our being that likewise pulses through the whole of existence. We begin to comprehend that although we are embodied creatures, we also possess a connection to something larger, which can be more tangible in this intuitive realm. It is important to distinguish that in some yoga traditions, we close the eyes in order to withdraw and numb the senses. In the Tantric approach, however, we soften the gaze in order to become more attuned to all of our senses. As we sharpen our ability to interact with life through various modalities including taste, touch, sound, and smell, our internal intuitive capacities are better informed and thus more refined. Like building a new muscle, strengthening vijnanamaya kosha takes time, and the process can be supported through dedicated introspection, mindful eating, yoga nidra, journaling, deep relaxation, pranayama and chanting. As Mary Oliver descirbes in *The Journey* sometimes we are required to leave the outer voices behind, cultivate and listen to our own inner wisdom as we walk deeper and deeper into the world determined to save the only life we can save, our own[41].

Inquiries

On the Mat: Enhance your relationship with the wisdom sheath through engaging in a more introspective sadhana. Regardless of which category of asana you utilize, each posture can be seasoned with the intention to awaken more fully from the inside out. Utilize the intuitive sense of the body, the power of the breath, and the support of routine mental tasks to make space for heightened sensitivity and awareness of how this sixth sense offers guidance. Practice postures with your eyes closed or a soft gaze to stimulate internal vision. Contemplate how softening the eyes and turning inward creates more sensitivity, expanding your ability to navigate from a rooted, subtle place. Focus on forward-folding asanas, and intersperse pranayama, chanting, and meditation into the body of your sadhana. Explore hip openers and forward folds with humble warrior, eyes closed in tree to engage proprioception, bound angle, baby cradle, knee to head, pigeon, parsvotanasana, seated forward fold, child, hero, seated yoga mudra, and cow face.

Off the Mat: Dedicate one day to making your food choices from the vantage of vijnanamaya kosha. Before sitting own to a meal, soften your eyes, take a few deep breaths, and ask yourself what it is you truly want. Contemplate whether the response is a habitual groove, a label of what is healthy or unhealthy, or truly the body's intuition.

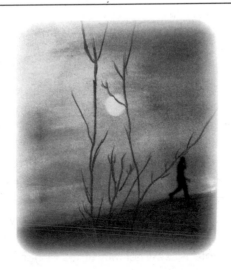

Practices

Supportive Words
innate knowledge, inner vision, insight, instinct, intuition

Visualization
Walking in the dark, vision obscured, feeling and sensing as you navigate from inside out.

Complementary Breath
ujjayi

Closing Ritual
Begin or end your practice with a circular walking meditation in which you repeat the walking route several times. Walk a total of seven cycles, and on your second round begin to soften your eyes. By the sixth or seventh round, experiment with walking part or all of the way with your eyes closed.

Teacher's Note
Lead a trust walk. Have students pair up. As one student walks with eyes closed, the other supports the experience minimally by guiding them around any obstacles. When they do offer guidance, instruct them to use clear words like "stop," "turn right," or "continue walking". After a minute, prompt the students to switch roles. Once the second student has had a turn, allow a few moments for them to process the experience by sharing what came up. Many share that they begin to feel more comfortable by engaging their underutilized senses and internal intuition as the trust walk progresses.

With faith, I listen to the subtle yet persistent messages from deep inside I tap into the depth of insight inherent to my nature I deeply trust the power of my intuition

Joy to the World:

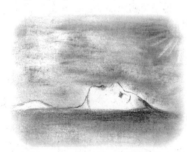

Our bliss layer pulsates at the core of our being while simultaneously permeating all the other planes of our internal and external universe. It is the eternal center of consciousness that is woven into both the primal instincts and structural components of our body. Ananda can be felt through all layers of our experience and is the catalyst for our ability to truly savor life. It can manifest in the most ecstatic experiences like riding a roller coaster, or it can seep into the most seemingly mundane moments like sitting on the subway. This idea that bliss is not only associated with high ecstatic energy states is key, as an experience of ananda is indeed possible at any moment. When we can open to the expanded vision of this sheath, we feel a deep sense of belonging and accept life as perfect in all its splendor, grace, messiness, and imperfection. As we attune more fully to each kosha, we can recognize each as a conduit to this space of recognition. Whether through a meal that piques the full range of our senses, a felt sense of the potency of the breath, a deep clarity and attunement to our mental workings, or a profound trust in the wisdom of our hearts, there are countless moments in our lives that offer us access to this state of being. Lingering in anandamaya kosha, we remember our essence as without beginning or end, ageless, all-pervading, and deeply infused with the wisdom and light of universal consciousness. Although the state of ananda is always in the background, it is natural for our relationship to this cycle to vary in intensity. At certain times in our lives, we will embody this kosha on all levels of our being with ease, while other moments might find us feeling disconnected from even the tiniest inkling of ananda. By becoming more present to the physical senses, the breath, the workings of the mind, and the presence of our intuition through yoga, we can ultimately recognize and appreciate more moments of bliss. Mary Oliver describes in *Happiness* the voyage of a bear, in its search for honey. As she finds her treasure among the swarming bees she becomes full, sleepy, and drunk with sweetness[42].

Inquiries

On the Mat: Notice whether the practice of yoga helps you become more sensitive, opens your heart, and strengthens the physical temple of your soul. Contemplate the particular potency of yoga a safe and sacred space where all the layers of being are honored and nurtured. Flow through a practice to review the four preceding koshas. Focus your exploration on each of the previous sheaths, sensing how ananda is accessible in every layer. Close your practice with a long savasana. Take time to transition back to a seated position, and allow a few moments to feel the integration of these sacred internal chambers as they pulse with seamless synchronicity. Explore an arm-balancing practice with pointer, knee-down lunge, high lunge, hands inside food in knee-down lung, quad stretch in knee-down lunge-, runner's stretch, tree, eagle, warrior one, cobra, locust, side plank, wild thing, down dog, leg twist in down dog, and child.

Off the Mat: Connect with a friend and take turns sharing what happiness and bliss mean to each of you. Utilize the following contemplations: What emerges as an image or a feeling when you think of bliss? Do you believe that this is something outside of yourself you need to attain, or is it inherently within? What are the feelings or emotions that block you from experiencing more joy? How do you react when ecstasy is not constantly present?

Practices

I awaken to the distinctive experiences of bliss unique to each kosha I affirm the multidimensional elements that comprise my being I honor the conduits to bliss that are present in every moment

Supportive Words
beatitude, bliss, ecstasy, gladness, happiness, joy, rapture

Visualization
Floating in the calm waters of the ocean on a beautiful day, taking in fresh air, sun, and simple joy.

Complementary Breath
analum valom
At each pause between nostrils, pause and savor.

Closing Ritual
ananda mindmap
On a blank piece of paper, write or draw your name inside a circle in the very middle. Next, draw four lines radiating out from the central circle, and draw a large circle at the end of each line. In each of these large circles, write the name of one of the previous four koshas. Fill in the remaining space with the ways you experience bliss through each of these respective layers of being.

The Chakras: {inspired by Anodea Judith}

The term "chakras," derived from the Sanskrit word meaning wheel or circle[43], refers to the seven known energy centers that exist in the pranamaya kosha, or energy sheath, of the body. They most directly correspond to the nerve ganglia and glands of the endocrine system on the physical plane, but these wheels of life are not actually physical locations in the body. Rather, they are overlaid like a transparent yet connected skin[44]. The three lower chakras represent the more primal energies of survival, sexuality, and personal power[45]. The fourth chakra is characterized by its location at the center of the chain, reflected in its qualities of balance, love, and compassion. Finally, the three higher chakras correspond to sound, intuition, and our universal nature, thus representing a subtler, more ethereal dimension. We can visualize each of these energy centers as an intersection of subtle energy tubes, referred to as "nadis," creating a lotus that blossoms or contracts as a result of our life experiences. The central nadi is the sushumna, and it is as thin as a single strand of a spider's web; it is superimposed along the central channel of the spine. Ida and pingala are the two other principal nadis. These lines of energy begin at the root chakra, and from there they extend upward crisscrossing at certain points along the sushumna nadi. Each place where ida and pingala intersect, an energy wheel or chakra is present. The chakras are depicted as circular symbols, each with its own symbolic shape, arrangement of leaf petals, and Sanskrit letter. Each energy wheel's shape and quantity of leaf petals holds a different meaning corresponding to the qualities of that particular chakra. Swami Sivananda writes: "The number of petals of the lotuses varies. Muladhara, Svadhishthana, Manipura, Anahata, Visuddha and Ajna Chakras have 4, 6, 10, 12, 16, and 2 petals respectively. All the 50 Sanskrit letters are on the 50 petals. The number of petals in each Chakra is determined by the number and position of the Yoga Nadis around the Chakra... The sound produced by the vibrations of the Yoga Nadis is represented by the corresponding Sanskrit letter[46]." From this description, it is easy to understand why the bija mantras *(or seed sounds)* of each energy center are vital in the exploration of chakra sadhana.

The chakras are imprinted on all of us whether or not we are aware of how they impact and or influence our path. When we are born, these energy wheels are apt to be naturally open and unobstructed, but over time they begin to mirror the cosmic pulsation of yin and yang, contraction and expansion, and concealment and revelation that underlies the intricate functioning of the universe. There are times when the chakras become congested and armored as we experience some of the harsh realities of the human path. When we partake in healing, root into our truth, and savor the sweetness of life, the wheels of life can be cleared and open once more. Thus transpires the ongoing endeavor of reconnecting with ourselves on this energetic level as we engage in practices that encourage the chakras to blossom and open, while honoring the times when they are in a more contracted state. Keep in mind that in some yoga traditions, the goal of practices focused on the chakras is to generate a state of eternal openness that eventually leads to permanent, out-of-body liberation. In the point of view offered below, the wheels of life instead serve as the basis for an ongoing inquiry as they fluctuate between more expanded and contracted states of being.

The chakras serve as wonderful contemplations for yoga sadhana. An especially effective approach for utilizing them is to work with them consecutively in a series of personal practices, beginning with the root and progressing all the way up to the crown. This sequence will give you an opportunity to physically and mentally embody each center, experiencing the symbolism of each wheel through various senses. Many of us are energetically disconnected from our lower halves and as a result feel estranged from our sensual, passionate, and sexual selves. Many are also increasingly disengaged from the energies of our hearts. With connections to family, friends, and community dwindling, the chance to embody heart energy and create a yoga family is an opportunity ripe with possibility. Similarly, many of us also experience detachment from the more subtle parts of our being. We struggle to hear our inner voice, trust our own intuition, or recognize our true nature as elements of a greater whole. By entering into relationship with these aspects of the self, though, we can utilize them as intelligent means to live a more conscious and joyful life. Like a flower which first roots into the earth for safety and stability and then rises slowly skyward before finally blossoming open, people who experience the progression of the chakras in their personal practice will likely encounter transformation in other realms of life.

Teacher's Note:

Focusing on one chakra per week tends to work well, even if you have students who come to your classes multiple times during this span. As you build the theme of a single energy vortex within each class, students have time to experience a gradual understanding and integration of the energies native to each of these centers. Allow your inner artist to weave together the various elements that will best illuminate the benefits and wisdom available in each wheel. For example, each of the chakras has a unique sound that stimulates its specific subtle energies. Experiment with inviting your students to use these sounds throughout the class or by simply replacing your usual "aum" chant with the bija mantra that corresponds to a given focal point. In addition, keep in mind that these contemplations have been written with the intent of summarizing the immense amount of symbolism and data available for each vibrating circle. Present as much information as is personally meaningful for you in one class, and save the rest for the next time you teach this series. The chakra system is vast, with each energy wheel containing literal and symbolic correlations to glands, organs, body parts and senses, psychological identities, developmental stages, and emotions. For further study of the chakra system, refer to Anodea Judith's *Wheels of Life* or *Eastern Body, Western Mind*. As you lead the following classes, practice dynamic language by diversifying the ways of saying the word chakra. Try: disk, focal point, energy center, energy hub, energy wheel, energy vortex, (the earth, water, fire, etc.) lotus, vibrating circle, and wheel of life.

Root Power:

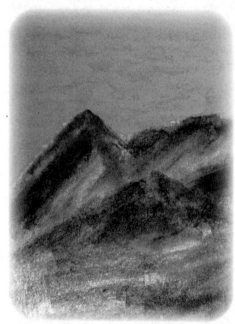

Muladhara Chakra, also known as root support, is the first chakra; it is located between the anus and genitals at the perineum for men, and in the cervix between the vagina and uterus for women. This energy wheel is our foundation and corresponds to the earth element[5]. Its seed sound is "lam," and its color is red. It addresses our need for safety and correlates to our earliest developmental stages of being in the womb and of requiring constant care in the first year of life. The first vortex helps us to feel grounded and to set clear boundaries so we can nourish ourselves physically, emotionally, and spiritually. The main purpose of muladhara is indeed to solidify, root, and stabilize. It supports us in knowing the earth, the natural world, and the material world. This vortex is the seat of concepts such as earth, roots, embodiment, and grounding[47]. "I cultivate safety and stability," is the phrase associated with its power and action. This hub holds our primal animal energies and is home to our survival instincts. Muladhara chakra has four petals, which can be related to the four corners of the feet or the four legs of a table to symbolize solidity[48].

When we cultivate this wheel of life, we hone and strengthen our vessel so that shakti (*creative energy*) and abundance will flow through us with more ease. Muladhara also encompasses trust and stability, which pair to form the foundation of asana practice, for it is only when rooted in these qualities that we can fully open to our poses. When we are rooted, steady, and feel safe in our bodies and in our communities, we can step into the full potential of our being both on and off the mat, as the sense of groundedness available to us in this chakra also supports us in cultivating openness and expansion in our lives. While building stability may initially seem like a solitary journey, it can also be enhanced through the support of our social relations. Consider the symbol of a mountain, which seems to stand alone and separate at its peak, but is almost always surrounded by a network of fellow mountains. Though the peaks, as individuals, garner the most attention, we cannot deny that they exist as parts of a greater whole. Moreover, it is from this sprawling expanse of connection with the earth that each peak draws its stability. This is true in our lives, as well, as often the support of a widespread network of family and friends is what enables us to stand on our own two feet and blossom in our individuality. Although we tread our own unique paths, we can rely on community as a source of support and strength for the journey.

Inquiries

On the Mat: Whether you are a beginner or a more seasoned practitioner, muladhara is a particularly useful concept for engendering awareness of safety and stability, as it evokes qualities of beginner's mind and steadiness. In this practice, utilize a slower pace, and focus on building a strong base for each posture from the ground up. Acquaint yourself with the four corners of the feet, the importance of activating the toes to engage the leg muscles, the stability available to knees and hips when the feet remain parallel, and the steadiness created when the hips remain squared in space. In addition, investigate the influence of lower body positioning on the health and stability of your spine, as the legs govern the entire length of the back. With regard to the breath, take time to hone the basics of three-part breath (or *dirgha pranayama*) by reclining in supine mountain with a cushion on your belly. Draw your attention to this subtle weight on the abdomen as well as the way the whole back body spreads onto the earth with each full inhale. Explore standing poses with mountain, standing half moon, tree, warrior one, warrior two, lateral angle, triangle, standing forward fold, goddess, standing wide-angle forward fold, down dog, and plank.

Off the Mat: Contemplate what comprises your personal foundation. On one side of a piece of paper, write down all of the things in your life that help you stay grounded and firm, thus providing the safety and stability for you to grow. On the other side, list any foundational cornerstones that are missing and therefore hindering your ability to expand. What are three ways in which you can create a more stable foundation today?

Practices

Supportive Words
earth, embodiment, grounded, steadfast, rooted

Visualization
A mountain as a beacon of stability, at once firmly rooted in the earth and deeply connected to its surroundings, or a temple with four stable cornerstones and a foundation of ancient stone.

Complementary Breath
dirgha

Closing Ritual
Individual or partner foot rubs at the beginning of practice.

I affirm that I have all I need in this moment to build, grow, and flourish

the safety I feel within

I source strength from

I draw energy from the earth and connect to my stability

Fluid Motion:

Rooted in the stability of earth, we travel upwards along the chakra path to the second energy wheel. Svadhishthana is the seat of sweetness, and it is located between the navel and genitals. From the steady, grounded energy of earth, we are able to access the more fluid, sensual energies of water. The contour of the earth serves as a container for this essential, sacred element. Svadhishthana's seed sound is "vam," and its color is orange[49]. It relates to our desire for pleasure and corresponds to the first two years of life when we begin to actively interact with the world around us and start to experience various sensations and emotions. This energy hub is fluid, formless, and is connected to the feminine qualities of yielding and softness. The primary purpose of thus vibrating circle is to liberate and nurture sexual and feminine energies, which enables circulation of the vital life force. Svadhishthana corresponds to pleasure, emotion, and sensuality. "I open to all emotion," is the phrase associated with its power and action.

This lotus flower is the wellspring of our life force and invites us to experience ritual, sexuality, pleasure, and the movement of prana. Igniting the second chakra supports us in freeing emotions through physical movement instead of harboring them inside, as motion and change stimulate a sense of possibility. Svadhishthana energy balances, renews, restores, and keeps our reproductive organs healthy. Connecting to our pleasure principle through this doorway, we can release rigidity within and begin to heal on a deep, internal level. This energy vortex affirms our desires and acknowledges that as embodied beings, conscious gratification is revered. Because the second wheel of life is related to goddess spirit and deep-rooted power, it encourages us to turn into the current of life and honor the sacred nature of our innermost self. When we block or repress this energy wheel, we disrupt our journey towards expanded consciousness and awareness. By softening into our fluid nature, we create space to nurture ourselves more fully, to reap the benefits of our feminine energies, and to remain present with the emotions surfacing in each breath[50].

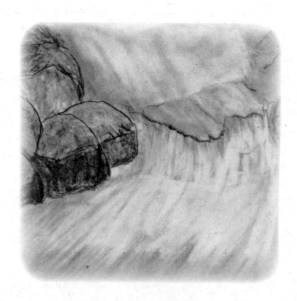

Inquiries

On the Mat: Svadhishthana can be a sensitive chakra for many people and is one of the most potent with regard to inner work. Many of us have had awkward or damaging sexual relationships, which tend to clog this energy wheel. Feel and be present with whatever surfaces during your practice as you engage this contemplation. This concept has the potential to be especially poignant for anyone working with repression in the sexual and emotional realms. In this practice, investigate postures that flow smoothly from one another, and hold for shorter periods of time to create a fluid dance through yoga asana. Originate the majority of your movements from the hips, lead with your senses as you follow the trail of the breath, and assume the qualities of unencumbered water. Focus on ujjayi pranayama, sensing its fluidity and noticing how it aids you in diving deeply into both the physical and subtle realms of your being. When you practice the ocean breath, plug your ears with your thumbs to connect to the potent hum of the breath. Finally, recognize the support you feel from the stability and safety of the first chakra as you excavate the range of emotions and feelings contained in this second vibrant vortex. Explore hip openers in reclining bound angle, fluid sun salutes, cobra, bound angle, half circle, gate, cow face, fire log, seated wide-angle forward fold, wide-legged child, pigeon, and frog (*The frog is symbolic of water, fertility, and abundance. Frogs are deeply connected to water, which is vital to their life processes of cleansing, healing, growth, and reproduction.*)

Off the Mat: Dedicate a weekend to fully pampering your sensual and emotional self. Explore your body, spend time in water, and wear clothing that feels good against your skin. Spend some time at the spa enjoying a massage, facial, or hot tub, or treat yourself to an experience of an art form that helps you feel connected (*such as going to the movies, the theater, a museum, an opera, live music, etc.*).

Practices

I allow feelings and sensations to move fluidly through the conduits

Supportive Words
delight, gratification, pleasure, sensuality, sexuality

Visualization
A spring that forms a pond of clear water and spills out of this container to create a lively stream.

Complementary Breath
ujjayi

Closing Ritual
Envision something that brings you genuine pleasure. Spend a few moments fully developing the image in your mind as you allow the felt sense of it to circulate and pulse throughout your whole body.

to me in each breath

of my body

I drink with

I open to the possibilities for change available

delight from the sweet waters of pleasure

Personal Fire:

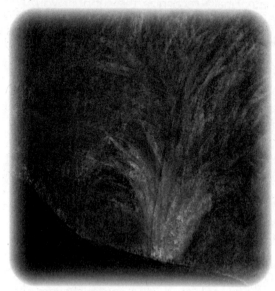

Manipura, or "lustrous gem," is also known as the third chakra, which is located at the navel and solar plexus. This wheel is a radiant, glowing vortex of the energy body that shines bright like the sun, and thus is related to the element of fire. The image of heated flames represents our internal digestive fires, which support our physical health by transforming our food into useable energy. This hub's seed sound is "ram," and its color is yellow[51]. Manipura encompasses our ability to cultivate self-esteem and correlates to the developmental period from eighteen months to two years of age, when we are asserting a sense of self. We have established stability, experienced fluidity within the container of safety, and now we can begin to channel and guide our life energy with more skill and intent. This chakra seeks and supports transformation as we gain clarity regarding our individual needs, power, and perspective. Manipura is dependent on the steady flow of life force or prana, which serves as fuel for the commanding flames associated with this chakra. As heat moves upwards, it alters form and transports matter to new dimensions, enabling us to awaken to a sense of purpose that we might have once deemed inconceivable[52]. This vortex is the center of action, vitality, will, and internal power, and "I can do it," is the phrase that reflects its actions.

The third energy circle asks us to embrace our personal value and assert our actions in the world with integrity and honor. As we align with our strength, purpose, and intentions, we are empowered to realize our dreams and visions. It takes tremendous courage and steadfastness to create a life that fulfills these conscious desires while also contributing to the welfare of society at large. By connecting to the unique potency of the third wheel of life, we can source the determination and will that are ever-present but often lie dormant. We can also rid ourselves of any and all limiting beliefs by offering them up to manipura's transformative flames, freeing ourselves to fully flourish. Indeed, this lotus invites us to consider that it is through mindful encounters with our internal fires that we can ultimately embody our greatest potential.

Inquiries

On the Mat: In yoga, we can consciously stoke our inner fire to cultivate self-esteem while honoring our greater purpose. Furthermore, the practice of postures and breath brings about transformation in the physical body, transmuting any hindering beliefs on a psychological and cellular level. As you step onto the mat, contemplate this question: What area of your life or practice do you most wish to transform? The physical postures of yoga literally serve as conduits that can shift our being from the inside out. Just like a young child asserting his personality and direction, we can utilize our exploration on the mat to embrace our individual presence. Each time you engage in asana practice, you are guaranteed to encounter inquiries that have the potential to enable deeper understanding of self. The true potency of the practice is that its effects continue to reverbrate long after we have left our mats, slowly but surely affecting shifts in our reality. As you explore manipura, take time to literally strengthen your outer shell in order to meet with the world with greater vitality. In this practice, honor the previous two chakras by blending holding poses symbolizing earth with faster vinyasa movements representing water; notice how both serve to stoke the inner fire of the third chakra. If possible, heat your practice space to simulate fire. Investigate skull-shining breath to stimulate digestive fire and cultivate personal power. As you experiment with this warming breath, place one hand at your solar plexus, and experiment with the effects of different speeds on the potency of this pranayama. Focus on accessing the heat of the core through reverse table, sun salutations, warriors one, two, and three, reverse warrior, chair, plank, side plank, core strengtheners, and upward boat.

Off the Mat: Once a month for six months, choose one adventure you've always yearned to have from afar *(remembering that adventure can be subtle as well as grand)*. Take active steps towards this experience, and notice how it feels to assert your will. How does stepping into your power in one area of your life evoke transformations in others?

Practices

I overcome inertia to act in accordance with my individual will   I use the

Supportive Words
action, inner power, will, vitality

Visualization
Volcanic fire: through the incredible heat, gemstones are unearthed.

Complementary Breath
kapalabhati

Closing Ritual
chant to Ram

transformation

postures of my yoga

practice to stoke the fires of inner determination   I offer all that isn't serving me to the fires of

Heart Space:

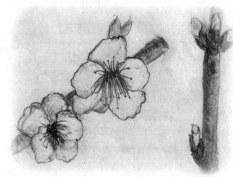

Anahata, which translates as "unstruck" or "unwounded," is the fourth chakra and is located at the heart center. From stability, fluidity, and will, we progress to a state of integration represented by the air element. Its seed sound is "yam," and its color is green[53]. This hue is one often associated with the wisdom and grace of nature. This energy wheel reflects our need for community and correlates to the childhood years from four to seven when we start to form authentic connections, learn to share, and begin to interact with greater society. The symbol of this hub is two intersecting triangles. One faces upward and the other faces downward, and together they form a shape similar to the Star of David. The downward facing triangle stands for the three energy centers below the heart; taken together, they represent more tangible realms of existence. The upward facing triangle indicates the three chakras above the heart, which comprise the more subtle planes of being. It is here at the heart that the tangible and the subtle intersect and unite their various energies. As these two currents connect, they remind us that true wholeness is the partnering of the physical aspects of our being with the less tangible energetic, emotional, and intellectual realms. When we understand this fully, the heart softens and its glow amplifies. The main purpose of this fourth spinning circle is to integrate and align the various layers that make up our complete being. This spinning vortex is the source of love, connection, healing, and optimal balance, and "I love myself and others," is the phrase associated with its power.

The heart is a phenomenal organ that pumps and circulates nutrients to every cell in the body. Although it is a single organ, the heart is split into two pumps; "The first pump carries oxygen-poor blood to your lungs, where it unloads carbon dioxide and picks up oxygen. It then delivers oxygen-rich blood back to your heart. The second pump delivers oxygen-rich blood to every part of your body. Blood needing more oxygen is sent back to the heart to begin the cycle again. In one day, your heart transports all your blood around your body about 1000 times[54]." In this same way, we can utilize the fourth energy hub and its qualities of air to circulate emotional love and remove beliefs and past wounds that are creating blockages. As circulation improves at this subtle level, we can find compassion for those who may have wronged us, breathe into the sensations of our own emotions, and offer healing to ourselves and others. When we open to the possibility of love as the essential force of life, we access a sense of fullness that bears within it the seeds of inner peace. Engagement is required, though, to pump this heart energy into daily life. To activate and support its flow, we can make time to engage in loving touch, spend a whole day frolicking with our beloved, or immerse ourselves in a nurturing activity without imposing any time constraints.

When we work with opening the heart center, we might realize that we have been conceiving of love as an elusive, preconceived quality. As we soften into the layers of anahata, we begin to recognize that we are in fact made up of love and that we can therefore experience it through every aspect of our being if we so choose. Once we immerse ourselves in this force by accepting all of who we are, we can open to the possibility of others offering their hearts to us, as this chakra encompasses self-acceptance as well as social identity. Opening the heart chakra doesn't ensure a smooth ride through life, but as we engage it more fully, we can cultivate an ability to savor and ride the various waves we encounter. We lead from our hearts and trust that whatever unfolds will provide valuable learning and deep expansion.

Inquiries

On the Mat: Utilize the many facets of the practice including postures, breath, and mindfulness to connect to your heart center. Take time to first and foremost cultivate self-acceptance and self-love. From that foundation, evaluate whether you feel ready to send your energy outward to others in your life. Experiment with a practice of back extensions to generate more spaciousness both physically and subtly around the heart center. Consciously channel the breath as a source of integration for both body and mind. Pay special attention to your hands and arms as pathways leading to and from the heart, and consider how you can utilize them to receive and give love to both yourself and others. Towards the end of your sadhana, practice alternate-nostril breath as a technique to support integration. Explore balancing and heart-opening poses with tree, eagle, standing half moon, balancing half moon, cobra, locust, standing forward fold, fingers under toes in standing forward fold, hamstring tie stretches, quad stretch in pigeon, camel, bow, bridge, upward-facing bow.

Off the Mat: For one week, choose to explore either the practice of giving or receiving. Pick the one that is less comfortable for you in this moment. In the inquiry of receiving, notice how often you eschew compliments or refuse help or support from others. Do you frequently decline gifts that are given from the heart? For an inquiry of giving, take note of instances in which giving makes you feel you have something to lose, moments when you close your heart to helping a friend because of lack of time, or fears that giving will result in dependency or expectation. At the end of the week, write in your journal about any learning that surfaced through this exercise.

Practices

I open to the flame of love that glows from within. I allow the

Supportive Words
balance, connection, giving, love, receiving

Visualization
A green bud opening in spring.

Complementary Breath
nadi shodana

Closing Ritual
metta meditation

Teacher's Note
Utilize the first half of practice to support students in cultivating self-compassion and love through self-massage and positive affirmation (*I am loved, I am openhearted, I am fabulous, I am worthy*). During the second half, shift the class to include more interactive partner poses and partner massage to allow students to explore their social identity and offer heart energy to fellow practitioners.

to seep into every cell of my body

As I offer my heart, I pause to receive the love that is

being offered back to me

verdant green of the heart chakra

Voice of Truth:

Visuddha chakra is the fifth in the series of energy centers and is located at the base of the throat. Visuddha translates as virtuous or honest[55], indicating the authentic creativity and self-expression we can access as a result of the self-acceptance and love we cultivate in anahata. With this energy wheel, which correlates to the voice, we begin to move into the ethereal plane of the body, which is less tangible but just as potent as the preceding hubs. Its seed sound is "ham", and its color is bright blue. It addresses our need for creative expression and correlates to the childhood years between seven and twelve, when we begin to express more of what we deem as truth[56]. This lotus flower's main purpose is to serve as a portal into the realms of subtle energy, awareness, and inner precision. This vortex is the hub of creative self-expression, communication, sound, and vibration. "I speak my truth," is the phrase associated with its power.

As we explore the fifth chakra, we can delve into more authentic and honest communication with ourselves and others. As Socrates notes, "The greatest way to live with honor in this world is to be who we pretend to be." When we become attuned to the sounds and vibrations that words and voice carry, the results can be transformational and healing. It is interesting to note that the thyroid—which is the gland associated with this wheel—is a common site of disease in people of Western societies. Yogic thought would offer that in addition to many other lifestyle factors responsible for thyroid dysfunction, our inability to speak our personal truth or be authentic in our creative expressions is also a significant contributing factor. Living in harmony with our fifth life center, we no longer allow our words to simply spill out, but rather imbue them with deep meaning and strong intention. In this way, we can resonate harmoniously with those around us and ensure that the conversations and words that surround us are truly life-enhancing. Clarity of communication is another step towards increased alignment with our innate nature, as sound is associated with the expression and manifestation of the creative aspect of consciousness. In Sanskrit, the words matrika[57] *(womb, mother)* shakti *(creative energy)* represent the idea that each sound of the alphabet is imbued with unique potential. When used, each one of these vibrations has the power to manifest a word or thought as reality. Or in other words our "words *do* things; they don't merely *say* things[58]." For example, when we pause to consider it closely, we can recognize that thoughts, words, and sentences combine to create meaning, which in turn implants an image in our mind. That image radiates through our whole being, generating a feeling of joy, for example, which then emanates a vibration that frames our current experience. If we constantly berate ourselves for being a certain way, we are, in a sense, creating a vicious cycle that leaves us mired in the same deflated reality. Although the term vibration is commonly used in the spiritual world, science supports the notion that all things, even atoms *(which are the smallest units of an element having all the characteristics of that element)* vibrate with sound. Therefore, it is logical to assume that rhythm and pulse affect our emotions, thoughts, and actions on both the physical and subtle levels. Hazarat Inayat Khan reminds us, "He who knows the secret of sound, knows the mystery of the whole universe."

Inquiries

On the Mat: Investigating a particular pose becomes a deep communication of your inner words, thoughts, and feelings to the world around you. A warrior pose may appear to be a picture-perfect asana, but depending on the inner feeling, the outer form can express numerous different messages. In practice, we have an opportunity to express ourselves in alignment with who we truly are. Just as with taste in music, we might each be excited by a different genre. Use this time to discern any rhythms that aren't speaking to you, and invite the sound of your own personal truth to be expressed. Source the courage it takes to step into postures with a sense of steadfast truth aligned with the internal beat of your heart; notice how opening the fifth chakra on the mat can strengthen your ability to speak your truth in daily life. Examine both verbal and nonverbal ways of communicating. Express sounds diverse in pitch, tone, and volume, and remember to tune into your inner conversation, as well. Notice whether you tend towards excessive talking or an inability to listen, or whether you instead struggle to speak your truth. Remain mindful of the idea that the way you approach every single posture creates a distinct vibrational communication with long-lasting effects. Work with bramari pranayama as the breath that awakens the sound and heat of this energy vortex while you utilize ujjayi breath as an anchor throughout your practice. Focus on making a connection with the throat center by placing a hand gently on your throat periodically. To aid in releasing tension around the throat, move into shoulder openers, neck stretches, and a slow massage of muscles in the face and jaw. Investigate postures that awaken the throat such as mountain with hands clasped overhead, mountain, tree, eagle, standing yoga mudra, warrior I, lateral angle, triangle, inclined plane, bridge, camel, fish, and shoulder stand.

Off the Mat: Spend one day taking an inventory of the words you use regularly in daily life, making note of them throughout the day. How would you describe their overall tone? Do you use disempowering words like "maybe", "I don't know," and "I am not"? Or is your language compassionately direct, serving as a means of embracing who you are and honoring your truth?

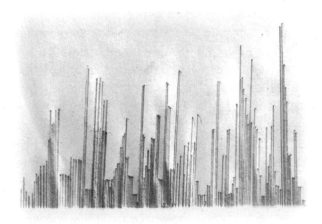

Practices

Supportive Words
creative expression, communication, sound, vibration

Visualization
Sound waves traveling through the ethers.

Complementary Breath
bramari

Closing Ritual
Chant, Aum Mani Padme Hum
The jewel of the lotus resides within

Teacher's Note
In partners, have students stand in front of one another and choose who will go first. Have the first speakers introduce themselves to their partner by saying, "Hi my name is _____, and I stand firmly in my truth," but guide them to voice these words in a wimpy, whispery way. Switch to partner B, and repeat. Now have partner B start, expressing the same statement again, but utilizing fifth chakra awareness. Change one last time back to partner A, inviting this person to repeat the introduction in an authentic way. Guide students to note the differences, thank their partners, and return to their mats.

Inner Knowing:

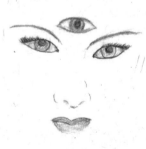

Ajna chakra is the sixth dynamic wheel of life. Ajna means "perception" and is located at the center of the forehead, just above eye level. This wheel also known as the third eye, is associated with deep-seated intuition, and relates to light. Rooted in our cultivated self-expression, truth, and creativity, we can embark on an exploration of our intuitive landscape. Ajna's seed sound is "aum" and its color is indigo blue[59]. It is the seat of inner knowing and thus corresponds to adolescence, when we awaken to our capacities for self-reflection and tap into greater insight. This energy hub is depicted as two petals representing the left and right sides of the brain or the ida and pingala nadis, which are the two primary energy conduits running through the body. Ajna's main purpose is to honor the gift of intuitive wisdom by reminding us that even in perceived darkness, our inner light can illuminate our path in subtle ways that engender heightened sensitivity. This vortex is the origin of energies related to seeing, intuition, light, vision, and imagination. "I see clearly inside and out," is the phrase associated with its power.

Light is an element that travels faster than sound, and everything we see in the world as concrete form is essentially reflected light. For this reason, two people looking at the same object could potentially see different things depending on where they stand and their own internal perspective. Our intuition and point of view have just as much impact on our interpretation as the object that is before us. As we surround ourselves with uplifting vibrations in the form of people, objects, and ways of living, we can attune to the inquiry of seeing versus simply looking by mindfully engaging the sixth chakra. When we can truly see as opposed to merely looking, we enter a new dimension of awareness. Seeing usually involves more than just the use of our eyes, and thus true vision emerges when we call upon our deep-seated instinct in the endeavor to understand something new. When we use our physical eyes, we perform the action of actively looking outward in search of external information, which is a vital and important function of human life. As we transition to seeing with our inner eye, we reach instead toward internal sources of increased sensitivity and heartfelt clarity[60]. In this way, ajna chakra allows us to move beyond surface judgments and superficial layers in order to connect to the divine light inherent in every being. With this recognition in place, we can skillfully use our physical observations as valuable sources of information, while at the same time exploring life and relationships in more than just this one apparent dimension.

Inquiries

On the Mat: Immerse yourself in the experience of movement and breath in order to clarify both your inner and outer vision. Honor the external forms of each asana, and then soften your gaze to access the internal realm of the pose. Follow your internal vision into the endless corners of your inner universe, and explore a relationship to yourself that expands your preconceived notions of existence. Remain aware of both your inner and outer gaze as you investigate the terrain of each posture. Engage in a more introspective practice focused on honing your internal vision even amidst the darkness. Awaken to your ability to become even more refined as you adjust each posture from the inside out. Explore eye stretches in your warm-up sequence, and focus your sadhana on twists *(twisting towards a larger, intuitive vision)* and forward folds *(to invite third eye to make contact with the earth)*. Practice aum pranayama both at the beginning of your practice and in moments of transition to repeatedly connect to the sixth energy vortex. Explore twists in standing yoga mudra, hands inside foot, thumbs to third eye in knee-down lunge, twisting warrior, twisting triangle, twisting chair, warrior two, humble warrior, easy pose twist, seated yoga mudra, marychiasana prep, and twisting cow face pose.

Off the Mat: If you were to lead your life from a place of intuition and imagination, what would this look like? Spend a few moments centering yourself in a way that serves you, and take the next several hours to express your internal vision through a creative medium of your choosing. Set your logical mind aside and approach this inquiry in a fluid, dream-like state.

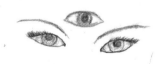

Practices

Supportive Words
intuition, insight, light, seeing, vision

Visualization
The third eye glowing with the light of deep knowing, illuminating the inner realms of being.

Complementary Breath
aum pranayama
Inhale to sweep the palms together overhead, and begin the "aum" sound on the exhale, continuing as you release hands downward towards the third eye; pause with thumbs touching the third eye, and repeat.

Closing Ritual
arti, ceremony of light
To perform this celebration of radiance and life, begin by lighting a candle. Place it on your altar or near your practice space. Begin to chant "saravam brahman maya re re[61]" (*Look, behold, God/Goddess/Spirit is everywhere*). As you chant, sweep your hands above the candle mindfully and draw the light into your third eye center and your whole being.

Teacher's Note
If you perform arti in class, inform students that you will be passing by with the candle and fanning the energy of the light towards them. Invite them to receive the light with a soft gaze, allowing it to caress their face, eyes, heart, third eye center, or any other area that feels appropriate. You may want to play a chant softly in the background, or you can invite students to chant the mantra above.

imagination as companions on my path

I open to the source of inner

With every breath, I honor my intuition and ... *wisdom that thrives within*

Web of Connection:

Sahasrara, meaning "thousand-petals" is the seventh chakra; it corresponds to the cerebral cortex and is often depicted as white, red, or multicolored. This energy wheel houses our connection to universal energy and the greater web of existence and is known as the seat of the soul[62]. It corresponds to our universal identity, which we interact with and explore throughout our lives. The main purpose of sahasrara is to serve as a portal to our ever-present divine intelligence and to encourage us to recognize our true nature. This vortex is related to expanded understanding, self-knowledge, universal connection, and the ability to dance in the current of life. "I know my individual and universal presence," is the phrase associated with its action and power. Although the chakras don't necessarily have to be experienced systematically, it can be of great benefit to establish safety, flow with the dance of emotions, anchor into our individual power, integrate and balance, explore our truth and self-expression, and illuminate our source of intuition; as we acknowledge and activate these vital dimensions of our being, we are better equipped to discover our innate and infinite consciousness. Sahasrara invites us to consider that we are inherently divine beings and to recognize that all that surrounds us is imbued with the same eternal life force that we are. When we are able to see every facet of life and sense the way it contributes to the greater tapestry, we can access a deeper understanding of our true nature. Rooted in this understanding, we can better comprehend our role in the world, the functioning of the cosmos, and the deeper meaning of all things.

In several Tantric-based Kundalini Yoga traditions, this last spinning circle is the pinnacle or goal we attempt to reach through transcending the lower energy centers. In other schools, the prevailing view equates life to an ongoing, fluctuating dance transpiring at all levels of existence; just like the other chakras, sahasrara opens and closes due to different experiences and events in our life and is not deemed superior to those vortexes below it. The adage "everything is contained in everything[63]" reminds us that all of the wheels of life are essentially embedded in each specific one. For this reason, recognition of our interconnected nature can come through exploration of any of the previous hubs. For example, when exploring the first energy wheel of safety, foundation, and earth, we might become aware of our greater connection to life on the planet. Although sahasrara is indeed enmeshed in the other wheels of life, it also provides us with a distinct and expansive perspective. It invites us to broaden our view and metaphorically zoom out to embrace a more universal vision. While this implies outward expansion, the seventh wheel also encourages us to contemplate the possibilities for growth within our own internal landscape. Science tells us that the body has thousands of receptors that enact trillions of synapses to relay messages to the mind. Thus the mind is as sensitive to its interior landscape and functions as it is to external stimuli. Indeed, there is a whole universe residing within us, and the mind is serves as the master mechanism of our embodied form, serving us on both the internal and external planes. Sahasrara encourages us to engage even the most minute levels of functioning on the internal plane to successfully cultivate a relationship to the universe from the inside out. As we bring about this inner awakening, the resulting change in our attitudes and behaviors profoundly affects the embodied experiences that comprise our days. As Hafiz reminds us:

> Running
> Through the streets
> Screaming,
>
> Throwing rocks through windows,
> Using my own head to ring
> Great bells,
>
> Pulling out my hair,
> Tearing off my clothes,
>
> Tying everything I own
> To a stick,
> And setting it on
> Fire.
>
> What else can Hafiz do tonight
> To celebrate the madness,
> The joy,
>
> Of seeing God
> Everywhere![64]

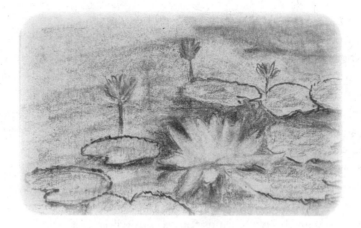

Inquiries

On the Mat: In the practice of yoga, we have an opportunity to connect our limited perception of ourselves with the infinite reality of the cosmos. As we hone our ability to engage in this profound act of paying attention, we open to the awareness of our vast, timeless nature. We can utilize the various elements of asana practice to both cultivate a more spacious outward vision and dive into the vast expanse of our interior. By holding these two different yet complementary visions, the thousand lotus petals of this wheel of life become enlivened with the immense possibility of our human form. In this practice, incorporate some of the elements of the previous chakras as a reminder that all is interconnected. Move through a series of open and expansive postures fostering connection to universal presence from the outside in. During the sequence, allow time to explore the internal universe that serves as a bridge to sahasrara and buoys your connection to both your individual and universal self. Practice viloma pranayama, varying the ratios to create the internal spaciousness related to sahasrara. Explore inversions in mountain, knee-down lunge, warrior one, warrior two, lateral angle, triangle, humble warrior, twisting warrior, standing yoga mudra, standing forward fold, parsvotanasana, seated yoga mudra, bound angle, and headstand. Complete your time on the mat with an intuitive flow to honor body and breath.

Off the Mat: Invoke the practice of samyama *(flowing of attention, deep concentration)* for one day. To practice, begin by immersing your attention for thirty seconds on inanimate objects. Pay attention to your breath in the background and honor any distractions, but attempt to stay fully present. Progress to longer holding times and a variety of focal points, like elements from nature, animals, or people. Notice if you sense the energy of each particular objectt of focus.

Practices

Supportive Words
interconnected, interdependent, interrelated, intertwined, interwoven

Visualization
A lotus buoyant at the surface of the water, with its petals unfurling gracefully even as its roots are bound by mud.

Complementary Breath
natural

Closing Ritual
Sit with your natural breath, and focus on the way it enlivens your individual body. After ten cycles of softly inhaling and exhaling, begin to follow the invisible thread of the breath and meditate on how it seamlessly binds all of existence. Start with objects and people near you, and then progress to individuals and entities that are further and far greater than you.

Teacher's Note
Have the students arrange their mats in a large circle to symbolize the interconnected nature of the seventh wheel of life. At the end of class, toss a ball of twine or yarn to one student, and then ask this student to toss it to someone else. Continue until everyone has had a chance, and admire the beautiful web of connection that emerges. Once the web is complete, have one person tug on the string to demonstrate how we are all interconnected and feel the effects of each other's actions.

Brahma Viharas:

The Brahma Viharas are teachings derived from the Buddhist tradition, and they encompass four divine abodes or practices of the heart. These four specific conventions are described as different aspects of a unified vision that can support us in living our lives to the fullest. They are metta *(loving-kindness)*, mudita *(joy for others)*, karuna *(compassion)*, and upekkha *(equanimity)*. Each of the Brahma Viharas offers a unique lens through which we can explore our world and our habitual behaviors. Loving-kindness invites us to identify the areas of our lives in which we have become overly fixated on our own needs. Joy for others illuminates interactions or relationships that are sources of resentment. The practice of compassion can reveal aspects of our lives infused with pity or even cruel intention. Finally, equanimity can help us recognize area in which we have become overly indifferent or, conversely, overly attached to various people or situations in our lives. The names of the four divine abodes are written in Pali, which is the language of the Buddhist scriptures. Note that only two of the divine abodes are discussed in detail.

Metta: {*inspired by Anne Cushman*}

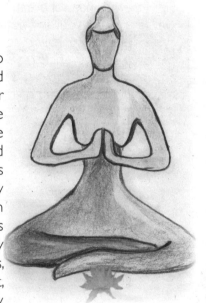

Yoga provides us with a platform for exploring our ability to cultivate loving-kindness. True and devoted friendship is a rare and special gift that is treasured for a lifetime. As we cultivate deeper friendship with ourselves, it is common to encounter hurdles. In the West, for example, many women and men struggle with body image issues, often as a result of advertising that communicates a standardized view of beauty. In yoga, we are invited to contemplate loving-kindness for both ourselves and others, recognizing that when we are personally uplifted, everyone benefits. One of the tools for cultivating support on all levels is that of Loving-Kindness Mediation. Traditional metta involves offering support to ourselves first *(May I be safe. May I be healthy. May I be joyful. May I be free.)* and then extending this well wishing to others, including loved ones, strangers, a person with whom we are in conflict, all planetary beings, and all of existence. In this way, we simultaneously affirm our own right to thrive as well as the prerogative of others to be as they are, learn, and grow to their fullest. Anne Cushman writes, "Metta helps us shift our focus from getting love to creating it, from improving our bodies to cherishing them, and from fixing life to embracing it[65]." The ultimate aim of metta is to shift our relationship with self to one of friendship and love, and then apply this to our interactions with rest of the world. As Sharon Salzberg shares:

> *Doing metta, we plant seeds of love, knowing that nature will take its course and in time those seeds will bear fruit. Some seeds will come to fruition quickly, some slowly, but our work is simply to plant the seeds. Every time we form the intention in the mind for our own happiness or the happiness of others, we are doing our work; we are channeling the powerful energies of our own minds. Beyond that, we can trust the laws of nature to continually support the flowering of our love[66].*

Inquiries

On the Mat: In this practice, use the tools of asana and breath to nurture a sense of loving-kindness both within and without. At the outset of sadhana, take time to establish the foundation of the breath, as it is the first step in crafting an atmosphere of loving awareness. Next, check in with yourself and acknowledge your present state, whether it is open, joyful, clenched, or withdrawn. As you set an intention for your practice, choose one particular metta phrase that resonates with your current state of mind. If you are struggling with a particular part of your body, one valuable strategy is to send love to the part that is aching, injured, or feeling abandoned. Throughout practice, listen carefully to what your body truly needs; if you encounter a moment of internal critique, gently return to your metta phrase, which will offer a more compassionate vibration. In addition to or instead of a personal focus, dedicate your practice to a loved one, affirming the power of metta to reach a wider circle. Feel the effect of this meditation as you immerse yourself or your loved one in the energy of loving-kindness. Explore back extensions, side stretches, and twists to open the heart and awaken to the possibility of fully thriving. At the end of the practice, take time to complete a full metta meditation. Alternately, incorporate this into the body of the practice, focusing on one metta statement during each segment of class; offer love to yourself at the outset, and progress through the various layers, completing with an offering to all beings near the end of class. Explore back extensions with high lunge, knee-down lunge, warrior one with back heel to the sky, warrior one, reverse warrior, twisting warrior, cobra, locust, bow, half frog, eye of the needle, wind-relieving, supine twist, bridge, and bridge with one leg extended skyward.

Off the Mat: During the span of a week, commit to four actions of loving-kindness. Let the first be towards yourself (*space, quiet, nature, or fun*), the second towards a loved one (*a meal, massage, quality time, or unexpected gift*), the third towards your immediate community (*volunteer, make food for a friend, watch a friend's child*), and the fourth for the benefit of the planet and all beings (*offset your carbon, invest in green energy, or use alternative modes of transportation*). Take note of how you feel at the end of the week.

Practices

I cultivate unconditional friendliness towards myself and others

Supportive Words
compassion, friendliness, love, loving-kindness,

Visualization
Hands clasped in anjali mudra, bowing to a little flower with kindness and love.

Complementary Breath
ujjayi

Closing Ritual
metta meditation

gift of my body

open to self-love as I cherish the

be healthy. May I be joyful. May I be free

May I be safe. May I

Mudita: {*inspired by Liam Beliveau*}

Mudita is translated as altruistic joy and exemplifies the state of being so full and well-nourished in ourselves that we allow our love to overflow and support the accomplishments of others. Parents experience the energy of mudita as they watch their children grow, succeed, and interact with the world. Teachers enjoy this current of altruistic joy as they guide and nurture students in external learning and inner discovery. When mudita is at work, we are able to draw inspiration from the beauty emerging along another's path. Altruistic joy helps us recognize that when others are fulfilled, there are far-reaching implications for society as a whole. Liam is a nineteen-year-old student who was participating in Kripalu's Semester Intensive program. Over the course of his five months of study, we cultivated a friendship that involved practicing yoga, rich conversations, and conscious sharing. After his time at Kripalu, Liam decided to travel to Thailand to embark on deeper study of Tantric Yoga Philosophy. When he told me of his upcoming plans, I was surprised that jealousy and envy didn't rear their heads, as I am an avid student of this same subject. Instead, I felt excitement and joy for his opportunity to engage in deeper learning and have new adventures. In my heart, I knew that his voyage would allow him to grow further, strengthen his character, and share himself more fully once he returned.

Mudita is a profoundly rewarding practice and yet also regarded as the most challenging of the Brahma Viharas. With students or children, the practice of joy for another is often quite easy to cultivate. As we contemplate altruistic joy for co-workers, acquaintances, and mere strangers, the fog thickens; jealousy, envy, and unproductive comparisons are likely to creep up when we believe that another's success equates to our own failure or lack of worth. As stories of blame and disbelief start to spin, we can capitalize on feelings of frustration, greed, and judgment as means of delving into our own patterning. It is common to compare our own achievements with someone else's when we feel a lack of clarity or trust with regard to what it is we want. We start to focus our attention on why they are privileged and why we are not, when in fact it is often our lack of belief in ourselves that is creating this misperception. For example, when someone else receives a promotion we desperately wanted, we can pause to contemplate whether it was truly the right fit or consider that not getting it may actually be a blessing in disguise that will be revealed later on. It is vital to draw on our capacity for trusting in ourselves and also to recognize the benefit we receive when those around us are vibrating at a higher frequency. In this way, mudita relates to the idea of abundance and fullness; if we approach our life with the perspective that the universe is constantly expanding, then there is enough room for everyone's successes. If we really want what our friend has, we can trust that we too can achieve it; it simply requires intention, conscious action, patience with timing, and the recognition that the aspiration might not manifest for us in exactly the same fashion. When we believe in this process and wholly embrace who we are, practicing mudita becomes much easier to integrate into our lives. Through stretching our ability to walk our own road with steadfastness and grace while sharing in the joy of others, we can honor the unique gifts that each and every one of us shares with the world. As Sharon Salzberg writes in *Loving Kindness*:

> *It is a rare and beautiful quality to feel truly happy when others are happy. When someone rejoices in our happiness, we are flooded with respect and gratitude for their appreciation. When we take delight in the happiness of another, when we genuinely rejoice at their prosperity, success, or good fortune rather than begrudging it in any way...Unlike a state of mere excitement or giddiness, the quality of sympathetic joy*

challenges our deep assumptions about aloneness, loss, and happiness, and shows us another possibility[67].

Inquiries

On the Mat: Take this contemplation into the yoga studio, and utilize your practice as a potent opportunity to exercise altruistic joy, as the light of other practitioners surrounds you on all sides. Notice whether there are times when the class becomes a competitive stomping ground in which you covet the most advanced postures. Sense your ability to hold space for others' experiences while recognizing your own beauty and abundance. Alternatively, practice on your own and mindfully cultivate mudita for someone in your life. Explore a potpourri practice with knee-down lunge, quad stretch in knee-down lunge, plank, down dog, lateral angle, wide-angle standing forward fold, star gazer, intense stretch, cobra, locust, bow, crocodile, pigeon, quad stretch in pigeon, and half camel.

Off the Mat: Over the span of a week, make a point of telling three people in your life how much joy you feel because they are thriving in their lives. Sense the energy that manifests as a result.

Practices

I trust in myself and in the path I am forging.

Supportive Words
benevolent, bountiful, generous, charitable, magnanimous

Visualization
A high five, raising both hands in a gesture of excitement on behalf of a friend.

Complementary Breath
nadi shodana

Closing Ritual
Sit in front of a photo of someone toward whom you feel a genuine sense of mudita. Use their image as a focal point for your meditation, sending them charitable thoughts from the space of the heart.

Teacher's Note
In this class, invite students to face a partner for the warm-up portion of the practice, and encourage them to draw inspiration from their mirror. Encourage them to linger in the inquiry of how it feels to honor the joy of someone else's practice. When you reach the peak of your posture flow, ask students to create a large circle. Clarify that the exercise is optional, and then invite two at a time to come into the center and do one of their most joyful poses. As they do so, invite the remaining students to simply observe for a few breaths. Next, ask them to share one word aloud as an expression of mudita for their fellow practitioners. Take turns until all students who wish to participate have stepped into the middle of the circle. Alternatively or in addition, lead an experience of mudita in pairs, as follows: have students find a partner and determine who will go first. Guide students into a soft breath meditation, and after they are settled, instruct partner one to open her eyes and witness the beauty and wholeness of her friend; encourage her to simply drink in her partner's light. After a few minutes, switch roles. Once the second partner has finished, instruct them to linger here for a few moments with their eyes closed to see if they can feel mudita taking root. Close the exercise with a soft "aum".

I cultivate joy for my loved ones' successes

With compassion, I experience the full spectrum of feelings within.

the wisdom of yoga 157

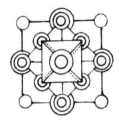

the
hindu
gods & goddesses

"You must understand the whole of life, not just one little part of it. That is why you must read, that is why you must look at the skies, that is why you must sing, and dance, and write poems, and suffer, and understand, for all that is life."

-J. Krishnamurti

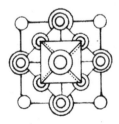

Hinduism, like many spiritual traditions, is difficult to clearly define. Depending on whom you consult and in what part of India, you will likely get a different spin on the beliefs and practices enacted on this spiritual path. With regard to the Hindu Gods and Goddesses, in particular, there are numerous interpretations of their symbolism and myths. One of the core principles underlying the nondualist school of thought is the belief that we are all interconnected and comprised of the same substance, while each still possessing qualities of uniqueness and individuality. As such, the Hindu deities represent the diverse aspects of the divine and likewise—according to the beliefs of the tradition—the various aspects of our inner selves. It becomes easier to engage an authentic inquiry of the deities once we understand this notion of them as embodiments of internal qualities rather than external, supreme beings.

The gods and goddesses are key characters in many of Hinduism's most prominent tales, which can be found in the four sacred hymns of Hinduism (also known as the Vedas), in ancient legends like the Ramayana and Mahabharata, and in the Puranas (ancient religious stories that provide an account of the deities most familiar to the West)[1]. The symbolism of these divine beings is embedded in both the events and details of their stories, as well as in their physical iconography. Bear in mind, though, that there are many myths and many versions of these tales depending on the specific source tradition. It is also important to note that the concept of myths within Indian culture encourages their creative application in the endeavor to bridge understanding of a greater truth. The implication of this definition is profound because it conveys the idea of deeply embedded, underlying wisdom being transmitted through the indirect means of mythology. There are two ways to work with these transmissions of information and their meanings. The first involves direct and literal interpretation with a single, clear perspective as the outcome. The Old and New Testaments are potent examples of stories that were initially interpreted in just one way. Whole religions are built on the literal writings without room for readers to mine a deeper understanding of the essence of the teachings. Because a single meaning is already prescribed in many traditions, readers don't have the opportunity to apply their own wisdom and reason; they are essentially confined to just one version of the myth and advised to follow this preexisting understanding or face dire consequences. In the Tantric world view and in many other mystical traditions, however, classical myths came to be approached in a new way. These traditions invite readers to interact with the stories, assign value, add personal interpretations, and ultimately recognize more than one view of the same event. In this way, they cultivate an openness to the possibility that these ancient stories hold more than solely the overt, literal meaning, and they allow readers to view the various characters in the story as different manifestations of themselves. This innovative relationship to myths thus expands the potential for deeper understanding of their messages by opening ancient ideas to exploration and inquiry in the context of daily life in the modern world.

The deities as a group comprise a rich and extensive realm of teachings. Each of the following sections, therefore, focuses on one specific thematic strand and several iconographical representations of each deity. You might consider closing or opening some of these sadhanas by invoking the deities through ritual chanting of their names. This is a particularly effective means of tuning into each deity's specific vibration and igniting that same energy within, whether it be confidence, acceptance, abundance, or dexterity.

The Gods:

The Puranas are split into three groups of stories, with each one focusing on the manifestations, consorts, and lives of one of the three primary gods still commonly worshipped today[2]. These three gods are representative of the three principal energies cycling both within us and in the world outside of us. The ancient stories tell us that Consciousness split herself into three distinct energies: Brahma to create, Vishnu to preserve, and Shiva to destroy and transform. In theory, these three gods are of equal importance, as each represents one aspect of the divine. When described by their respective devotees, however, a hierarchy does often emerge with the favored god assuming the post as the superior of the three. Often, this god is even credited with playing all three roles of creator, preserver, and transformer by those who identify most strongly with him. Although these primary figures are most well known for their roles as creator, sustainer, and transformer they also offer many other contemplations through their symbolism, iconography, and myth.

Brahma the Creator: {inspired by Israel Milikovski & Leon Arguetty}

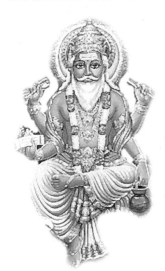

According to the Upanishads, there was an all-pervading divine essence that was all of everything but was without form. Into the waters of the unknown it planted a seed, which slowly grew into a majestic golden egg, resplendent as the sun. When this egg hatched, Brahma—the creator of the Universe—was awakened and made manifest in form. In Hindu cosmology, time is tracked by the days and years of Brahma's life. When he awoke and opened his eyes, the universe and everything in it was created, and when he closes his eyes, all of creation will cease to exist. Luckily for us, one day in his life is 4,320 million human years. In Hindu myth, Brahma is often described as the beloved grandfather of the worlds, representing the wisdom of those who have journeyed before us across the landscape of life. Brahma is usually depicted with four heads and four arms, and he is either seated on a lotus or riding a golden goose. In his hands, he holds a spoon, a water jug, mala beads, a lotus flower, and sometimes a book (the Vedas)[3].

As human beings, one of our most remarkable gifts is this ability to create ourselves as we emerge from our own golden egg. A single imaginative seed sparked the whole universe, and in that seed existed the potential for all that is. Nature reminds us of this innate power, as one tiny walnut has the potential to manifest the grandeur of a mature tree. How do we as humans create our universe day-by-day? When we open our eyes on any given morning, we too, have the power to sculpt our reality. We can make choices that not only lead us in the direction of the next phase of our journey but also allow us to actively co-create the process. The journey of life is to remain steadfast on this path while gaining expanded knowledge of all its aspects through experience, exploration, and risk.

The symbolism associated with Brahma provides us with reminders of the tools we already possess to aid our endeavor of creative co-participation. The image of an elder grandfather indicates that others have walked this path before and thus that we needn't reinvent the wheel. His presence reminds us to call upon the wisdom of our elders, particularly when we embark upon a new endeavor. At the same time, the beloved grandfather also urges us to acknowledge our own wisdom, drawing contrasts and recognizing that some things that worked in the past will not serve us in the present. Brahma's four hands relate to the four points of a compass, which serves as a tool of guidance and direction on a physical journey. In life, we can cultivate a clear sense of direction for the next step by tuning into the internal compass of our intuition and taking time to consider this existing wisdom. When using a compass to find true North, we have to utilize careful precision to get the little red line into a small box. The compass is calibrated by the magnetic pull of the Earth, representative of the greater power at the root of our wanderings. As we explore our creative vision, we may encounter a multiplicity of possible paths. In these instances, we must pause for contemplation and make those choices which most genuinely reflect our own unique way of being while also attuning to this deeper knowing. Brahma's four heads represent the four Vedas (*or books of knowledge*) and illustrate the capacity to watch, observe, and adapt to the movement of life with clarity and ease. Choosing a definitive direction, we initiate a new experience that will provide us a foundation of firsthand knowledge and understanding for that which will naturally follow. Finally, his water jug is a symbol which honors the sacred and life-giving power of water and serves as a reminder of how we must nourish the seeds of our internal vision[4].

Inquiries

On the Mat: There are many diverse paths available to us in yoga, and it is through our creative power that we can craft a mélange of personal practices to optimally support all parts of our being. As we gain more knowledge over time through personal practice, we are better able to utilize our internal compass to tend to each creative seed in the most fruitful way. Investigate how a single asana could be the origin of this root system, as it might lead you through feelings of struggle, understanding, awareness, softness, and strength. When you step onto the mat, you can connect to a deeper sense of yourself, which in turn initiates imaginative sparks. Just like Brahma, utilize all of your diverse tools to guide the depth and direction of your sadhana. Acknowledge the value of the gifts you bring into each pose while staying open to whatever may surface when you engage with awareness and purpose. Choose which aspects of yourself you will nurture in your practice, and—just like a seed—this object of your attention will indeed develop and grow. Choose to nurture a particular posture, a specific breath, an internal relationship, or a creative aspect of yourself. Investigate how you can hone your connection to your inner compass, develop an ever-expanding base of knowledge, and cultivate the capacity for choosing which creative sparks you nurture, all through the vehicle of your practice. Explore standing forward fold, standing splits, down dog, three-legged dog twist, runner's stretch, parsvotanasana, standing hand to big toe, marychiasana twist, fire log, twist in fire log, twist in high lunge, knee-down lunge, hands inside foot in knee-down lunge, heron and sundial.

Off the Mat: Spend time with your grandfather(s), or make an effort to learn more about them if they have already passed. Journal about what aspects of their personalities can support you in nourishing the creative vision of your own life path.

I acknowledge the latent power of the many seeds I plant each day. I trust that

Supportive Words
beginning, bud, concept, notion, nucleus, spark, start

Visualization
Brahma's golden egg, resplendent as the sun.

Complementary Breath
dirgha

Closing Ritual
Plant a seed of intention for the week ahead.

I utilize the tools I already possess to fuel my

my creative vision, the more it will expand

personal creativity

the more I nurture

Vishnu the Sustainer: {*inspired by Ann Greene*}

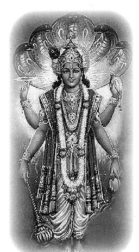

Vishnu is known as the all-pervading one. He is considered omnipresent, and his is the energy that keeps the universe running smoothly. This sustaining essence can be thought of as all the elements of the universe, nature, and life that stabilize us and allow us to thrive, including the sun, Mother Earth herself, the five elements *(ether, air, fire, water, earth)*, societal structures, relationships, technology, and spiritual practices to name a few. According to classical myth, there are times when Vishnu must incarnate as other beings known as avatars. These avatars descend or cross over into this realm, assuming embodied form to aid in the unfolding of worldly events. Vishnu is depicted as a four-armed man with a blue or black complexion who wears a crown on his head and is guarded by a protective canopy of cobras' *(Shesha)* heads. He is typically depicted holding a discus, a lotus, a conch shell, and a thunderbolt[5].

As we move through our lives, we are constantly juggling different responsibilities, carefully maintaining balance as we fulfill our many obligations to ourselves and others. To this end, we must engage a certain amount of endurance and wisdom to skillfully maneuver our path. At times, we may have to assume different or unexpected roles to sustain the necessary balance. We become avatars, taking on new responsibilities in order to support someone or something of value in our lives. This can occur in the realms of family, relationship, and livelihood, among others. If a parent dies suddenly, we might have to put work on hold and return home to help out for a few months. When a baby is born, life completely transforms as we become responsible for sustaining and nurturing another's life. In essence, these are instances of fulfilling our duty as we step in to the realities of embodied life. These duties may not align with our true desires of the moment, but deep down we know that engaging them will facilitate the situation at hand and serve the greater good.

Vishnu's blue or black complexion indicates his omnipresence as related to the complete cycle of daytime and nighttime. His sankha, or conch shell, represents a call to action and the fullness of the breath. This is a reminder of the vital support oxygen provides us in each moment, even though we do not always see or recognize that we are, in fact, immersed in an ocean of breath. Furthermore, the conch shell teaches us how we can employ the breath to engender steadiness, vitality, and internal focus as tools in the effort to sustain the various activities of our lives. The chakra, or discus, spins on the horizontal plane, symbolizing our ability to interact skillfully with intimate partners, peers, and everyday situations. The vajra, or thunderbolt, moves up and down on the vertical plane, symbolizing the times when we are called to respond quickly to forces or relationships outside of our typical daily routines. The padma, or lotus, is another widely used symbol associated with Vishnu, representing the beauty, happiness, and eternal renewal that manages to flourish even with roots deep in the mud[6]. In relationship to Vishnu, the flower represents the beauty that can emerge when we work hard, persist, and thus boost life force both for ourselves and those around us.

Inquiries

On the Mat: Notice where there are times when you want to release a pose because it simply feels too laborious to sustain. You've assumed the role of yoga practitioner, but the little voice inside generates obstacles that keep you from reaping the full benefits of this endeavor. What occurs when you stay with the experience of the posture? As you hold longer and enter new depths, does a surge of energy arise that expands your capacity for staying centered and strong? Explore a practice with longer holdings, and feel the energetic imprint of sustaining poses at the edge of what you would normally deem as comfortable. Use the symbol of the conch as a focus, drawing attention to sustenance of your breath and its ability to aid you in staying with the asanas. Notice if holding a pose slightly beyond your own preconceived limit actually sparks your vitality. Explore arms clasped overhead in mountain, eagle arm rotations, shoulder stretch in cow face, plank, plank on forearms, down dog, standing yoga mudra, locust, upward boat, dolphin, and supported headstand.

Off the Mat: Go on a longer walk or bike ride than usual, going the extra mile to build the muscle of sustaining. Does this practice deplete you in any way? What aspects of going the extra mile offer you energy and vitality?

Practices

I utilize the vital force of the breath to sustain myself both on and off the mat

Supportive Words
sustain, maintain, uphold, bolster, bridge, support, augment

Visualization
Vishnu, with his four arms, golden crown, and canopy of snake heads

Complementary Breath
ujjayi

Closing Ritual
journal contemplation

How do you embody the energy of Vishnu in your daily life?

Teacher's Note
At the end of the practice, instruct your class to form a large circle. Have students turn to face the back of the person in front of them. Guide them to take one step closer towards the center so that they are very close together. When they are close enough, invite them to sit down on one another's laps to form a chair pose circle, powered to sustain.

companions in my journey

I honor the roles in my

I model stability for those who are

life that require me to be steady and strong

The Epic of Rama: {inspired by Isaac Arguetty}

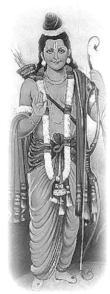

Ramachandra is the seventh incarnation of Vishnu and one of the most popular heroes in Hindu mythology. The word "ramachandra" literally translates to "pleasing," "delighting," "rejoicing," and "beloved." This incarnation of Vishnu represents the essence of courage, strength, steadfastness, and determination. Rama is one of the key characters in the Ramayana or *Celebrated Poem of the Journey of Rama*, in which he is joined by his consort Sita, his brother Lakshmana, and the monkey god Hanuman on an exhilarating adventure. According to legend, Rama relinquishes his claim to the throne and goes into exile with his wife Sita and brother Lakshman for fourteen years in order to honor his father. Surpanakha, sister of the ten-headed king Ravana, develops an interest in Rama and attempts to seduce him without success. She then attempts to seduce his brother, who also refuses her wishes. In anger, Surpanakha tries to attack Sita, but Lakshman saves her by severing the evil demon's nose and ears. Infuriated, she returns home to Ravana, who vows to destroy Rama and take Sita for himself. One day, Rama and Lakshman are drawn into the forest, leaving Sita alone in their hermitage. The demon Maricha disguises himself as an old man and appears at her door begging for food. Sita decides to help him, and as soon as she steps outside, Ravana captures her and takes her to the island of Sri Lanka. Rama and Lakshman thus embark on a search for Sita, and along the way they are joined by Hanuman, who offers his skillful service to Rama in her rescue. Rama, Hanuman, and an army of monkeys build a massive bridge over the water and cross to Sri Lanka, where they engage in a fierce, prolonged battle leaving many dead and wounded on both sides. Towards the end of the skirmish, Rama faces Ravana in a duel, and he defeats the evil demon after many hours of combat[7].

As this first part of the narrative demonstrates, Rama is a man of integrity and clear determination who is constantly surmounting new obstacles. Through his honorable actions in the roles of son, husband, brother, prince, and citizen, Rama embodies virtue. Not once does he give in to fear, hesitate in his commitment to his father, or pause in his journey to rescue Sita. As Jon Kabat-Zinn alludes to in his book *Full Catastrophe Living*, life can often feel like an epic of ever-renewing challenges. These arrive in the form of a new job or relationship, a death in the family, or mounting financial responsibilities, among other things. The skill comes in facing what is before us with the heart of Ram, knowing there is wisdom to be gained through every episode of our life's story. The essence of Rama is related to the Sanskrit word "karma," which is translated as "action." In the embodied plane, we enter into relationship with life in an abundance of manifest forms and thus encounter many realities of existence. As we make decisions that lead us one way or another, we must pause to recognize the direct outcomes of our actions. As Rama demonstrates, karma is not a problem to transcend but rather an opportunity to maneuver the voyage of life as skillfully as possible. As we navigate through life, it is valuable to remember the range of resources available to us. Just like Ram, we can turn within to source our innate power and skill, call upon our family (*Lakshman*) for help, and befriend new supporters (*Hanuman*) as our journey progresses. Even though the Ramayana eventually comes to an end, the essence of Rama's story lives on and communicates the power of approaching life as a constant practice of savoring each experience in order to know the full richness of our humanity. As Edward Abbey writes in *Benedicto*:

May your trails be crooked, winding, lonesome, dangerous, leading to the most amazing view. May your mountains rise into and above the clouds. May your rivers flow without end, meandering through pastoral valleys tinkling with bells, past temples and castles and poets' towers into a dark primeval forest where tigers belch and monkeys howl, through miasmal and mysterious swamps and down into a desert of red rock, blue mesas, domes and pinnacles and grottos of endless stone, and down again into a deep, vast, ancient, unknown chasm where bars of sunlight blaze on profiled cliffs, where deer walk across the white sand beaches, where storms come and go as lightning clangs upon the high crags, where something strange and more beautiful and more full of wonder than your deepest dreams waits for you—beyond that next turning of the canyon walls.

Inquiries

On the Mat: Carve out space to practice yoga for three full hours, and prepare a long sequence in advance. Notice whether you feel as though you are entering into the Ramayana, sensing that the journey of posture and breath is going to be arduous and long. Take this opportunity to step into the experience with total commitment and courage in spite of your apprehension. Honor even the most challenging and awkward postures, moments of disbelief or frustration, and times of low energy. Remember that in your sadhana, there are many resources at your disposal to help make your adventure life-enhancing and authentic. Utilize the soft strength of your breath, connect to mindfulness, trust in the energetic support of your community, use a prop to enhance an asana, or in the studio call on a teacher to aid you in a difficult posture. Just like Rama, we are the ones who must ultimately complete the endeavor, and yet there may be times when we need added motivation to set us in motion or someone to back us up along the way. Stay conscious and fully notice how your actions on the mat affect the overall outcome of your practice. To connect to the energy of Rama, chant "ram" during moments such as transitions or extended holdings. Explore standing half moon, standing forward fold, standing yoga mudra, knee-down lunge, hands inside foot in knee-down lunge, runner's stretch, warriors one and two, hands clasped in lateral angle, sleeping Vishnu, crane, and visvamitrasana.

Off the Mat: Sketch out a timeline of your own life, making sure to include any significant events that have shaped, nourished, or challenged you. Use collage, drawings, or words to elaborate and affirm your own unique epic.

Practices

I hug into the strength of my heart as I courageously traverse the path ahead

Supportive Words
grand, heroic, legendary, majestic, narrative, saga, tale

Visualization
Rama standing in wholeness and strength, with Sita, Lakshman, and Hanuman by his side.

Complementary Breath
ujjayi

Closing Ritual
chant
Shri Ram Jai Ram Jai Jai Ram, Sita Ram
(beloved Ram, victory to Ram)

The Divine Play of Krishna: {inspired by Douglas Brooks}

Krishna (black or dark blue one) is the eight incarnation of Vishnu and is worshipped by millions of people in India and around the world. Vishnu plucked a single white hair from his own head and placed it in the womb of Rohini and also one black hair, which he placed in the womb of Devaki. Krishna was born from the black hair and his older brother, Balarama, from the white. In his youth, Krishna enchanted the young gopis (the girls who tended cows) with his skills on the flute. During his lifetime, he defeated many enemies who threatened the equilibrium of life on Earth. He is probably best known for the guidance he offered to Arjuna on the battlefield during the confrontation between the Pandavas and the Kauravas, as recounted in the Bhagavad Gita (the Lord's song)[8].

Another name for Krishna is Krishnalila. In Sanskrit, lila is defined as play, or—more specifically—divine or cosmic play[10]. Tantra states that the universe (in this case represented by Krishna) enacts what it does simply for the joy of it and does so spontaneously, without seeking to fulfill any need, lack, or desire. The energy of Krishna is one of playful devotion, as consciousness delights when we revel in the miracle of life and don't take ourselves, our lives, or our work too seriously. In the stories of Krishna as a young man, he is depicted as a mischievous fellow, stealing the gopis' clothing, enchanting them with his flute, and hiding their milk. He embodies the qualities of surprise, intoxication, and sensuality and invites us to engage with these facets of life. This realm of divine play also encompasses the notion of entangled randomness, as there are many occurrences in our lives that defy the scientific predictability of cause and effect. In these instances, it is our perception and response that makes all the difference. Indeed the universe is largely rooted in a matrix of probability, and as we work hard and act skillfully to cultivate and share our unique gifts, we will most often achieve our established goals. Yet in a universe of seeming certainty, nothing is exclusively bound by cause and effect due to this element of lila or randomness. In a grand-slam tennis final, for example, there are two top professionals playing against one another. No matter how strong their skills are, the lila of the day is always a factor in the outcome. A sudden sprained ankle, heat exhaustion, or loss of motivation sometimes usurps skill and determines the winner. How do we react when this random energy of the universe steals our clothes and leaves us swimming naked in the river? Can we encounter this moment with the same lightness as those times when lila is seemingly more aligned with our desires?

In yoga and other forms of conscious movement, we ideally approach our practice with a concentrated dose of skill and dedication coupled with an intention for lightness and joy. In many styles of yoga, though, the essence of the practice easily becomes lost in exaggerated details or overly serious forms of discipline aimed at punishing the body. Osho, a spiritual teacher who was active in the 1970s, wrote that when we enter into a relationship (be it with our practice or a loved one), we often feel a need to fit everything perfectly into place. He equates this to locking the doors and shutting all the windows of a house. When we erect this same kind of stormproofing within, the natural currents of vitality are impeded, and we lose our ability to swim playfully amidst the spontaneous flow of life.

As Hafiz writes:

Everything is clapping today.

Light,
Sound,
Motion,
All movement.

A rabbit I pass pulls a cymbal
From a hidden pocket
Then winks.

This causes a few planets and I
To go nuts
And start grabbing each other.

Someone sees this,
Calls a
Shrink,

Tries to get me
Committed
For
Being too
Happy.

Listen: this world is the lunatic's sphere,
Don't always agree it's real,

Even with my feet upon it
And the postman knowing my door

My address is somewhere else[9].

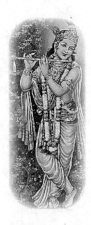

Inquiries

On the Mat: Invite a friend to practice with you as you cultivate your lighthearted side by brewing joy and ease in the internal realm. Even as you surrender to the play of lila, acknowledge the foundation of skillful action and safety in your practice. Some ideas to stimulate playfulness include: seated contract and release; making meow and moo sounds in cat and cow; moving into lion's breath facing a friend and teasingly scaring one another; sitting back to back, interlacing arms, and attempting to stand up together at the count of three; allowing yourself a lively tantrum *(in bridge prep, fists and feet pummel the floor like a wild child as you make lots of noise);* leading sun salutations facing your friend; and vocalizing throughout the practice. Explore plank, one-legged plank, side plank, pigeon, runner's stretch, crane, core strengtheners, reclining hero, dwi hasta bhujasana, eka pada koundinyasana, and bhujapidasana.

Off the Mat: Spend time engaging in an activity that will connect you to the energy of play; finger paint, ride a rollercoaster, do cartwheels, throw a party with stuffed animals, play pickup sticks, pull out old board games, build a sand castle, or fly a kite. Notice what shifts within as you immerse yourself in the play of life.

Practices

I open to a sense of lightness even when life delivers the unexpected

and remember to play

Supportive Words
romp, jump, revel, enthusiasm, intense love, passion, glorify, zest, zeal

Visualization
Krishna playing enchanting music on the flute.

Complementary Breath
bramari

Closing Ritual
chant
Shri Krishna, Govinda Hare Murare, He Natha Narayana Vasudeva
praise the beloved Krishna

I romp and revel

I soften around the serious aspects of my day

in the blessings thriving in my own heart

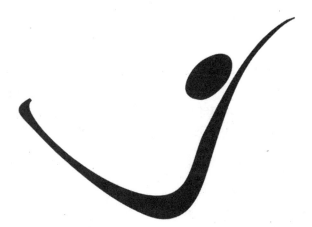

The Delight of Concealment & Revelation: {inspired by Douglas Brooks}

Shiva is depicted in many forms and is thus an icon representing a range of rich and intricate concepts. One of Shiva's most captivating and ubiquitous forms is Lord of the Dance, symbolizing the great pulsation of the universe wherein all of life, natural laws, and entangled randomness swirl and interact with one another. Shiva dances the Anandatandava (*Dance of Bliss*), which is an illustrative metaphor for the five core manifestations of perpetual energy—creation, destruction or transformation, preservation, veiling, and revealing. In most depictions of Nataraja *(as the Lord of the Dance is known),* Shiva's left hand is elongated and curved towards the right side of his body, covering his heart and signifying our tendency towards forgetfulness regarding our true nature. At the same time, though, his left fingers are pointing to his raised left foot in a gesture that represents the power of revelation, as this is what we first notice when we approach him from the side. These two complementary yet contrasting forces are evident and ever-present in day-to-day life, nature, and the universe at large. The frog emerging from and disappearing into camouflage, the sun and moon playing hide-and-seek as the light transitions, and the flowers opening to the brightness of the sun and hugging back into themselves once darkness settles…each of these is an example of the dance of concealment and revelation embodied by Shiva.

Working with my nutrition clients, I have the opportunity to both observe and participate in this magical process as it applies to the world of whole foods. When clients taste or cook quinoa for the first time or begin experimenting with unfamiliar leafy greens, something shifts for them. They are exposed to a whole new realm of food possibilities, and the joy that ensues is powerful. Upon first contemplation of the idea of things being cloaked or hidden, we may be inclined to label this phenomenon as one to avoid. But imagine the world without this energy of concealment. What if you woke up one day and knew all that there was to know about life or your future? Wouldn't something be lost? One deeply potent aspect of the Tantric world view is this recognition and valuing of concealment as well as revelation. In fact, Tantra claims there is always more concealed than revealed at any given time. Even when we awaken to greater awareness of ourselves or a broader understanding of the universe, there is always even more still waiting to be revealed. As such, the purpose of our lives and our practice of yoga is not to arrive at some final destination, but rather to simply participate in the dance and recognize the gifts inherent in acknowledging both concealment and revelation. A song is forgotten and then rediscovered months later to be thoroughly enjoyed anew. We lose touch with a friend only to encounter them after a number of years and reawaken a loving friendship. We forget about the practices that soothe us and then go on a retreat that reminds us of our innate tools for mining deep inner peace. Instead of thinking about the typically negative connotations of concealment, consider adopting the metaphor of a wrapped gift, which holds the promise of joy among its contents. Through the act of opening this gift, we access the magic of discovery as we experience new facets and flavors of our embodied human experience. As Diane Bergstrom shares in *Remind Me*:

Darkness always births the light. There is no insanity
without surfacing reason. Apathy can give way to
conviction and action.
Remind me.

There is no suppression without eventual uprising.
Public silence unleashes individual voices.
Where there is death, there must be life.
Remind me.

Where there is waste, growth will be forged.
Narcissistic leaders incense empowered communities.
Censorship spurs collective voices.
Remind me.

Senseless occupations cause people to question.
Unjustified spending arouses investigations.
The pendulum always swings.
Remind me.

Hopelessness, despair, intolerance and fear can debilitate.
Belief, anger, purpose, education and faith can facilitate. What can I do?
Remind me[10].

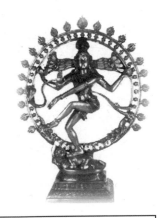

Inquiries

On the Mat: Investigate the areas of your practice that feel more concealed. Is there subtle functioning of particular muscles with which you are not familiar? Or do you lack refined sensitivity to certain areas of your body? Notice whether you are veiled with regard to a particular posture. As you acknowledge these areas of not knowing, remain open to the notion that revelation can occur in subtle ways. Remind yourself that fireworks aren't necessary for an experience of recognition and growth. An experience of revelation can be equally as powerful for someone reaching his fingers to the floor for the first time in standing forward fold as for someone finally getting into side crane. Identify the places where you feel cloaked and shadowed, and remember that a shift is possible in any moment if you simply honor these areas of contraction. Explore pigeon, fire log, baby cradle, marichyasana three, heron, lord of the fishes, bharadvajasana one, head to knee, rotated marichyasana, and revolved head to knee.

Off the Mat: Gather a few friends for a revelation party. Choose a topic of interest about which you know very little (*i.e. wine, tuning a bike, raw desserts, baking bread, canning jams/pickles, building a raised bed garden, knitting, or pruning a tree*). Do some research on this topic prior to the gathering. When guests arrive, take time to share what you've learned with the group, and ask others to contribute their insights. Culminate the evening with a hands-on activity that relates to the topic, followed by a final group sharing to integrate this newfound wisdom.

Practices

Supportive Words
Conceal: *camouflage, cloak, cover, veil, wrap*
Reveal: *bare, disclose, expose, open, uncover, unearth, unmask, unveil*

Visualization
Clouds condense into a fog cloaking a valley; slowly, as the curtain of clouds begins to lift, the brilliant colors of the morning are revealed.

Complementary Breath
ujjayi, with breath retention
Exhaling, hold breath out for a few moments to experience contraction and concealment, then inhale to relish the breath more fully in its expansion and revelation.

Closing Ritual
journal contemplation
What, if anything, was revealed to you during your practice today?

Teacher's Note
During the course of the practice, ask students to pair up, and guide a few simple partner postures as well as some physical assists and adjustments. Often, it is when we are assisted that we experience something new in our yoga. Make sure to remind students to communicate clearly regarding their needs and any injuries when assisting one another. Lead a cobra assist, a partner down dog press, and a simple seated twist assist. Before beginning this exercise, ask them to share any areas of concealment regarding each particular pose with their partner. Remind them that the simple act of verbalizing the places where they typically feel contracted in a given asana can effect a huge shift in their practice. At the end of the last partner-assisted posture, ask them to share briefly with one another any revelations that may have surfaced during the partner experience.

is always more to be discovered

I recognize the gift of disguise

I revel in the idea that there • *and the joy inherent in the ritual of unmasking*

The Dynamic Dance of Culture & Nature: {inspired by Mitchel Bleier}

Ganesha is the son of Parvati and Shiva and is rich with iconography and symbolism. He is typically depicted as a being with a young man's body and an elephant's head and is often in a seated position. There is usually a bowl of ladus, or Indian sweets, near his feet, along with a little mouse. Ganesha holds a noose, a small ax, and a lotus in one hand. His other hand is shown in the "fear not" mudra with the marking of an aum tattoo. One version of Ganesha's birth describes his mother, Paravati, taking a bath and forming him from a mixture of her oils and scents sprinkled with water from the Ganges River. Once she forms Ganapati *(as Ganesha is also known)* in this way, she instructs him to guard the entrance to her bathroom so she can finish bathing. Shortly thereafter, Shiva returns home unexpectedly and wants to enter the room, but—adhering to his mother's request—the boy refuses to let him in. In his indignant rage, Shiva decapitates Ganesha, and Parvati becomes inconsolable. In his haste to appease her, Shiva asks his brother to go out and quickly bring back the first head he finds. His brother ventures out and stumbles upon a sleeping elephant. He brings this elephant's head back to Shiva, who puts it on the boy's body to remedy the situation[11] .

In this story, Ganesha is born of both his mother's oils (culture) and the water from the holy river (nature) and thus reminds us we are all comprised of composite elements blending together to create a unique form. More specifically, we are also by-products of culture and nature; at conception and throughout gestation, we are nature in its simplest, purest form, but we begin to be sculpted by culture the instant we enter the world. We are influenced and shaped by our parents, educators, religious institutions, cultural traditions, and society at-large. This dynamic dance between our primordial self and our cultural self is one that ebbs and flows in every moment of our lives. What does it mean to be a by-product? How often does our desire to act from the heart get reigned in by our beliefs, which have been so deftly crafted by custom? In Western culture, in particular, it can be so easy to get swept up into the currents of majority thought. The endeavors of constantly upgrading our lives and maintaining a certain image in the world are two forces of society that are extremely powerful and can easily seduce us. As we consider human history, we see that there has always been a majority of mainstream thought augmented by smaller groups expressing more intuitive views considered counterculture. Instead of engaging skillful action and dialogue, many of these groups have elected to sequester themselves from society at-large, thus allowing the status quo to grow and proliferate. Ultimately, even these small groups are ruled by their own kind of culture, but it is often the case that their beliefs are more welcoming, expansive, and responsive to the natural, intuitive self.

In the dance of customs and essence, we must contemplate the consequences of acting only from our most basic, natural instincts, as interactions with others could easily deteriorate in the absence of the structures and etiquettes of culture. This is one of the reasons why extremists are rarely given any real attention, as their message is so outlandish and abrasive that people have a hard time relating to any part of their cause, yet even they are needed to make a point. Discovering what is most appropriate in a given situation by being deeply engaged in the world while also listening closely to our intuitive selves is a delicate and challenging endeavor. Through cultivating this balance, though, we can both live in our truth and thrive within the shifting boundaries of society at-large. Ganesha's hybrid form is indeed this very notion of the dance of convention and natural constitution embodied. Interestingly, the young man's body represents nature, because as children we are closer to the universal source and the wisdom of the heart. The elephant's head stands for the intelligence and refinement of culture, as the elephant is a wise, socially adapted, and well-regarded animal in India. Ganesha's mouse serves as a reminder that when we get wrapped up in the belief systems of others, we can become obstacles to our own personal joy. Because of its talent for moving easily in constricted places, the mouse symbolizes our ability to get out of our own way. For this reason, Ganapati is often called the remover of obstacles and is invoked before a new venture or journey.

A good friend of mine attended an advanced yoga workshop which by its very essence carried a particular culture, as highly developed practitioners gathered to play, expand, and dive more fully into their sadhana. As she settled in, she noticed a feeling of vulnerability in her physical frame, a sense of shadow in her heart, and a desire to slow down. During the practice, she could feel herself being swept away by the energy in the room. The prevailing customs of the workshop took the lead in her yoga, dimming her internal voice of reason. By the end of the class, she felt diminished rather than energized and was even experiencing a minor sensation of nausea. In this way, the dance between nature and culture enters the realm of our asana practice as we endeavor to balance the instructions of a chosen teacher with those of the teacher within. The dance of nature and culture is always transpiring in the background as we lead our lives. It is up to us to determine when each will serve us best and apply our wisdom accordingly.

To build up
Dismantle first
To expand
Contract first
To attain clarity
Allow confusion
To become civilized
First live in the wild.

The balance of all things
Is in their opposites;
The truth points in both directions.
Thus the clenched fist holds weakness
*   within*
And the open hand offers the hidden
*   power of suns...*[12]

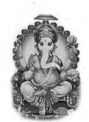

Inquiries

On the Mat: Many of us have experimented with different yoga traditions. At times, the variation can be confusing and can leave us debating which system to follow more closely or which one is "right." A true marvel of our practice lies in our ability to absorb teachings from different traditions while at the same time connecting to our natural intuition, which ultimately guides us in selecting what is most optimal for the inquiry at hand. Take this inquiry of nature and culture into the studio, identifying the culture of the yoga system to which you adhere. Do you come into postures a certain way because it is part of your inherited yoga culture, or because the movement is intuitive in your body? How can we take care of ourselves without caving in to the pressure of the group or culture at-large? Cultivate the ability to listen to the calling of your heart instead of the external voice delivering a barrage of "shoulds." In this class, become more conscious of the fact that your teacher represents a kind of culture. Utilize his or her offerings to your advantage, while at the same time listening to your innermost knowing in order to craft an optimal experience.

Off the Mat: Take a few hours to experience a culture with which you are unfamiliar. Explore an immigrant community, spend time with the elderly or little kids, or take part in a holiday or ritual outside of your religion or regular spiritual practice. As you immerse in new conventions , notice the contrasts they offers to your own. Acknowledge areas of similarity and places of difference. What aspects of this culture challenge your innermost nature? What characteristics enable you to see your own circle in a new light?

Supportive Words

Culture: *civilization, conventions, customs, habit, lifestyle, society*

Nature: *being, constitution, essence, substance*

Visualization

Ganapati, with an elephant's head and boy's body, a mouse and sweet treats at his side.

Complementary Breath

nadi shodana

Closing Ritual

chant

Ganesha Sharanam

taking refuge in or respect and reverence for Ganesha

Spirit of Hanuman: {*inspired by Jennifer Goldberg*}

Hanuman is the monkey god who loyally aids Rama during his voyage to rescue Sita from the evil demon Ravana. He is revered for his agility, strength, and unwavering courage. Hanuman is depicted with a monkey's head and a muscular human body, and in many images he is shown carrying a mountain. Legend has it that during the battle in Sri Lanka, Rama's brother Lakshmana is seriously injured, and Hanuman is entrusted to acquire healing herbs from the Himalayas. Upon arrival, though, he is unsure which herbs to pick, so he decides to return with the whole mountain to ensure Lakshmana will be well cared for[13]. In the case of Sita's rescue, Ram asks Hanuman afterwards why he was so eager to come to his aid. As they hug, the monkey god replies that Ram is his friend, which was motivation enough for him to help.

Seva, or service, is a simple yet powerful concept with the potential to change lives and the world. In the process of service, not only do we give to others, but we also bask in the joy of cultivating more splendor in the world around us. In Western culture, it can be easy to get caught up in our own private world and forget we are connected to a much larger web of life. We tend to overlook the profound effects of every one of our actions on the quality and vibration of the larger whole. Service occurs when we find ways to give without asking anything in return, even though we do inevitably still receive by virtue of the act of giving. What we receive is the inner joy accessed through our participation and engagement in those endeavors and relationships we have deemed important. Seva is often translated as selfless service, but Dinabandhu Garrett Sarley interprets it instead as "self-full" service. When we offer our time and our energy, we do so from a place of loving desire and an inward call to action. We are invested in the outcome of an event or the flourishing of an organization because we identify with the greater, collective energy manifested in these forms, and our own hearts are bolstered as we acknowledge this interconnectedness through our participation.

The yogic interpretation of service invites us to acknowledge the varying degrees and different guises this kind of action can take. There are those who start nonprofit organizations or dedicate their whole lives to volunteer organizations, while others leave a secret gift for a friend, buy flowers for a loved one, or share food with a stranger. Consider the range of forms service takes in your life, and awaken to the array of instances in which seva is being offered to you by others. Just as Hanuman is endowed with various powers used to aid Rama on his quest, we too, possess powerful skills we can share with others to create more beauty and abundance in the world. Lawyers volunteer their legal services to battered women or the poor, doctors go abroad to aid citizens of developing countries, and individuals mentor young boys and girls, providing them with strong role models for the future. We all possess skills that can be shared to uplift those around us. Yet in our culture, it is easy to fall into the mindset of every person for himself and forget that inaction is in fact an action contributing to the environmental degradation, violence, and poverty pervading our communities. There is tremendous value in both recognizing the many simple ways service can be integrated into our daily lives and understanding that what benefits others ends up enhancing our own lives, as well. To do this, though, we must first shift our way of thinking and, like Martin Luther King or Mother Teresa, open to seeing the ways in which all of culture is interconnected. What would change if we embodied the mantra "That which I am doing for someone else, I am doing for myself?" When we serve from a place of fullness, we can effect monumental shifts rooted in the simple act of being authentic to our heart. A mere moment infused with service could ripple out and have a long-lasting effect we might never be able to track or trace, and so its power is undeniable. As George Bernard Shaw expresses:

> This is the true joy in life, being used for a purpose recognized by yourself as a mighty one. Being a force of nature instead of a feverish, selfish little clod of ailments and grievances, complaining that the world will not devote itself to making you happy. I am of the opinion that my life belongs to the whole community and as long as I live, it is my privilege to do for it what I can. I want to be thoroughly used up when I die, for the harder I work, the more I live. I rejoice in life for its own sake. Life is no brief candle to me. It is a sort of splendid torch which I have got hold of for the moment and I want to make it burn as brightly as possible before handing it on to future generations.

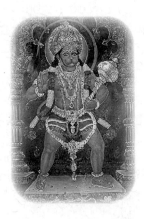

Inquiries

On the Mat: Investigate the ever-renewing opportunities to source your inherent power for contributing to the greater good. Take time to fill your own cup through the mindful and vital action of sadhana. Notice whether there is a category of postures or aspect of the practice in which you feel most at ease because this is where you shine brightest. Take advantage of these moments to drink in affirming energy and nourish yourself so that you may serve the world more wholeheartedly when the opportunity arises. As you progress through your postures, hold in your heart a person, organization, or cause with which you desire to be in "self full" relationship. It is often easier to play it small on the mat or in the world, but—just like Hanuman—you can embrace the powers and skills that are uniquely yours and employ them to effect shifts both within yourself and for the benefit of those around you. Rooted in stability and self-affirmation, you can give of yourself fully, knowing you are making a positive offering to the world through your actions. Remember to be "self-full" in each posture, and notice how this focus of nurturing yourself floods out into your home, surroundings, and community. Explore standing forward fold, runner's stretch, tree, standing hand to big toe, warrior two, parsvotanasana, lateral angle, yoga tie in standing hand to big toe, pigeon, down dog, knee-down lunge, hands inside foot in knee-down lunge, quad stretch in knee-down lunge, runner's stretch, and hanumanasana.

Off the Mat: Volunteer your time to an organization or a cause with which you feel aligned. Take note of what you receive through the act of giving graciously.

Practices

I attune to the potential and value of all I have to offer

Supportive Words
aid, avail, benefit, employ, help, labor, supply, use, value, work

Visualization
Hanuman and Ram embracing in the love of heartfelt friendship and service.

Complementary Breath
ujjayi

Closing Ritual
Listen to and/or chant the Hanuman Chalisa.

Teacher's Note
partner share

In pairs, guide students to share a story of a time when someone offered them loving service or assistance. Ask them to share how it felt to receive this kindness and whether the incident motivated them to offer the same to someone else.

capable beyond belief

I take a leap of faith as

I open to the possibility that I am

I share my beauty from a seat of fullness

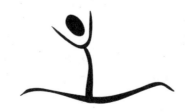

The Goddesses:

Devi, which means "goddess," is the general term in Sanskrit used for the many manifestations of the feminine divine. She is often referred to as "Ma" and is worshipped by at least 1008 different names, if not more. The Goddess represents the creative energy of existence and the physical manifestations that comprise the cosmos. She assumes immense and minute proportions, is responsible for creation and dissolution, and is the embodiment of shakti (universal energies)[14] in her role as the mother of the universe. This comsic energy is made manifest in the diverse forms of the various goddesses, including Lalita, Durga, Ganga, Kali, Lakshmi, Parvati, Radha, Rati, Saraswati, Sati, and Sita, to name a few. Each Devi has her own unique story and symbolism, which can support us in excavating a deeper understanding of our inner embodied nature.

Sacred Protection of Durga: {inspired by Bella Arguetty}

Durga's name translates to "impassable" or "a difficult or narrow passage," both of which allude to her immense strength and power[15]. One of the stories of her origin involves the evil demon god Mahisha, who took on many forms—including that of a buffalo—in an attack on the gods. Mahisha was immune to the powers of the male gods, and thus only the goddesses could defeat him. With little maneuvering room left, the gods were forced to retreat to the earthly plane. There, they engaged in serious consultations with Vishnu, Shiva, and Brahma and decided to take part in a sacred fire ritual wherein they brewed a concoction of herbs, chanted mantras, and offered blessings into the flames. After hours of ritual, Durga emerged equipped with the power, illumination, and consciousness of each of the gods. Shiva gave her his trident, Vishnu a discus, Varuna a conch shell, Agni a dart, Vayu a bow, Surya arrows, Indra a thunderbolt, Kuvera a mace, Brahma a rosary and water pot, Kala a shield and sword, and Visvakarma a battle axe. Durga proclaimed she would aid the gods in their conflict, but reminded them all that she did not belong to any one of them. After a long, fierce battle, the fearless goddess severed Mahisha's head and stabbed him in the chest, returning peace to all realms of existence[16]. Durga is usually depicted wearing a bright red sari (which represents passion, strength, and potent life force)[17], armed with weapons in her ten hands, and accompanied by a lion with a bright, golden mane[18].

Durga is extremely potent, as she cradles the world with intention and heart. She is different than Kali, who is fierce and protects by eliminating that which is not serving us. Durga is not a consort of any one god, as she brings forth her identity through her own will. She is deep, primal, maternal energy that will transform her into a vicious warrior if anyone tries to harm her creation. Her power is always present and only comes out to strike when danger is imminent or near. Her attack is poignant, acute, and full of passion, as she is protecting that which is of highest value to her. Durga is invoked when we need to shield ourselves with the loyal muscle of a mother. She might erupt if someone is trying to assault us, if we see a loved one in danger, or if injustice is staring us in the face. The lion accompanying Durga mirrors her deep-seated connection to our inner power and represents her demeanor and intent. Lions are calm but strong; they utilize their mane as a tool of intimidation and only join the hunt when the lioness needs aid in tackling larger prey. The lion's color symbolizes the radiant sun, which can bring light to a potentially frightening situation[19]. When a threat emerges on our path, we can literally embody Durga's multifaceted power and intimidate those who would do us harm with a shift in energy and demeanor. In much the same way as an animal's scent changes in the moments before battle, we can communicate our intention of power and self-preservation. Arming ourselves in this way, we are responding to heightened sensitivity and affirming our right to exist. Durga supports us in these instances so we can move forward in our endeavor to honor beauty and light in the world. As Haven Trevino writes:

> We spring forth from the All,
> Fed by light
> Clothed in matter,
> Sculpted by streams of inspiration,
> We shape Love like the eagle shapes the wind.
> Returning at last to the Sun,
> We bring only our joy of flight.
>
> When the Mothering Spirit gives birth,
> Her light effortlessly feeds, shelters,
> Nurtures, and uplifts.
> So the true healer
> Nurtures but does not control
> Shelters but does not imprison
> Guides others to the edge of the cliff
> But does not force them to fly[20].

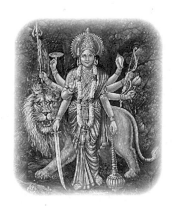

Inquiries

On the Mat: For most of us, moments that draw upon our internal wellspring of Durga-intensity surface rarely. As such, our yoga sadhana is a perfect place to stir and reconnect to this vital energy, as doing so can prepare us to access this potent force more readily when the need does arise. Typically, we either run or fight in a panicked way when we are unjustly attacked. Durga, however, encourages us to align the composite of energies of presence, intellect, spirit, and strength to generate a dominant force poised to strike if need be. She invites us to embody directed, contained, and focused power that isn't easily disseminated. Connect to this sense of strength in the heart, embodying the essence of the sacred mother willing to do anything to protect her loved ones. Utilize hara breaths from deep in the belly, investigate structured moments of low, vibratory sounding, and focus on the potency of muscle activation and the stability of the physical body. Incorporate lion's breath, and practice invigorating standing poses to source your innate ability to channel the mighty vitality of Durga. Explore warriors one and two, reverse warrior, twisting warrior one, lateral angle, hands inside foot in lateral angle, goddess variations (*pulsations, tai chi, eagle arms, free flow*), warrior to goddess to warrior to goddess flow, up and down pulsation in goddess with lion's breath, and holding in goddess.

Off the Mat: Take part in a karate, aikido, self-defense, or kickboxing class. Notice the effects of cultivating skillful power.

Practices

I connect to the innate mother energy residing within. I utilize my multi-faceted power to emit a stream of courageous intimidation when necessary. I hold my loved ones close and offer them the protection of Durga.

Supportive Words
backbone, clout, durability, fortitude, hardiness, might, potency, power, vigor

Visualization
Durga riding her lion, with weapons outstretched in all ten hands.

Complementary Breath
kapalabhati, bhastrika, lion's breath

Closing Ritual
chant
Baja Mana Ma, Ma, Ma, Ma; Ananda Mayi Ma Ma
reverence to the great mother, bliss to the beloved mother

The Flowing Essence of Saraswati: {inspired by Douglas Brooks}

Saraswati was first identified as the river goddess, who descended to Earth to offer fertility, bounty, and riches. Over time, she also came to be known as the celestial guardian of knowledge, sacred speech, and creative arts. Saraswati embodies the process of acquiring proficiency and refining skill while staying open to the fluidity of the moment. Revered artists and musicians are deeply steeped in the sara[21] *(essence or marrow)* of their practice, yet they have the capacity to improvise with their own individual creativity and heart. When people embark on the path of learning a musical instrument, writing literature, or sculpting clay, they must first learn the fundamentals before progressing into the more free-flowing realm of their chosen practice. The dynamic balance represented by this sacred goddess is not only limited to the arts, as lawyers, doctors, or businesswomen also have to achieve a certain level of competence before they can begin to experiment with expanding the boundaries of their profession. Saraswati encourages us to embrace the seeming contradiction that both essence and flow can exist in the same breath. The cultivation of sara provides us with a deep sense of stability and a feeling of relative consistency. At the same time, Saraswati's identity as river goddess invokes and nurtures flexibility, speed, and constant change. If we get stuck in the theory or structure of a practice and never release into the flow of the waters, we miss out on the opportunity for fuller, richer understanding. Alternatively, if we only play freely and never take the time to slow down, acquire deeper knowledge, and integrate our learning, then we miss out on another vital aspect of experience.

When illustrated, Saraswati is depicted seated on a lotus and playing the vina *(stringed musical instrument)*, with a swan and/or peacock by her side, the Vedas in one hand, and mala beads in the other[22]. The white swan is one of the most significant symbols for understanding Saraswati's nature, as it conveys the paradox of essence and flow simply and clearly. Swans migrate along a relatively similar route each year as they follow familiar paths. The knowledge of migration is passed from generation to generation, partly learned and partly genetic. The changing of light creates an internal shift that prepares the swans' bodies for the long journey ahead. The birds travel mostly along the north/south axis and follow coastlines, river valleys, and mountain ranges in order to take advantage of updrafts and avoid wide areas of open water. The migration process supports the birds in maximizing the daylight hours *(and thus food potential)* of the summer months, while ensuring a reliable source of sustenance in southern latitudes during the colder ones[23]. Although the swan exemplifies deep-rooted knowledge and consistency of action, it also demonstrates an ability to respond to the flow of the journey. Often, these remarkable birds will stop at the same exact ponds each year, but on some trips they will break at a different body of water due to weather conditions, predators, or human influence. As their voyage unfolds, there is always a backup plan poised as their instinct guides them through the sky. Thus, the completion of their annual expedition requires innate knowledge coupled with creative flexibility. Saraswati's other symbols include the Vedas, which are representative of the importance of foundational knowledge as we endeavor towards creative expression; the vina *(Indian lute)*, which illustrates her love for rhythm, the power of vibration, and the dedication required to become fluent in a creative art; and the peacock, which represents seeing with multiple eyes and taking a broader view. Finally, Saraswati wears a white sari, which represents wisdom, a clean slate for learning, and abundant knowledge.

Inquiries

On the Mat: Explore the relationship of structure and flow as you follow the inherited landmarks of your sadhana, while also leaving room to be creative with the body and breath. Draw support from the time-honored structure of poses, breath, and sequences and simultaneously create personal interpretations of these concepts, sculpting them from the inside out. Notice how you may rely more on the established structure when you first encounter a given posture, which will often mean fully assuming the role of the student by listening closely to the instructions, ascertaining the basic principles, and feeling your body in relationship to the asana. Honoring received knowledge, cultivating skills, and being in the company of teachers who show us the way are all essential and vital parts of the process. Over time—once you have developed a relationship with the pose—sense how your ability to establish the basic foundation quickly can free you to spend more time opening to the possibilities and inquiries of the posture.

Begin each pose by internally reviewing detailed instructions to establish the essence of each asana, and follow this with a few moments of creative flow within the established construct. As an experiment, focus on utilizing this technique in tree pose. First build the posture from the ground up and stabilize your pose. Once you are anchored, notice the freedom and lightness in your upper body and move into a personal exploration by freeing the torso and arms into creative variations. Explore hands clasped overhead in mountain, yoga-mudra arms in mountain, quad stretch in mountain, back heel to sky in warrior one, chair, standing wind-relieving, standing marichyasana, upward boat, bound angle, hands inside foot in knee-down lunge, and tree.

Off the Mat: Treat yourself to quality performing arts *(such as a symphony, an opera, a dance performance, or theater)*, fully witnessing the masterful skill and fluid creativity of these highly refined performers.

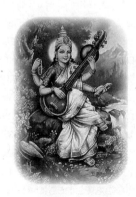

Practices

Supportive Words
Fluid: *flexible, flowing, fluent, malleable*
Essence: *base, being, core, entity, root, soul, spirit*

Visualization
Saraswati seated on a lotus, playing the vina, book in hand.

Complementary Breath
ujjayi

Closing Ritual
mantra meditation
Hamsa, or 'hum-su,' translates as both "swan" and "I am that." For the swan to fly, it needs to balance its wings through both structural integrity and creative flow.

Teacher's Note
In this class, begin with clearly guided instruction to establish the essence of the practice, and then lead students into the flow of each pose. When guiding tree pose, instruct the pose in great detail. Rooted in this foundation of skillful stability, invite students to notice the freedom and lightness in the upper body. Encourage them to flow into a unique exploration of the pose by freeing the torso and arms to explore creative variations. As a related take-home assignment, ask students to choose one pose with which they are extremely familiar and spend time investigating improvisational movements rooted in this chosen posture.

The Radiant Abundance of Lakshmi: {*inspired by Sudha Carolyn Lundeen*}

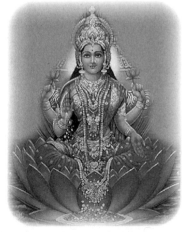

The Sanskrit word "lakshmi" is defined as value, good fortune, riches, beauty, splendor, and luster[24]. Hence Lakshmi is known as the goddess of light, auspicious beauty, and prosperity. She is often referred to as Shri, and she is Vishnu's consort, manifesting in earthly incarnations as Rama's wife Sita or Krishna's Radha. Lakshmi's good fortune is not limited to the material realm, as she also symbolizes wealth of character, health, and wisdom. She embodies these vast riches, hinting at the value of sustaining respectable and noble qualities even as challenges materialize along our path. Lakshmi is the embodiment of fullness evidenced in the splendor of the full moon, the crest of a wave, or the abundance of a summer garden in bloom. She is depicted sitting in or standing on a lotus flower, with coins dropping out of her palms as she offers lotus petals from her hands. She is usually accompanied by two elephants either pouring water or holding the flower garlands that surround her[25].

The story of Lakshmi's birth involves the devas (*gods*) who were in conflict with the asuras (*demons*) in the struggle to obtain amrita (*the nectar of immortality*). The gods consulted Vishnu, and he suggested they churn the oceans to gather amrita. They created a churning mechanism by threading the serpent Vauki around Mt. Mandara. Taking the form of Kurma, the tortoise, Vishnu balanced the mountain on his back, and fourteen treasures emerged from the ocean floor as they churned. Lasksmi Devi was one of these gifts; she rose from the ocean floor seated on a thousand-petal lotus. Lakshmi then picked Vishnu as her consort and proclaimed her power to bestow abundance upon all who ask for it[26]. In this story, the ocean can be interpreted as representative of consciousness, with the churning symbolic of the journey many of us undertake once we recognize we are more than just physical beings. As we enter a deeper exploration of our selves, numerous gifts and challenges begin to surface, all bearing their own unique teachings.

In life, it is easy to succumb to scarcity thinking or dwell on what is not working. Lakshmi reminds us of the abundance always within our reach and reveals that we are the ones who choose to pinch ourselves off from the wealth and beauty of our lives. As we turn a blind eye to the truth of prosperity, our attention instead becomes fixated on lack. To rediscover and cultivate internal wealth, we can begin by acknowledging the simple things that contribute to our happiness and well-being. This may take the form of being thankful for the breath, acknowledging nourishing foods, savoring time with family and friends, or fully recognizing the gifts of being in nature. By activating feelings of appreciation for what we already have, we generate an energy of gratitude and abundance that is self-perpetuating. The more appreciation we cultivate, the more wealth and prosperity we attract; the more we recognize riches in our lives, the more grateful we feel. The culture of advertising in which we live sends us a very different message, as it encourages us to measure our happiness according to our material possessions and feeds the desire to constantly upgrade to the next best thing. According to Tantric philosophy, these material possessions and desires do have a place in our enjoyment and experience of the world. When materialism swallows our ability to be thankful for the simplest joys of life, however, Tantrikas maintain that we can wind up stranded amidst feelings of emptiness and dissatisfaction with little recourse to maneuver our way out. Lakshmi invites us to enter into a relationship with abundance by generating a sense of fulfillment rooted in our existing blessings and then contemplating how much we really need to live in the world. The lotus upon which Lakshmi sits and the petals she offers are reminders that beauty is always present and blossoming, even amongst roots anchored in darkness. The coins dropping from her hands are a clear representation of the constant and infinite flow of resources available to each of us. Our work comes in the process of lining up to receive this wealth by eschewing limiting beliefs and cultivating an ever-increasing capacity for gratitude. The elephants surrounding her represent wisdom and faithfulness, inviting us to remain steadfast in our exploration of inner light and shadow, which always contributes to internal prosperity and expansion. Lakshmi's four arms or hands indicate the four aims of life: dharma (*virtue*), artha (*prosperity*), kama (*desires*) and moksha (*freedom from self-limiting beliefs/habits*). Lastly, she wears a green sari representing the ever-renewing bounty of the Earth [27].

Inquiries

On the Mat: Sense any temptation to focus on where you are lacking or which postures challenge you most. Call upon Lakshmi to support you during these moments of self-limiting thought. By shifting the focus instead to gratitude for all that is going well in your sadhana, you can generate more energy for manifesting greater abundance. Identify the various riches of your own unique practice, whether they take the form of the body's range of motion, the bounty of the breath, or the determination and steadfastness of the heart. Locate your personal well of abundance for every pose, and notice the gifts offered by each asana. Extend your fullest effort in each moment, each movement, and every breath as you tap into the bounty of yoga. Invoke the true spirit of Lakshmi by first acknowledging and appreciating the many gifts already in your possession, both spiritual as well as material. Explore knee-down lunge, high lunge, pigeon, half frog, cobra, locust, bow, seated eagle arms, eagle pose, lateral angle, triangle, standing wide-angle forward fold, mermaid one, and mermaid two.

Off the Mat: Practice the rampage of appreciation (*described below*) every day for a week, and write about anything that results.

Practices

I admire the lotus petals in bloom, rooted in the mud and yet open to life

Supportive Words
bounty, fortune, plentitude, plenty, prosperity, riches, wealth

Visualization
Gracious Lakshmi perched elegantly on her brilliant, beautiful lotus throne.

Complementary Breath
dirgha

Closing Ritual
Rampage of Appreciation, by Abraham and Esther Hicks: At the end of practice, spend two to three minutes in a "rampage" of appreciation. Begin by visualizing something in your life for which you feel grateful, and then continue the exercise by allowing this image to morph into another, and then another in an organic and fluid way. Remember to simply return to the prompt of gratitude if your thoughts drift to something else during the meditation[28].

boundless flow of prosperity

I acknowledge and receive the

churn the ocean of consciousness to access the depths within

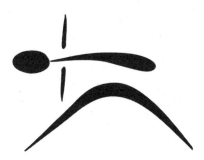

The Discerning Nature of Kali: {inspired by Maya Weintraub}

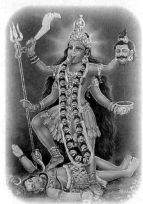

Closure is an aspect of life that is often hard to grasp or welcome. Certain endings are extremely abrupt and can literally leave us feeling as though a vital part of ourselves has been unexpectedly severed. When we encounter this kind of experience, we are in the realm of Kali. She is a powerful goddess who represents the devouring of cloaks hampering our lives, thus crafting fertile ground for something new to arise. She cuts with scalpel-like precision and might take the form of an unexpected death or a partner suddenly packed up and leaving. There are many tales describing the origin of Kali ma. In the Markandeya Purana, legend finds Durga in the midst of battle with the two demons Sumbha and Nisumbha. In a bind, Durga decides to create Kali from her third eye in order to bring an end to the battle[29]. Kali is traditionally depicted with dark blue or black skin, red eyes flaring, blood dripping from her extended tongue, and four to ten arms holding an array of weapons, severed heads, and mudras. She is often adorned with a necklace of skulls and is sometimes depicted with ten heads [30].

Kali's untamed hair represents unrestrained power and boundless freedom. Although endings in life are often accompanied by a sense of grief, they can also bestow an immense sense of freedom. Many of us face life situations that drain our energy, like being stuck in a dead-end job, staying in a stagnant relationship, or living in a place that doesn't resonate internally. When we can step wholeheartedly into the place of closure and let go, we can regain our internal autonomy and open ourselves to what lies beyond. Kali's four hands convey important messages to support us in the process of dissolving that which is not of service. In one hand, she creates a blessing mudra to invite us to take refuge in her cleansing power. In the other hand, she extends the "fear not" mudra, inviting us to soften our existential fear of endings. Her sword reminds us that her wisdom can slay our illusions of smallness and separation, which often accompany challenging life transitions. Finally, the severed head is a symbol of deep softening and an acknowledgement that we can stay present even in the company of the most uncomfortable or gruesome feelings. Kali is essentially communicating that even though she has come in like a fierce tornado and seemingly wrecked our lives, we can still find solace in her arms.

The tiger is considered to be Kali's vehicle and is an additional symbol of her tremendous power. This majestic creature is a nomad who prefers to stalk and observe its prey before it leaps in for an easy meal. In our lives, certain situations might brew for months or even years before they culminate in a turbulent storm. Furthermore, the tiger "embodies unsurpassed power (and) a sense of vicious freedom as at times it kills simply to kill and acts in an impulsive and opportunistic manner, exerting the least amount of effort[31]." When a tiger rears its head on our path, we typically flee from its wrath, but Kali encourages us to take refuge in the storm itself. As nature demonstrates, that which isn't pruned will cease to bear fruit, and thus the process of pruning is vital to nurturing the ground of possibility and growth.

As David Whyte writes in the *Well of Grief*:

Those who will not slip beneath
*   the still surface on the well of grief,*

turning down through its black water
*   to the place we cannot breathe,*

will never know the source from which we drink,
*   the secret water, cold and clear,*

nor find in the darkness glimmering,
*   the small round coins,*
*   thrown by those who wished for something else[32].*

Inquiries

On the Mat: Instead of just watching or trying to figure out a response, Kali asks us to yield to the initial cut and to fully immerse ourselves in the darkness. How often do we give ourselves permission to feel the anger or deep pain that has accumulated inside? Are there knots held internally that haven't been fully integrated because we won't allow time and space for their unraveling? Our yoga practice can take us to these sharp edges within, and we can access new realms of understanding and integration when we are able to take shelter in the intensity of a posture or in the potency of the breath. Seek refuge in the intensity of your practice, literally offering yourself back to yourself even as the seams unravel and the world turns upside-down. Create a stormy experience that will evoke your relationship to loss or endings by making use of the intensity of pranayamas to generate energy and stir an internal squall. Utilize some of these breathing practices during posture holdings, and intersperse them throughout your practice. Honor your skills of observation, but spend more time honing your ability to dive headlong into the feelings you hold inside. Sense what shifts when there is no need to formulate a conscious response to the emotions that arise. Instead, simply ride the waves that may emerge from deep within your cellular, mental, and emotional strata. As a cautionary note, bear in mind that Kali energy is intense; remember to take care of yourself as you embark upon this journey. Modify postures or soften your breath at any time in order to honor your needs in a given moment. Explore mountain, eagle, warrior one, goddess, eagle arms in warrior two, quad stretch in mountain, high lunge, twisting high lunge, knee-down lunge, hands inside foot in knee-down lunge, chair, and chair with kapalabhati.

Off the Mat: Spend time excavating any unresolved endings in your life related to old relationships, loss of family or friends, or other challenging life situations. Intentionally confront these areas of your psyche. Hold space for them, journal about them, and see what shifts when you engage rather than repress these less desirable yet valuable artifacts of life. As an expressive ritual, make a bon fire and dissolve letters, journal entries, or pictures that will help you release emotional holding.

Practices

Supportive Words
conclusion, decay, disbandment, end, evaporation, release, resolution

Visualization
Kali's red flaring eyes, extended tongue, and necklace of skulls.

Complementary Breath
dirgha, ujjayi, kapalabhati, alternate-nostril kapalabhati, bhastrika, bramari, anulom vilom, and nadi shodana.

Closing Ritual
chant
Om Ma Kali Ma Sada Guru Sri Mata, Parashakti
Om Ma Kali, Sada Guru Shri Mata

tenderness and courage

sensations that arise in the

I fear not as I engage in inquiry holding the heart in a state of

process of dissolution

the
alchemy
of
nature

"A human being is part of the whole called by us 'universe', a part limited in time and space. We experience ourselves, our thoughts and feelings as something separate from the rest. A kind of optical delusion of consciousness. This delusion is a kind of prison for us, restricting us to our personal desires and to affection for a few persons nearest to us. Our task must be to free ourselves from the prison by widening our circle of compassion to embrace all living creatures and the whole of nature in its beauty."

-Albert Einstein

Elements of Life:

Due to the structured movement of asana, conscious focus on the breath, and intentional mindfulness, we often emerge from our yoga chemically and physically more attuned to our surroundings. The five basic elements of earth, air, fire, water, and ether comprise everything in nature and are likewise intricate components of our own physical and energetic makeup. If we examine the human body, for example, we will see the subtle dance of these five fundamental materials in its composition: bones and muscles *(earth)*, breath *(air)*, digestive system *(fire)*, blood *(water)*, and ether *(spirit)*. As we flow through our lives, there are times when one of these elements begins to overwhelm the others. This can occur as a result of genetic predetermination, work stress, relationship drama, negative self-talk, weather, or the type of food we consume. When we become mired in these imbalanced states for too long, our light dims, and we are rendered unable to align with the grand pulsation of life. We get so distracted and caught up in the whirlwind of our days that our ability to nourish ourselves and extend support to others is diminished. The beauty of embodied form, however, is that we are energetic matrixes; we are never truly stuck, and thus we are always able to effect change in order to live our lives from a fuller place. Going to a yoga class or partaking in other mindfulness practices are among the most effective ways to reintegrate our elemental framework.

Keep in mind that yoga practices based on the elements will best serve you if you tailor them to your own individual nature. For example, as you consider a practice centered on fire, you might realize that you already gravitate towards heat in daily life. For you, the practice for this concept is cultivating a balanced relationship to fire. On the other hand, if you are overly lethargic or cool, you would be best served by opening to the intensity and heat offered by this element. It can also be powerful to bring the actual substance you are working with *(or an indication of it)* into your sacred space; a container of soil, a bowl of water, a candle, or a feather can serve as vivid symbolic representations of these essentials of life. Finally, practicing outside—if at all possible—can be especially effective, as it will allow you to see and be in the company of all of these profound substances at once.

Spacious Expanse:

One of the workshops I teach is called "Untangle Your Stress." In this workshop, I lead participants in breathing exercises, simple movement, journaling, art making, partner listening, and a sampling of yoga poses. Over the course of a few years teaching and refining this workshop, I came to realize that the principal aim of all of these activities is to create a sense of spaciousness. As humans inhabiting a busy world, we can easily become overly condensed in our body, mind, and heart. The body loses its ability to move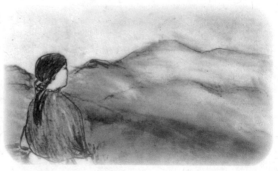
freely in space, the breath becomes constricted, the mind gets overly cluttered with various stimuli, and our world contracts as we become isolated from community. By investigating the qualities of ether, we can reconnect with our innately expansive nature and live our lives with greater perspective. Space, or

ether, is the medium for all of existence. It is infinite, transparent, celestial, and without dimension. As such, when we connect to ether in a balanced way, we can experience freedom in the body, expansiveness in the breath, open-mindedness, access to our intuition, and increased perspective. If the qualities of space become overly active, however, we might experience a sense of disconnection from the body and be left feeling ungrounded. To cultivate a healthy relationship with this vital aspect of our constitution, we can engage in prolonged meditation, connect to sound through chanting, and create rituals that summon awareness of our interconnectedness with all life. As Pierre Teilhard De Chardin writes:

> Blessed be you, universal matter, immeasurable time, boundless ether, triple abyss of stars and atoms and generations: you who by overflowing and dissolving our narrow standards or measurements reveal to us ether dimensions of (something greater)[1].

Inquiries

On the Mat: Explore a fusion of postures, mantra chanting, and pranayama. Concentrate on expansive poses that will enable you to feel a sense of boundlessness, connect to the hollow spaces inside your body, and attune to the larger energy that exists internally, externally, and as your embodied form. Focus on opening the hips by experimenting with standing yoga mudra, standing wind-relieving pose, easy pose twist, knee-down lunge, hands inside foot in knee-down lunge, runner's stretch, twisting high lunge, pigeon, pigeon backbend, quad stretch in pigeon, cobra, locust, bound angle, baby cradle, half lotus and full lotus.

Off the Mat: Spend time in a place that offers an extensive view, such as the edge of a body of water or a mountaintop. Take time to simply absorb the energy of the wide expanse. Notice how it resonates in your body and what effect it engenders for the rest of your day.

Practices

I recognize the benefit of expanded

Supportive Words
breadth, expanse, field, room, scope

Visualization
Sitting at the summit of a mountain on a clear day, resting, meditating, and chanting there. From here you can see for miles and thus fully absorb the big picture both literally and figuratively.

Complementary Breath
ujjayi

Focus on holding your breath following each inhalation. Feel the sense of spaciousness invoked as the breath is retained inside the body.

Closing Ritual
A softly rocking meditation. Instead of sitting still, allow yourself to sink into the space around you and be gently rocked by its encompassing energy.

it pulses through me

I connect to my

I open to the vital energy of life as

intuition and the spaciousness that resides within

perspective

Swift Air:

Air is ether in motion, or spaciousness that has begun to flow in its invisible form. It provides the creative energy of the universe a vehicle for travel and an instrument through which to infuse life into the world. This element is agile, buoyant, dynamic, and responsive. In the body, it is both the conduit for energy transfer and the breath of life enabling our existence. The element of air stirs things up, as evidenced through leaves dancing on trees or the waves of a stormy ocean. It can have the finesse of a gentle breath extinguishing a candle's flame, or it can assume the power and velocity of a massive hurricane. Likewise, air can be invigorating and energizing like an autumn breeze that draws goose bumps to the surface of the skin, or it can become agitating like the insistent prodding of a fan blowing for too long.

In yoga, there are five primary vayus, or functions of air, each with its own unique attributes. Doug Keller writes: "In each case this specific function is called a 'vayu,' which is sometimes translated as 'wind.' The root 'va' means "that which flows"—and so a vayu is a vehicle for activities and experiences within the body, or a 'force' that moves in a specific way and in a specific area of the body that it governs. The practices of yoga—both asana and pranayama—are meant to optimize the functioning of these vayus[2]." Prana vayu is related to inhalation and can thus be illustrated by the upward motion of liquid filling a glass from its base to its rim. Since inhaling is the process of taking in energy, this aspect of air is responsible for assimilating information and experience from the physical, mental, and emotional realms. Apana vayu corresponds to exhalation, symbolized by the downward motion of a leaf floating towards the earth from on high. The release of the breath corresponds to the act of letting go, so this aspect of air is responsible for elimination of unnecessary toxins from all levels of our being. Samana vayu resides in the solar plexus and is related to the fiery air that separates nutrients from toxins or uplifting emotions from draining ones. Udana vayu circulates around the throat area, is related to the production of sound and speech, and is fundamental to our creative expression. Vyana vayu encompasses the whole body. According to Doug Keller "It has no specific seat, but rather coordinates all the powers such as sensory awareness, and runs through the whole network of the 72,000 nadis or passageways of prana in the body, connecting the functions of the nerves, veins, muscles and joints[3]."

When these various characteristics of air are in alignment, we experience innovative thought, creative expression, and focused direction. People who are in harmony with air as a whole exhibit traits of quick thinking, swiftness on their feet, and a capacity for providing ground-breaking solutions. If vayu is aggravated, though, we might encounter bouts of restlessness, agitation, flightiness, and unproductive multi-tasking. To cultivate greater dexterity with the air element, we can change our routine, practice yoga poses or sequences in a quicker and new way, embrace the effects of a warm breeze or take in the energy of wind as we drive with the windows down. As John Lame Deer shares:

> Listen to the air. You can hear it, feel it, smell it, taste it. Woniya wakan—the holy air—which renews all by its breath. Woniya wakan, waniya wakan—spirit, life, breath, renewal—it means all that. Woniya—we sit together, don't touch, but something is there; we feel it between us as a presence[4].

Inquiries

On the Mat: Move through a vinyasa flow to heighten the sensation of air moving around the body. Utilize each part of the practice to focus on a different aspect of the air element *(or choose to focus on one or two aspects if working with all five feels overwhelming)*. Remain light on your feet and sense the flow of air as you dance with fluid rhythm from pose to pose. Even though you are moving quickly, make sure to build each posture from the ground up to cultivate stability. While vinyasa is normally associated with a fast-paced practice, know that you can flow from pose to pose more slowly and still experience the tangible qualities of vayu by focusing your awareness. Explore balancing by practicing standing sun breaths, half circle, pointer, lion's breath, sun salutation, plank, high lunge, twisting high lunge, warrior one, warrior three, lateral angle, triangle, tree, baby dancer, standing splits, and balancing half moon.

Off the Mat: Go outside on a warm, windy day, and allow the wind to caress your entire body. Feel it fully, and sense your relationship to this element.

Practices

Supportive Words
creative, focused, innovative, quick, sharp

Visualization
Wind blowing through the trees, leaves moving in all directions

Complementary Breath
bhastrika
Use the bellows breath to generate wind.

Closing Ritual
Prepare a blank piece of paper, a few crayons or markers, and something hard to write on. After relaxation, fold your paper in half. On one side, draw the air element as it appears when it feels balanced in your life; on the other, illustrate it when it is out of alignment. Note the difference.

With lightness, I flow in the direction of my heart.

movement or thought

I embrace my intellectual agility.

I use my breath to maintain focus and steadiness amidst rapid

Heated Fire:

Fire is the element of transformation, embodying vast creative potential as it burns one substance thereby morphing it into another. In our journey of seeking fulfillment, skill is essential in order to ignite and maintain a fire that is hot enough to support our intentions but does not burn out of control. Agni the Sanskrit word for fire is connected to vision or sight, as fire can illuminate new possibilities as we travel along our path. When we actively engage an exploration of fire, we can locate the deepest knots within and watch as air draws them up to the surface. Once there, we can allow them to blaze and transmute, utilizing the ash of the old to nourish and sustain the new. At those times when we become stagnant, we can benefit from "lighting a fire under ourselves" in order to awaken our genuine potential. Opening to the possibility of being transformed by this primal element, our spirit brightens as we align with the intentions of the heart. When we live firmly rooted in this ripe, embodied state, our internal luster becomes readily apparent as it begins to manifest outwardly. Warmed by the flames of our inner fire, we can actively connect to our most deeply held passions, which in turn propel us forward to live our ultimate vision. Indeed, the flames of desire are not viewed negatively in an awakened, conscious state, but are instead recognized for their capacity to illuminate our steps as we traverse our path. As our fire element comes into balance, we experience clear vision, brightness, drive, self-confidence, passion, and courage. Contrarily, when agni becomes overly dynamic and intense, we might experience rage, egocentricity, impoliteness, and feelings of superiority. To cultivate fire, we can intensify our daily rhythm and dedicate ourselves anew to the life-enhancing practices that fuel our drive, which may be as subtle as gathering with others around a bonfire or fireplace or taking time to light candles, receive their warmth, and bathe in their glow. Inspired by the Hebrew poetry of Yannai

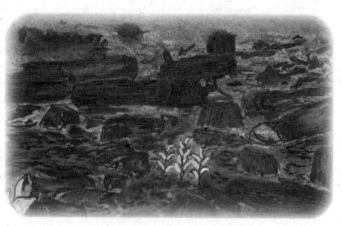

The celestial fire is upon us
a fire that devours fire
a flame that is like a crouching tiger
an inferno that remains burning without wood
a fire that sparkles and roars
a blaze that reveals itself in many forms
a fire that is, and never expires.

Inquiries

On the Mat: Utilize longer holdings and more rigorous postures to build heat and sensation in your practice. Light candles all around your space, and turn up the heat to stimulate the fire element. Weave core strengtheners into your practice, and contemplate your relationship to this particular force. Are you disconnected from this internal source of heat because it has the capacity to burn? Are you afraid of your inner power? Or are you instead so fiery that imbalance is prevailing in your life? Explore eye stretches, mountain, quad stretch in mountain, knee-down lunge, twisting high lunge, warrior one, warrior two, triangle, lateral angle, goddess, reverse warrior two, standing wide-angle forward fold, chair, and flying chair *(arms in T, torso moves forward, lower body weight remains behind)*

Off the Mat: Gather a group of friends for a bonfire or around a fireplace. Take note of the qualities invoked by the fire, and burn an object or piece of paper as an indication of something you wish to transform.

Practices

Supportive Words
change, evolution, rebirth, reformation, shift, transfiguration

Visualization
A raging forest fire and its aftermath; new wildflowers, shoots, and saplings begin to sprout in the charred landscape, bringing hope and new life in the weeks that follow.

Complementary Breath
kapalabhati & bhastrika
Raise the internal temperature during poses through the power of these breaths.

Closing Ritual
While seated, rub your palms vigorously together to generate heat. Place them onto the eyes, allowing the warmth to energize the whole body.

I embrace the heat of fire as a means of fueling my inner essence

that glows in my heart

I tend to the firelight

I hold space for all that surfaces from deep within

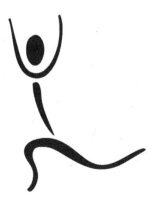

Enchanted Water:

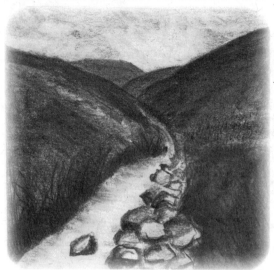

Water is fundamental for human life and is one of the most important elements for health and optimal functioning, as it regulates our body temperature, lubricates the joints, cushions organs and tissues, dissolves and carries nutrients to the cells, and helps flush out waste products[5]. It is formless, feminine, fluid, and transparent, and it corresponds to the sense of taste, representing our capacity to savor the various flavors that characterize a lifetime. Apas the the Sanskrit word for water is a symbol of our ability to flow with the river of constant change and adapt to the ever-evolving nature of life. For both plants and animals, water serves as a conduit for life by aiding in circulatory activity. Furthermore, water has connections to the womb *(the locus of individual life)* and to the oceans *(the origin of human life[6])*. This life-giving liquid has the power to cleanse, dissolve, and revitalize our core. When our water element is well-balanced, we experience flexibility, kindness, a nurturing spirit, spaciousness, and fluidity. Conversely, when apas is over-stimulated, we experience hyper-sensitivity, compromised limits, and excessive sympathy. To cultivate the qualities of water, we can make time for soothing relaxation, dance, and creative movement. Furthermore, we can immerse the body in this element by staying hydrated, taking long baths, swimming, or playing in the rain.

As one of life's most essential substances, water is also a potent theme for building awareness of one of the most serious environmental issues humans face today. Currently, there are over one billion people on the planet who live without access to potable water. In the U.S., the average person uses over 100 gallons of water a day, while this figure stands at only about 39 gallons for developing nations like India[7]. This troubling fact is further exacerbated by the amount of effort required to obtain those gallons of water versus the ease of simply turning on the tap in the West. Jeff Young, a reporter for *Living on Earth*, states, "We take this resource so much for granted, it's almost invisible to us. And the people around the world that go without water, they're pretty much invisible to us, too. It's kind of like water itself; you see through it until the light catches it just right, and then you see yourself reflected in it[8]." As we awaken to the power of this fundamental resource, we can begin to acknowledge it as an invisible thread connecting all of humanity. This recognition can motivate us to consider how more conscious action in our daily lives might uplift our brothers and sisters the world over. As Ralph Metzner writes:

O Great Spirit of the West,
Spirit of Great Water,
Of rain, rivers, lakes, and springs.
O Grandmother Ocean, Deep matrix, womb of all life.
Power to dissolve boundaries,
To release holdings,
Power to taste and to feel,

To cleanse and to heal,
Great blissful darkness of peace[9]...

Inquiries

On the Mat: Tailor a playlist of music to serve as your soundtrack for exploring the fluidity and changeability of water. Connect to this sacred element as you envision your whole being pulsing as embodied liquid. Notice and honor all of the vital functions water performs in your physical form. Utilize circular and repetitive warm-up motions before each pose, and keep the postures moving to the rhythm of the music and breath. Sequence a potpourri class that focuses on the fluid characteristics of each posture. Connect to this life-giving and nurturing element that cleanses, reflects, and serves as a vital connection among all beings. Explore back extensions with sun breath arms in warrior one, hip circles in table, dolphin waves, down dog to child back to down dog flow, flying chair to chair to twisting chair, backstroke in camel, and arm pulse in half circle.

Off the Mat: Dedicate at least thirty minutes to immersing your body in water. Take a bath, soak your feet, or go for a swim in an ocean, river, lake, or pond. Feel the effects of contact with this primal, life-giving element.

Practices
I connect to the fluid parts of my being   I allow the power of this essential

Supportive Words
ease, elasticity, fluidity, flexibility, motion

Visualization
A gentle mountain stream flowing over rocks and around boulders.

Complementary Breath
ujjayi

Focus on the breath having no real beginning or end as it ebbs and flows in its fluid cycle.

Closing Ritual
Play a recording of water sounds, or sit in the presence of a waterfall *(whether it be one in nature or an indoor miniature version)*. Listen carefully and absorb the quality and essence of water through its vibrations.

natural environment

substance to revitalize me

I use the reflective quality of water to highlight my connection with the   at the core

Grounded Earth:

Prithivi or the Sanskrit word for earth is associated with steadfastness, stability, groundedness, and vitality. Earth embodies nurturing energies, as it is the womb of our beloved planet. Seeds are planted in the ground of Mother Earth for cultivation, and they draw on her rich nutrients for growth. The mothering qualities of earth reflect a sense of foundation and solidify her role as abundant provider of life-sustaining nourishment. When we stand on or look at a patch of earth, we don't often pause to acknowledge the marvel that is right beneath us, but there is much more under the surface than meets the naked eye. In one tablespoon of soil, there are more living organisms than there are people on the planet. Microorganisms found in topsoil aid in the development of nutrient-rich medicines, and soil also reduces the risk of floods while filtering and storing water[10]. Earth energy has a weighty quality; it is firm and bulky and corresponds to our sense of smell, which supports us in distinguishing the gifts and dangers among Mother Earth's offerings. Although prithvi is solid, it is not completely impenetrable, as it takes in moisture, holds water, and softens around its apparent boundaries. When our earth element is balanced, we experience compassionate consistency, solid patience, steadiness in action, and an openness to giving. When our earth element is too rigid, we experience inflexibility, sluggishness, stubbornness, and an unyielding approach to life. To cultivate qualities of earth, we need to create structure and consistency in our lives from which we can expand and grow. Creating sustaining and nourishing rituals allows us to feel more connected, grounded, and stable. To build a relationship with this element, we can go outside for a meditative walk, place our bare feet or hands in the soil, and envision the ground below us even when standing in manmade structures. As Ralph Metzner writes:

> O Great Spirit of the South,
> Protector of the fruitful land,
> And of all green and growing things,
> The noble trees and grasses,
> Grandmother Earth, Soul of Nature.
> Great power of the receptive, of nurturance and endurance,
> Power to grow and bring forth
> Flowers of the field,
> Fruits of the garden[11].

Inquiries

On the Mat: Harvest the steadfastness that abounds in earth energy. Use the postures to settle and ground. Investigate stable standing postures as well as hip openers and forward bends, which will allow you to feel a tangible connection to Mother Earth while calming the nervous system and soothing the soul. Explore hip openers with bound angle, baby cradle, cow face, fire log, hands inside the front foot in knee-down lunge, pigeon, easy pose twist, head to knee, reclining hero, seated wide-angle forward fold and revolved seated wide-angle forward fold.

Off the Mat: Take twenty minutes to connect to the earth. Either rest on the ground, place your feet in sand or mud, or do a full-body clay mask.

Practices

Supportive Words
consistent, grounded, rooted, stable, steadfast

Visualization
A mountain; strong, stable, and rising up from its broad foundation of earth.

Complementary Breath
dirgha
Focus on apana, the element of the breath that flows downward and outward, grounding the body.

Closing Ritual
Prepare a small container of fresh soil before you begin your practice. As you complete your sadhana, take a few moments to examine the soil as though it were a foreign substance, taking note of its tactile, visual, and aromatic qualities.

I am always supported

of the ground to cultivate inner patience

With a sense of certitude, I affirm that

Remaining strong, I open to the supple nature of the earth

I use the stability

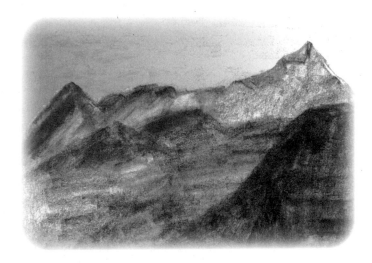

Natural Economy: {inspired by Douglas Brooks}

The natural world is abundant with wonder and beauty, and many of the functions of the planet seem almost magical. What is fascinating about this living organism, our planet Earth, is that it contains a plethora of natural treasures, and yet it sustains them with utmost efficiency and effectiveness. The Earth as a living, breathing system uses only as much as is necessary to fuel its functions and ensure its health. Human beings, though, have lost much of their connection to the natural environment. As a result, many of us lead lives that are disconnected from nature and we are therefore desensitized to the concept of natural economy. Because of this, we use more resources than we really need at the expense of the planet's well-being. The notion of becoming functional and efficient in our daily actions is not about squashing our desires. Instead, it is a matter of meeting our wants in more balanced, sensible, and economical ways that will create a win-win for both us and the environment. In an effort to asses our impact, we can consider the question, "How can we get the most out of the least amount of effort and use as much as we need, but not more than we need, if we don't need to?[12]". Natural economy can infuse every part of our lives with greater awareness of the impact of even the smallest actions. When I first arrived at Kripalu, I used two napkins per meal without much thought. Often, my second napkin would end up going into the trash unused. As time progressed, I started to recognize that one napkin would meet my needs, and that I could even save that same napkin and use it for a second meal. Later on, I began using a cloth napkin (which some members of my family still believe is a biohazard). The notion of economy not only reminds us to use just as much as we need, but also compels us to acknowledge the truly inestimable worth of the gifts Mother Earth offers. The precious resources of our planet have been and will continue to be the sources that fuel our world economy, provide healing medicines, and offer joy unconditionally through their natural brilliance. To honor those precious resources and to cultivate natural economy in our daily lives, we can be mindful of the amount of energy we use at home, think about alternative means of transportation, take canvas bags when we shop for groceries and other goods, compost our food waste, and donate money to an organization to offset our carbon footprint. As William Ellery Channing writes:

> To live content with small means; to seek elegance rather than luxury, and refinement rather than fashion; to be worthy, not respectable, and wealthy, not, rich; to listen to stars and birds, babes and sages, with open heart; to study hard; to think quietly, act frankly, talk gently, await occasions, hurry never; in a word, to let the spiritual, unbidden and unconscious, grow up through the common—this is my symphony[13].

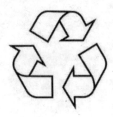

Inquiries

On the Mat: Since we are a part of nature, the idea of natural economy is ingrained *(although often forgotten)* in every cell of our being. At times, asana can become addictive, and spending too much time on the mat or stepping into a more vigorous practice turns into a depleting experience in the realms of energy and time. We buy into the idea that a longer sadhana will provide us with more vitality, yet our bodies are able to optimize and refuel in a very short amount of time. Especially if you typically practice for over an hour, take one week to experiment with shorter sadhanas. Spend no more than thirty minutes on your mat *(no more then four times during the week)* and notice how much you can accomplish in that amount of time. Dive into the quality of each posture and breath versus the quantity of how much you accomplish in this span of time. Investigate how you can get the most out of your yoga in a conscious way while putting forth only as much effort as you need. Honor times when you notice the urge to do more than would truly serve you. Feel the energetic effects of one minute of pranayama or the imprint of a single posture done with your full attention. As you practice with natural economy, notice whether you generate more vitality with a smaller amount of effort. Rooted in this awareness, we can engage our practice with greater efficacy and share more of ourselves in life off the mat without the draining side effects of overconsumption and overexertion. As you practice, consider how you use the various resources available to you, including breath, muscle strength, capacity for relaxation, mindful listening, skillful movement, internal conversation, and intention. Explore sun salutes, high lunge, knee-down lunge, hands inside of front foot in knee-down lunge, quad stretch in knee-down lunge, runner's stretch, plank, warrior one and two, lateral angle, balancing half moon, and warrior three *(either freestanding or against the wall)*.

Off the Mat: Explore some of the strategies mentioned on the previous page for cultivating and practicing natural economy.

Practices

I use only as much as I need to meet my needs   I cultivate natural economy for my own health for the wel-

Supportive Words
thrifty, sensible, economical, practical, far-sighted, functional

Visualization
The Reduce, Reuse, Recycle, symbol. A little bit can go a long way.

Complementary Breath
viloma *(inhale & exhale)*
Extract the most energy out of each pause in the breath.

Closing Ritual
Savor the power and presence accessed through a single chant of "Shri" the Sanskrit word for beauty, abundance and auspiciousness .

by the sustainable

-being of others, and for the prosperity of future generations   I affirm the wisdom demonstrated

Sacred Nectar: {inspired by Douglas Brooks}

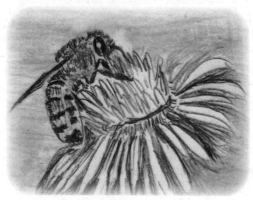

Bees are phenomenal creatures, with around 20,000 known species spread out among all the continents except Antarctica. Bees have existed between ten and twenty million years, and these insects are ultimately responsible for about one third of mankind's food supply because they perform the all-important task of pollinating blossoming flora. The average worker bee makes one-twelfth of a teaspoon of honey in its lifetime through a very labor-intensive process. As a bee makes rounds collecting pollen and nectar, it stops at as many as 50 to 100 flowers during a single trip. It may fly as far as one to two miles from the hive in order to seek out the treasure of nectar. The bee collects this food, takes it inside the hive for processing, and then offers it back to nature in the form of honey. More specifically, the process involves the bee regurgitating the nectar several times until it becomes partially digested. It is then stored in the open honeycomb, and the bees fan their wings to create a draft in order to expedite the evaporation of the excess water in the nectar. This in turn raises the sugar content and results in the concentrated, viscous liquid we know as honey. The wide range of flowers from which the bees harvest their nectar is what leads to the diverse flavors of honey we consume[14].

In Sanskrit, the word madhura[15] means "sweetness" or "syrup" and is one of the concepts we can use to savor the full spectrum of experience in the embodied realm. As we traverse our path and encounter different events and interactions, we have the ability to choose what is of value in each experience and assimilate this into our lives. Once we absorb this "nectar", we can utilize whatever means serves us best to process and digest it, whether this is journaling, yoga, meditation, drawing, prayer, or conscious conversation. After a period of time, we can offer this nectar back to ourselves and the world as the honey we've made through our own process of digestion. Douglas Brooks says the bee is a natural-born yogini because she imbibes nectar, processes it, and offers it back to nature in a sweetened form. We can take emotions and incidents labeled as negative and process them in a similar fashion. Elizabeth Gilbert, author of *Eat, Pray, Love* and Byron Katie, author of *The Work* are two women who took dark life experiences, distilled value from them by digesting them internally, and offered them back to the world in the form of inspirational writing and transformative teachings. Each one of us has this capacity for generating sweetness from our experiences as human beings. Furthermore, we can entertain the notion that the gift of life is, in a sense, incomplete when we receive it; it has to mature within us—by virtue of our willing engagement—in order to fully ripen. As such, we are an intricate part of the process of the manifestation and flowering of grace, in much the same way that the bees are responsible for generating energy in the form of honey as an offering of their experience[16].

Inquiries

On the Mat: Sense the possibility of absorbing the various experiences that surface in your practice, and contemplate how each yoga session offers its own unique nectar. Just like the bees, we revisit the same sequences, try new variations, or travel further afield to classes or workshops to deepen our personal inquiry. Each experience enables us to engage different parts of our being. We might spend one sadhana digesting our feelings of low energy or lack of motivation, the next exploring struggles with imperfection, and yet another processing the ecstatic sensations of coordinated breath and movement. In each instance, we are ingesting our experience, assimilating it, and then offering it back out into the world. Whatever flower you encounter, take the opportunity to find value in its distinctive nectar, drink it in, and then share the sweetness you distill from it with family, friends, and community.

As you step onto your mat, identify your most predominant state in the moment, whether it is anger, lethargy, sadness, or joy. Draw this feeling into your practice and become aware of how yoga refines your state of being from the inside out. Sense how the postures and breath help digest the nectar, and notice that one pose might fuel your current emotion while another might quell it. At the end of practice, assess what stage you have come to in processing this particular emotion or experience. Observe whether you have already tasted honey or whether you are still in the churning process, and make space for either as vital and worthwhile. Check in with yourself over the hours and days following your sadhana, and acknowledge when you feel the completion of offering sweetness back to yourself and the world with regard to this particular inquiry. Realize that the honey might take a form that is subtle yet profound. Explore down dog, side plank, high lunge, core strengtheners, crane, cow face, knee-down lunge, head to knee, standing forward fold, dwi hasta bhujangasana, and firefly. Utilize the arm balances in particular to experience short bursts of transformation akin to the work of creating honey, and then take time to process and digest your experience.

Off the Mat: Choose a recent experience that touched you, nourished you, and created a sense of sweetness in your life. When you feel it has been fully digested, find a creative way to offer it back to those around you in the form of a letter, card, poem, art piece, or e-mail.

I honor the multiple sources of nectar along my path   I welcome opportunities for absorbing experience, digesting it, and offering the fruits of this process back out into the world   I acknowledge my own unique ways of assimilating life's events

Supportive Words

absorption, assimilation, digestion, transmutation, taste

Visualization

A bee gathering nectar from a multitude of flowers, processing it, and transforming it into honey inside the hive.

Complementary Breath

bramari

Closing Ritual

Acquire a jar of raw, organic, local honey *(if you live near beekeepers, get it directly from them)*. Take time to be in mindful meditation with the smell, taste, and texture of honey. Savor this nourishing food on all levels of your being, bearing in mind the amount of energy expended by the bees to create this sweet nectar for your enjoyment.

Adaptation: {inspired by Anjali Budreski}

The power to adapt and the strength of the spirit residing within all living beings is truly astounding. After my little sister Leonie passed, I was astonished by the resolve of my father and stepmother to continue living life with optimism and hope. Seeing Knavin, my three-legged dog, walk around is always a reminder of grace, and thinking back on my own experiences of moving around and settling into a number of new environments reminds me of the incredible capacity we have to adapt to change. In nature, there are myriad examples of this ability to acclimate to the shifting conditions of life. As we hike up a mountain, we can witness the changes in landscape as it has adapted to increase the probability of sustaining life at higher altitudes. Plants and trees become smaller so as to better tolerate high winds, lichen spread more widely on the face of rocks to create more surface area for making food through photosynthesis, and animals living in these areas burrow under rocks or the ground to keep safe and warm. Even in the alpine zone, we find tremendous beauty, along with expansive views and fresh, crisp air. In spite of the blazing heat of the sun, freezing rain and snow, and high winds, life-forms here adapt remarkably well and indeed surmount the various obstacles

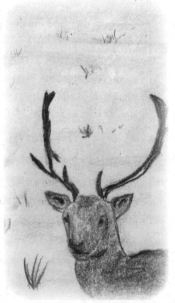

presented by their environment; they do so because their individual survival as well as that of their future generations depends on these adaptations. In daily life, we might think of adapting to change as an inconvenience, but indeed this process is often a source of incredible beauty and diversity; the butterfly adapted its wings to blend in with surrounding plants and to provide a safe camouflage from predators, jellyfish formed fluid, liquid bodies to thrive in the realm of the ocean, deer and moose developed thick winter coats that emerge as the days grow shorter and winter cold sets in, and whales have a blowhole enabling them to breathe even in their vast ocean habitat. The process of adaptation honors uniqueness, as it allows various life-forms to be more fully and truly what they are. As humans, adjusting invites us to be both realistic and ingenious as we engage and respond to the circumstances presented by a new or unfamiliar situation. In life, there is immense benefit in maintaining flexibility, as even a simple lunch plan could be delayed, postponed, or change, and our ability to acclimatize to the shift can determine whether our day is frustrating or pleasant. When we choose to delve more deeply into a situation that will require us to adapt, we are taking a risk. It is much easier to remain in familiar, protected territory, but we open to the possibility of seeing the world in a new way when we forge ahead knowing full well change will be necessary. As an anonymous soul writes:

The survival of the fittest is the ageless law of nature, but the fittest are rarely the strong. The fittest are those endowed with the qualifications for adaptation, the ability to accept the inevitable and conform to the unavoidable, to continually harmonize with the existing and changing conditions of the universe.

Inquiries

On the Mat: Yoga offers us many opportunities to hone and practice the skill of adaptation. When a substitute teacher shows up unexpectedly to class or we accidentally end up in gentle yoga instead of our usual vigorous vinyasa, we encounter occasions for growth. Our first inclination might be to turn away or complain that we didn't know our favorite teacher wasn't going to be around this week. But when we work to adapt to the unexpected, we often end up realizing gentle yoga was just what we needed or find that taking a class with a new instructor was refreshing and thought-provoking. Similarly, we can change to meet the needs of the moment in a difficult posture by modifying it to the realities of our situation instead of bowing out completely. In this practice use props, the aid of a teacher (*if taking this inquiry into class*), or personal experimentation to find a supportive stance. Instead of trying to adapt to a perceived image of how the asana should look, focus on the key actions for alignment, safety, and opening without worrying about the overall appearance of the pose. Investigate other ways to welcome adaptation in your practice including shifting the intensity and length of the breath, coming out of a pose to regroup, using a wall, increasing or decreasing the amount of muscle strength you are utilizing, and asking for help from a fellow student or teacher. Explore using a rolled mat under the feet to stretch hamstrings in standing forward fold. Also try leg at wall in three-legged down dog, a tie around the front foot in head to knee, a block or cushion under the knee in fire log, a block or blanket under the sits bones in hero/reclining hero, a tie in baby cradle, a blanket under the hip in pigeon, a tie in heron, and your foot to a friend's foot or to the wall in hanumanasana.

Off the Mat: Find a box and decorate it. Brainstorm and then write or illustrate the various tools for adaptation you possess on small pieces of paper. Place the adaptation box in a visible location, and when life requires you to shift, choose a tool from the box and utilize

Supportive Words
acclimate, accommodate, accustom, adjust,
habituate, harmonize, shift, tailor

Visualization
The changing landscape on a mountain hike,
or any of the animal adaptation examples
used in the contemplation.

Complementary Breath
ujjayi

Closing Ritual
Draw the tools of adaptation that you have in
your tool bag right now.

Hidden Oasis: {*inspired by Joshua Rosenthal*}

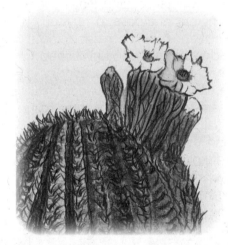

Deserts are described as arid, often sandy expanses with little rainfall, extreme temperatures, and sparse vegetation. They are found in the Middle East, northern Africa, Australia, western North America, and western South America. Not all deserts are the same; some are hot and sandy, others are cooler and rocky, and a few are found in vast canyons like the Colorado Desert. Their features include expansive plains, dry lake beds or sand seas, valleys, and abrupt, rocky mountain slopes. The desert is the domain of the sun's light and heat during the daylight hours, while temperatures become quite frigid at night. These landscapes convey a sense of timelessness, and they seem uninhabitable at first glance. Yet history shows us that many great civilizations, including the Egyptians, Native Americans, and the people of Peru's Coastal desert (*one of the driest in the world*), have taken root in these seemingly hostile landscapes.

Looking only at the surface, we might assume there is no life or vitality in these dry climates, and yet they hold countless treasures merely hidden from the untrained eye. Numerous animals make their homes here, including sheep, hawks, bats, wolves, camels, and iguanas. Wildflowers like desert chicory, dandelions, and sunflowers manage to sprout with beauty, while trees like the desert willow and cottonwood offer their nourishment to those who are aware of their gifts. Many inhabitants of the desert are nocturnal, coming out to play and hunt when temperatures are cooler and conditions calmer. One of the most renowned symbols of the desert is the cactus, which stores water within to be able to endure intense heat for prolonged periods of time. Cacti are beacons of perseverance amidst the harsh landscape of the desert. They grow in diverse shapes and sizes, and when they bloom, the landscape changes dramatically.

Their flowers beckon to passing birds and provide an array of color that transforms the surrounds. In the midst of an extreme environment, they are breathtaking beacons of life inspiring awe and reverence.

At times, we may feel as though life, or some aspect of it, is barren or infertile. In these moments of despair, we are often able to see only the emptiness that is immediately before us. As the desert demonstrates, though, what at first glance seems bleak often holds immense possibility and vitality. By carefully tending to these areas that feel disconnected or abandoned, we can begin to ease the discomfort and determine whether we have unconsciously deserted ourselves in some way. It is wholly up to us to become re-inspired and infuse promise into areas within that have grown lifeless. The arid climate of the desert landscape reminds us that even in areas of severe drought, the ground is fertile for the cultivation of beauty. Just like us, the planet is a living entity inextricably connected to energy and life force, even if part of her appears to be devoid of life.

Inquiries

On the Mat: As time passes and our yoga practice evolves, we may start to feel that certain poses, breathing exercises, and common sequences have lost their luster. Down dog might begin to feel like a ghost town, with little feeling or inspiration to be had. Yet with a single intentional breath, we can experience a reawakening. Notice whether going to a workshop, practicing with a friend, changing your usual sadhana time, or doing yoga with a new group of people infuses you with renewed zeal and energy that ignites even the most practiced poses. Experiment with creating variations through personal exploration or by combining new breaths with a familiar pose, and see if this revitalizes your sadhana. Additionally, you can generate fresh and inspired motivation on the mat by being fully present to your experience, softening around edges, and seeking the beauty in the mundane. See if something new can take root in a place you might have deserted. Investigate which postures quench your soul by providing nourishment and energy from within. At the same time, hold the space for the barren and dry aspects of the poses. Recognize your ability to constantly evolve, and notice how an area that feels infertile can become infused with life. For a change, begin your practice in a different position, lying in supine mountain or supine bound angle. Discover variations for some of the most commonly practiced poses. Explore flying warrior (*torso folded forward with arms extending behind like wings*), warrior one-*cactus arms*, warrior two-*eagle arms*, scorpion dog, flying chair (*same arm position as flying warrior*), tai chi goddess (*with the lower part of the body pulsing, arms explore the space with fluidity*), back bend in triangle, twist towards foot in pigeon, legs up the wall, and tie on upper thighs in savasana.

Off the Mat: Is there an area of your living space that can be revitalized to nourish your creative soul? Choose a room, corner, or nook to make your own. Think of it as an oasis, and allow it to serve as a wellspring of creativity flowing in the form that most resonates with you, whether this is sewing, knitting, dreaming, meditating, potting plants, journaling, painting, or reading.

I identify the places inside of me that feel arid and lack vitality

Supportive Words
fountain, haven, sanctuary, sanctum, source, wellspring

Complementary Breath
sitali
Bring moisture to the dry, deserted places.

Visualization
A bright pink saguaro cactus blooms amidst the barren, arid landscape of the desert.

Closing Ritual
Journal contemplation
What area of your life have you deserted? What is one thing you can do to revitalize this barren realm of your internal landscape?

devoid of color and light

infuse the deserted areas

I empower life to thrive in the places that feel most

of my being with the life force of breath

With the Flow: {inspired by Kelli Adams}

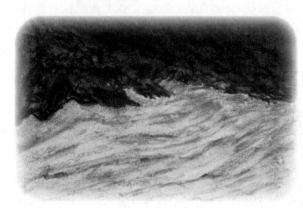

The river is one of the most powerful forces working its magic in the alchemy of nature. Rivers are symbols for the great current of life and also represent the energy of divine consciousness, as legend holds that Shakti flows down from Shiva's hair as the Ganges River. Much like a human life, a river is subject to constant evolution and change. No living being can ever step in the same river twice because it is constantly flowing. My sweet friend Anjali described a month long journey along the Allagash River in Maine co-leading a group of teenage girls as deeply transformative, in large part due to her observations of the river. At various points throughout the month, the river presented the group with tiny rapids, huge rolling waves, dangerous and chaotic currents, beautiful views, debates, internal struggles, fear, and joy. In time, she came to realize the key to making it through the experience was to go with the flow of all they encountered. There were instances in which the group chose to return to land to walk their canoes around a demanding obstacle, while at other times they decided to forge ahead and trust in the flow of the waters. Because Anjali's co-leader had more experience navigating the river, she was able to offer her wisdom and ask for the group's trust during some of the most pivotal moments of their journey. While she, also, was having a unique experience of the river, her past encounters with the body of water allowed her to intuit when a risk was truly significant, and likewise when an obstacle that appeared insurmountable was, in reality, one they could navigate with skill. Indeed, part of going with the flow is gaining familiarity with potential obstacles and utilizing this experience to hone our abilities.

In life, there are times when we embody the easy flow of a river as we sail smoothly through the day. On other occasions, we confront various challenges in the realms of work, emotions, relationships, and family. In these moments, we have the opportunity to emulate the river's adaptability as we meet the challenge at hand and still manage to flow. At times of real difficulty, we might want to go against the flow of the river, doing everything in our power to resist the present situation. We can become easily impeded by the surface currents of habitual patterns in these moments, and we might grasp for the safety of the banks, clinging to what feels sturdy and stable. Ultimately, it takes tremendous courage to step into the middle of the river where the deeper currents pull us and begin to carry us at an unpredictable speed. Once we do, though, we find ourselves on voyage of softening and releasing control while also steering around obstacles to keep from capsizing. As the The Elders of the Hopi Nation in Oraibi, Arizona, write:

There is a river flowing now very fast. It is so great and swift that there are those who will be afraid. They will try to hold onto the shore. They will feel they are being torn apart and they will suffer greatly. Know the river has its destination. The elders say we must let go of the shore, and push off and into the river, keep our eyes open, and our head above the water. See who is in there with you and celebrate. At this time in history, we are to take nothing personally. Least of all ourselves. For the moment that we do, our spiritual growth and journey comes to a halt. The time of the lone wolf is over. Gather yourselves! Banish the word struggle from your attitude and your vocabulary. All that you do now must be done in a sacred manner and in celebration. We are the ones we've been waiting for.

Inquiries

On the Mat: Become the vessel navigating the currents of your practice. Investigate the anticipation of an upcoming rapid in the form of a challenging pose like warrior three that stimulates the senses. Feel your heartbeat quickening and notice your awareness sharpening. Do you tip over and learn from the experience as you get back into the boat and continue to journey onward? Or do you ride the rapids fearlessly and savor the excitement of the moment? Move in a continuous posture flow to simulate the movement of a river. This faster pace can heighten the challenge of the practice and also offer you deep rewards at the same time. Consider whether you approach your postures cautiously or just sprint through them. Trust your skill as you travel downstream, and pause if a posture feels insurmountable. Recognize the options to either go around the obstacle or attempt to pass it with mindfulness while continually honoring where you are. Remember that courage, dexterity, experience, and awareness are essential for attempting a pose safely. Engage in the flow, whether yours is a fast-moving current or a slower and less intense one. Explore mountain with hands clasped overhead, eagle arm circles, standing yoga mudra, high lunge, knee-down lunge, dolphin, forearm pushups in down dog, L at the wall, and pincha mayurasana.

Off the Mat: Take three days to notice any resistance that comes up when other people make suggestions or when group energy is leading towards a certain decision. Do you overtly or quietly insist on being in control? As moments of resistance arise, try simply going with the flow of what is present. Write in your journal about your experience.

I tap into the fluid nature of life

I sense the profound wisdom

Supportive Words
current, drift, flux, outflow, stream, surge, tide

Closing Ritual
Drink a tall glass of water, and then simply sit and feel as it naturally flows downstream through the inner landscape of your body.

Visualization
The ever-shifting current of the river.

Complementary Breath
ujjayi

I trust that going with the flow holds the possibility

enduring coursing of the river.

of the unexpected

embedded in the vital

Against the Grain: {inspired by Me}

Animals are intrinsically connected to the energetic flow and intelligence of nature, and yet some of their behaviors seem counterintuitive at first glance. Salmon are born upstream in the waters of a river and soon after begin to follow the current, traveling downstream to eventually feed and live for four to seven years in the ocean[17]. Towards the end of their lives, the fish feel an instinctual call to reproduce, and they embark upon what many might consider an unusual journey. With fierce determination and vigor, they begin to swim upstream against the powerful currents of the river. An innate sense guides them to the exact place where they were born so they can spawn, lay their eggs, and then die where their lives began. In another example, male penguins spend many days protecting their eggs from harsh weather conditions in the sub-zero temperatures of the Arctic. As they persevere against the odds, their mates travel for miles to the water's edge to obtain food for the newborn chick. Both salmon and penguins model incredible determination as they live their lives in ways that defy ease but bring the deep and nourishing rewards of acting in alignment with the genuine intent of the heart.

In life, there are times when we have to source inner strength to pull ourselves upstream against majority perception, daunting odds, or common assumptions. We choose to act contrary to the norm because we know it is the only way to stay true to our intuition and internal values. When we travel in a direction opposite of the norm, we can expect to be bumped, harassed, and challenged both externally and internally. It takes great effort to stay on course and trust in what is to come. Human history abounds with individuals who have decided to go against the grain. The call to abolish slavery, the women's rights movement, and the push for equality for the GLBTQ (*gay, lesbian, bisexual, transgender, queer*) community all represent steadfast resolve to infuse new ideals into an ongoing conversation. When we swim against the current, we do so to bring about change, to create more options, and to infuse the world with added beauty. As with climbing a mountain, the majority of the journey is an uphill effort, but the rewards of the summit make the climb worthwhile. As Gandhi so gracefully modeled, the key in any movement to challenge the status quo is not to declare war, but rather to hold firm with a soft heart. Indeed, standing rooted in our own truth (*acknowledging that some opinions are more valuable and resonant for us than others*) while also respecting the right of others to have different ways of seeing the world is a most challenging yet rewarding endeavor.

Although yoga has been growing in popularity and has become quite common in many parts of the world, it is a movement practice that ultimately requires us to shift some of our common perceptions and stereotypes. The practice seeks to reawaken the innate integration of the physical, mental, and spiritual, and many of the activities invoked to this end might challenge our ideas of what is comfortable or acceptable in a public setting. Making loud noises, turning upside down, assuming odd-looking positions, lying supine in corpse pose, sitting still for meditation, and bowing to one another at the end of a session are a few examples of practices that might feel strange to us initially. Yoga, however, is an earnest invitation to connect to our innermost nature, and the practice empowers us to follow the calling of our truth even if doing so means challenging established norms. As Kirstin George writes:

I walk on the precarious edge
of the new and the old,
wanting to shed
the locks and lies of a mechanical world,
eager to dive into the smooth cool water of abundant life.

I am young,
I am a woman,
I live in a land where I can choose.

There are disco lights
and magnetic forces
pulling me into The Tunnel—
The Tunnel where everyone goes.

Almost everyone.

It vacuums up mall shoppers
and telemarketers,
executives and bartenders.
It promises clean sheets and Mickey Mouse vacations,
automatic garage doors
and cell phone communications.
If you choose The Tunnel
you will never have to be cold
or hungry or alone.
There are pills to erase headaches
and drinks to drown heart aches.

There are movies to make you laugh
and cars to move you fast.

If you don't like your face,
surgery will change its shape.

There is no need for God,
The Tunnel will keep you safe.

But if you stop believing,
oh! If you stop believing
The Tunnel will disintegrate
and leave you swimming in a septic tank.

My choice is clear.
I am stepping slowly
into the quiet open land beyond.

There are no roads, no maps, no guides.
There is no insurance coverage, no training school.
Edible vegetation is sparse.

Rain trickles down my back
as I fumble with reeds to make a hat.
Through the mist
I catch a thread of song
and rise to see a band of barefoot sisters
approach with open arms.

With nothing more than faith and grace,
our dance has just begun[18].

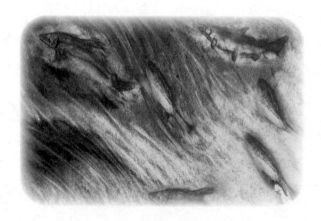

Inquiries

On the Mat: Explore your freedom to respond authentically to your genuine desires; feel free to yell even if you've always been told not to, express your love even if you've been told it's not appropriate to do so, and stick out your tongue even though it flies in the face of what is considered appropriate behavior. Practice swimming against the flow in your yoga, but remember that your goal is not merely to incite wonder or awe. Instead, you do so with awareness that this authentic action is an effort to create more brightness in your experience and in the world around you. In our culture, one of the most aberrant things we can do is simply slow down and pause. Common practice urges us to continually jump from one stimulated state to the next until we fizzle out completely. In the realm of yoga, meditation and restorative yoga might be considered the most resisted activities, as they stand in stark contrast to frenzied living. Begin with deep engagement and amplified courage to evoke the determination needed to initiate action in contrast to the greater tide. As the practice takes shape, slow your movement to create more space for nourishing and rejuvenating yourself. As you explore headstand, remember the benefits of inversions and thus the power accessed through non-habitual ways of moving *(in this case, increased lymphatic circulation, improved blood circulation to the upper body, energized endocrine and immune systems, and strengthening of small back muscles)*. Close your practice by utilizing a restorative posture during relaxation. Explore inversions with standing forward fold, standing yoga mudra, flying warrior one, warrior two, lateral angle, core strengtheners, triangle, standing wide-angle forward fold, block under sacrum in bridge, shoulderstand, supported headstand, and tripod head stand.

Off the Mat: The next time you are among family, consider whether you would be served by going against the grain. Notice any tendencies you might have to go along with something that does not truly resonate with you. Does this create internal bitterness or external conflict later? Explore going against the grain and staying true to you. Take note of whether this approach engenders more life force for all involved.

Practices

I acknowledge the areas of my life in which I have to paddle upstream   I trust

Supportive Words
counter to, facing, in contrast to, into, opposed to

Visualization
Salmon swimming upstream with steadfastness and determination.

Complementary Breath
viloma *(inhale & exhale)*
Tanslates as "against the grain" or "against the natural flow of things".

Closing Ritual
journal contemplation
In what realms of your life do you feel like you are treading against the grain? Who are your supporters? What enables you to persevere?

from a different vantage point

that going against the grain wi.

I notice what shifts as I turn upside down and see the world

I create more beauty

Holding Space: {*inspired by Kathy Budreski*}

Lakes are large, inland bodies of fresh water. Essentially, they are containers filled with the sacred element of life, and yet they are subtly imbued with the qualities of release and freedom brought by the waters spilling into their vast, spacious expanse after a long journey. Lakes relate to masculine energy, as they represent the notions of boundary and containment and are literally vessels holding within them the inspirations and activities of life. Unlike the constant, flowing nature of the stream, the lake gets to experience, feel, and hold many diverse states of being. One moment the waters are dead calm, and then suddenly winds roll in and whitecaps are visible all around. The next instant the winds subside, and gentle rain caresses the surface of the water. A few hours later, the sun returns, its resplendent rays reflecting off the bright blue surface. The lake, with its fleeting transformations, can serve as a rich symbol of our own constantly shifting experiences and emotions. We are all comprised of a balance of masculine and feminine energies, but in our culture masculinity is often associated with anger, the role of the provider, and constant activity without pause for self-care. Masculinity, though, is really much more than this limited set of characteristics, as it also encompasses a capacity for holding space, unwavering endurance, easeful tranquility, and concentrated mindfulness. As a symbol of this energy, the lake invites us to be open to what is arising, hold what is inside, see the larger perspective, and explore the clarity represented by the fresh, clear water.

As we move through various life experiences, there are times when tapping into this masculine steadfastness is vital for supporting both ourselves and others. When my friend's mom broke the news to her family that she had just been diagnosed with breast cancer, my friend's first inclination was to react and succumb to the waves of building emotion. Instead, she chose to simply pause and hold space for the situation as an act of respect for the energy of calm sadness she sensed in her mother. Instead of immediately trying to fix the situation, troubleshoot, or change what was going on, she merely tapped into her ability to be steady and present while keeping a soft heart. When we or someone close to us is struggling with an illness or challenging life situation, what awaits is often unknown. It is during those times that we can connect to the aforementioned male attributes to support us. Furthermore, just as the lake reflects its surroundings, we have the capacity to mirror to those around us their ability to make space for themselves. A Buddhist teaching reminds us that salt is extremely potent when dissolved in a small glass of water, but the same amount of salt in a larger body of water becomes diluted and thus has significantly less impact. In keeping with this principle, we can cultivate our ability to expand and hold more internally in order to dissipate the intensity of stressful situations. When we expand our awareness and pause to simply hold space, the pungent qualities of a particular moment can mellow and begin to dissipate. As Wendell Berry writes:

When despair for the world grows in me
and I wake in the middle of the night at the least sound
in fear of what my life and my children's lives may be,
I go and lie down where the wood drake
rests in his beauty on the water, and the great heron feeds.
I come into the peace of wild things
who do not tax their lives with forethought
of grief. I come into the presence of still water.

And I feel above me the day-blind stars waiting for their light. For a time
I rest in the grace of the world, and am free[18.5].

Inquiries

On the Mat: Envision your practice as a lake offering a greater perspective of your bodily experience. As the practice progresses, you encounter movement, breath, mindfulness, relationship, reflection, and a range of emotions. Continuously expand through your sadhana to become more spacious, periodically retreat to see the larger view, and cultivate an awareness of your surroundings throughout. At the beginning of practice, attune to any sounds entering your space from outside, whether they take the form of a gentle stream, singing birds, or the flow of nearby traffic. Witness the din of any chatter issuing forth from your internal landscape, as well. Tap into your masculine energy, bringing endurance, mindfulness, and tranquility into your poses as you create space for yourself. Explore the sequence below as an inquiry of holding space with steadiness, transitioning from one pose to the next without releasing your leg back to the ground. Practice warrior one, warrior two, standing wind-relieving, cobra pulsations, half frog, bow, balancing half moon, quad stretch in knee-down lunge, tree, tie in king dancer, and warrior three *(with arms by the sides or extended out in front)*.

Off the Mat: Ask a friend to take part in a co-listening experience with you. Co-listening is an opportunity to hold space for one another while sharing verbally in a stream-of-consciousness way. Sit shoulder to shoulder with your friend facing opposite directions, and touch shoulders if it feels right. Notice that sitting this way cuts off non-verbal communication, which is intentional. Designate who will begin. Take turns vocalizing anything you are aware of in the moment for a period of five minutes. The physical body is often a great place to start. From there, the sharing can extend to any other realm. When it is your turn to listen, hold the space silently, focusing full attention on the practice of active listening and directing the mind back to your partner's voice if it wanders. Afterwards, each take a few moments to share your experience of the exercise. How does it feel to simply hold space without trying to offer empathy, opinions, or solutions?

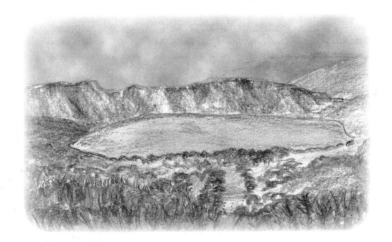

Practices

Supportive Words

Holding: *bear, bolster, sustain, uphold*
Space: *expanse, gap, interval, void*

Visualization

View of a lake from afar, the contour of the land forming a natural vessel to hold the water.

Complementary Breath

kapalabhati

Focus on the space created by holding the breath out at the end of each round.

Closing Ritual

Wrap your arms around yourself in a warm embrace, and pause here to hold space for whatever is arising for you in the moment. Hold this quietly for a few breaths.

Teacher's Note

If your space allows, guide the peak posture in a circle so students can form a container of support for one another in addition to making room for themselves energetically. Have students return to the circle at the end of class, creating a comforting boundary and holding space for the body of shared energy. Chant three rounds of "aum" to complete the practice.

Surfing the Waves: {*inspired by Jyoti Danika Kuhl*}

Oceans cover three-quarters of the earth's surface. Although they appear relatively calm when viewed from afar, they sustain a whole universe of living creatures and dynamic processes. The surface currents driven by prevailing winds keep the waters of the ocean circulating and therefore in constant flux. Due to complex weather patterns and storm conditions, there are times when the calm waters churn as massive, pulsating waves. Surfers choose to interact with this changeable nature of water in its most threatening yet magical form. Instead of fighting the waves, they cultivate skills that allow them to glide with the water in an effortless way while still honoring the intensity of the forces at work. Learning to surf requires significant time, dedication, and effort. It can take many days to simply stand upright on the surfboard and much longer to learn how to balance for an extended period of time without falling over. Long after the essentials are in place, these skills are continually refined as surfers head into ever deeper waters, experiment, fall, and get back up, learning from each experience.

Engaging in a relationship with an entity of this scale amplifies our ability to extract and appreciate lessons emerging amidst tumultuous surf. Waves of emotion carrying anger, joyfulness, anxiety, love, and jealousy wash over us on a daily basis. Cultivating the skill of how to remain present with such intense moments requires much effort and perseverance. When we choose to surf these waves, we must first swim out into the greater unknown, away from the safety zone of the shore. The bigger the waves that are approaching, the more tempted we will likely be to surrender and return to the refuge of the beach. Our experience can shift dramatically, however, when we can soften and recognize that the wave is actually a part of us that holds immense potential for learning. We must remain steadfast as we build the muscles and skills to stay on the board and develop a relationship with the force before us. Rather than allow the wave to overpower us, we can hold tight to our support and use its pure, raw momentum to recharge and empower our own active participation. As we develop skills for navigating bigger waves, there will likely even be moments of excitement as the waters begin to rise. In these instances, we recognize that a new, more challenging wave equates to a unique opportunity to dive more deeply within. Some waves will subside quickly, while others will linger and eventually carry us closer to shore and back to the comfort and safety of the sand. As John Welwood writes:

> A skilled surfer is aware of exactly where he is on a wave, whereas an unskilled surfer winds up getting creamed. By their very nature, waves are rising fifty percent of the time and falling the other fifty percent. Instead of fighting the down-cycles of our emotional life, we need to learn to keep our seat on the surfboard and have a full, conscious experience tof going down…Relative human love is not a peak experience nor a steady state. It wavers, fluctuates, waxes and wanes, comes and goes, changes shape and intensity, soars and crashes[19].

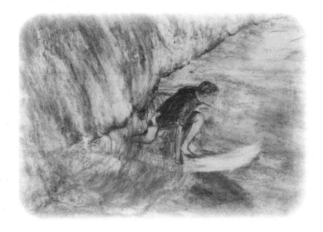

Inquiries

On the Mat: In the realm of formal education, most of us have little exposure to real learning regarding our relationship to inner self. The practice of coordinated movement and breath can begin to fill this void, teaching us how to better deal with the intensity guaranteed to escalate as we flow through life. Moving into the unknown, internal realm is much like stepping into the waters of the ocean. This endeavor requires the skills to surf the daunting waves of life, the courage to honor our singular mental and emotional identity, and the physical strength to sustain the voyage. When we first learn a new pose or pranayama, it can feel like an overwhelming wave, but it soon becomes effortless as we develop and hone our ability. Luckily, just as with surfing, our practice continually offers more to learn and unanticipated challenges to navigate. Each wave serves as a fresh opportunity to play with the posture and explore the subtle nuances therein. Envision your mat as a surfboard of sorts, and observe how yoga provides you the tools to be more mindful and skillful when waves of emotion or physical sensation surface. Seek support in the little adjustments that help you stay afloat, such as extending arms for balance,

flaring the toes, or utilizing the breath as an anchor amidst the energy of movement. Use postures that face towards the side plane of the mat in order to simulate a surfer's stance, and discover how more challenging poses or new asanas can symbolize the larger waves of life. Explore standing and balancing with eagle arm rotation, warrior two, lateral angle, triangle, balancing half moon, top leg in bow in balancing half moon, lateral angle, and revolved lateral angle.

Off the Mat: Spend three days in active contemplation of the notion that present moment experience undulates and shifts like the waves of the ocean. Notice moments of your day (*conversations with others, bouts of negative self-talk, or unexpected events*) when you feel like huge waves of emotion are crashing down upon you. Utilize the following three days to begin actively surfing any moments of intense experience that arise throughout your day. Reach into your tool bag of resources (*breath, support of others, healthy food, journaling, awareness, compassion, etc.*) to skillfully ride any waves that appear.

Practices

I welcome each new wave as an occasion to dive more deeply within

Supportive Words
surf: *cruise, drive, ride, journey*
wave: *ridge, ripple, surge, swell, undulation*

Visualization
Riding luminous ocean waves atop a surf board.

Complementary Breath
ujjayi

focus on the ocean-sounding and wave-like qualities of the breath

Closing Ritual
Place one hand on the belly and one hand on the heart, and feel the waves that pulse within.

exhilaration and ease

I sustain my courage, even if I fall off the board

I build the skill to ride each wave with a sense of

Sea Glass: {inspired by Anjali Budreski}

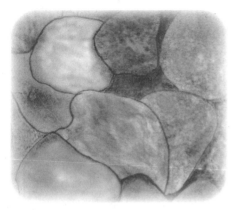

A bottle breaks at the seashore; sharp and hard, it is greeted by the graceful flow of the gentle waves. As the days pass, the ocean washes over the jagged edges of the glass with its rhythmic dance of tide and surf. Each day, the waves pound the fragments, transforming their shape and smoothing their sharp edges into softer lines. At the shore, there are always some pieces of glass that are spiky and new, others which appear jagged but have already been gently worn down, and those that have been pummeled by water and jostled by rocks and shells for many months. These latter pieces have already undergone transformation and can be handled without concern, but one that has recently broken must be handled with great care. The power of time, the steady caress of the ocean, and the engaging pulse of life combine to create a force that sculpts even the sharpest glass in a potent and profound way.

As we sow a deeper understanding of who we are, we are better able to recognize the places inside and out where our edges have been softened as well as those still characterized by sharp protrusions. Just like the diverse life stages of the sea glass, we are all at different stages in the various realms of our lives. If grief or tragedy strikes, we can honor our vulnerability and ask others to embrace us as our healing process takes place, holding us as delicately as they would a newly broken shard of glass. It is vital to remember we don't have to weather these times alone and to recognize that there is a natural timing to the smoothing of our jagged edges. One day the heart just feels lighter; often, one edge seems smoother while another is still sharp, and one part is healed while another still needs nurturing. Over time, the gifts of support and erosion allow us to move ahead and return to a more easeful flow. When an extreme life situation arrives, we tend to retreat into solitude and often think we are the only ones experiencing this level of pain. The truth is that most every person has experienced grief and has been emotionally vulnerable at some point. It is a universal part of life, and we all need to allow ourselves the experience and let others hold our sharp edges as we heal. The challenge is often giving ourselves permission to be exactly where we are and trusting our edges to transform as the ocean waters dance. In addition to times of grief, the sharpness of life may manifest when we enter a new relationship, embark on a new professional path, or start to build a new social network. At first, there is underlying apprehensiveness, nervous excitement, or slight instability, which over time begins to erode and disperse. Richard LaMotte writes:

> The goal of every collector is to find as rare a treasure as possible. In sea glass, the prize is a highly sought-after color in a softly rounded form. The value of an extraordinary piece of sea glass is unlikely to compare to a flawless diamond, but the relative beauty of each justly remains in the eye of the beholder. A diamond is created by nature and arduously refined by man, while sea glass is what man creates and nature refines for us[20].

Inquiries

On the Mat: These feelings of sharpness are encountered in our yoga practice, as well, when learning a new posture, attending a class for the first time, or practicing in a raw emotional state to name a few examples. Placing our body in an unfamiliar position or taking class while challenging our habitual patterns usually results in acute and heated sensations. As we practice the same pose over and over again, get to know people in our community, and honor our internal process, everything starts to take on a softer, more easeful quality. Our edges won't likely smooth in just one practice, though, as the process takes ample time to find completion. Set a deeper focus by using ujjayi breath and its ocean-sounding qualities. Move through a practice that is physically more rhythmic to simulate the movement of ocean waves washing over sea glass. Imagine yourself as piece of sea glass, allowing the breath, poses, connection with community (*if taking this inquiry into the studio*), and personal intention to be the factors which smooth and soften them like the caress of the waves. Engage the following poses in a soft, fluid way, coming in and out several times before pausing to hold: cat and cow, standing forward fold, runner's stretch, warrior one arms, chair, triangle to reverse warrior flow, bridge with arms over head, and easy pose twist.

Off the Mat: Next time a sharp edge arises along your path, step on your yoga mat, rug, or bed and curl up in a restorative fetal position. Make use of props to support the head, fill in space between the knees, and engage the ujjayi breath for a few deep rounds. Remain here for at least ten minutes, letting the breath soften and wash over you. Journal about what has transpired once you return back to a seated position.

Practices

Supportive Words
calm, comfort, ease, gloss, polish, round, sand, soften

Visualization
Sharp and colorful ocean glass being caressed and smoothed by the rhythm of the waves.

Complementary Breath
ujjayi

Closing Ritual
Carefully hold a jagged piece of ocean glass, and take a few deep breaths. Replace the sharp glass with a smoothed piece and take a few more rounds of deep breath.

Teacher's Note
Lead a back-to-back twist in pairs at the end of class to symbolize our shared humanity and the support we can offer one another in the process of smoothing our edges.

I allow myself to be with the sharpness of the moment. I trust that time will aid in healing my heart. I reach out to the love and support surrounding me.

The Pearl in the Oyster: {inspired by Kathy Budreski}

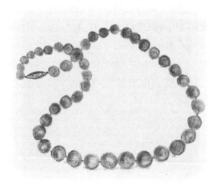

The splendor that emanates from a genuine pearl necklace is imbued with profound grace. Pearls have been revered by mankind for many centuries and are found near the coasts of India, Sri Lanka, the Persian Gulf, and the Red Sea. One Hindu story tells of Krishna offering the very first pearl, which he had acquired from the ocean, to his daughter Pandaia to wear on her wedding day[21]. Known as the queen of gems, pearls have traditionally played an important role in Chinese, Roman, Egyptian, and Arab cultures, and over time this reverence has migrated to European, South American, and North American societies. Some ancient cultures believed pearls were the tears of the gods, and others thought them to be dewdrops filled with the luster of moonlight that had descended into the waters and were swallowed by oysters[22].

A pearl is a natural jewel formed by a living organism, the mussel or oyster. When an unfamiliar entity enters the interior space of the organism, it responds by coating the irritant with a material called nacre, which is the same substance it uses to form its shell. As time passes (anywhere from a few months to a few years), the sheaths of nacre accumulate and gradually form the pearl. The longer a given aggravation remains inside the mollusk, the more layers of nacre are secreted, creating an even more brilliant drop of moonlight. "Nacre is not just a soothing protection for the mollusk. It's made of tiny crystals of calcium carbonate, perfectly aligned with each other, so that light passing along the axis of one is reflected and refracted by the other to produce a rainbow of light and color. Only when something becomes lodged— like a piece of shell, bone, coral, or parasite does the oyster start nacre production[23]."

In life, we experience many situations, people, and emotions that could be labeled as irritating. Annoyance and frustration can bubble up when we want to have things our way, or when we try to change the other person instead of finding a way to shift internally or simply be with what is arising. The irritation arrives from outside, but in reality it triggers something deep inside of us that already exists. Our first instinct might be to expel the sensation, but if we pause instead and focus on building brightness, we initiate a process of transformation. Kathy Budreski reflects, "My recent bout with cancer has been like a grain of sand which has truly transformed into an exquisite pearl. The strength of the pearl that evolved from the sand endures and brings forth courage, wisdom, and a very special grace that I hadn't experienced to this degree or level in the past. It is difficult to find words to adequately describe this intangible but very real feeling." It takes tremendous courage to own an irritation and to allow it to be inside of us while at the same time acknowledging our desire to blame another or push the feeling away.

In my own life, my relationships with both my grandma and stepmother (or bonus mom as my friend Jyoti likes to call herself) have felt like an adventure spanning two decades. In my youth, I was not able to see how I was choosing to cultivate agitation and difficulty through my interactions with them. Luckily, I was able to shift my vision and actions as I matured. Although it took time, introspection, and effort, these two relationships have transformed into striking pearls of equanimity and beauty. When we encounter an irritating situation or person in our lives, we can choose to respond with compassion, love, and commitment as the agitation gets soothed, assimilated, and allayed from the inside out. Just as the oyster takes the light and refracts it in the making of the pearl, we can also infuse light into frustrating situations. By aligning like the tiny crystals of calcium carbonate, we can cultivate respect for the other person, simply allowing them to be, instead of fighting or trying to change them. We can step into the experience of our interactions with a willingness to soften and actively seek beauty. Irritation is part of life, but we have a choice to engage, transform, and build understanding as we utilize it to slowly produce a beautiful strand of pearls. As an anonymous person shares:

There once was an oyster whose story I tell
Who found that some sand had got into his shell.
It was only a grain, but it gave him great pain.

For oysters have feelings although they're so plain.
Now, did he berate the harsh workings of fate that brought him to such a deplorable state?
Did he curse at the government, cry for election,
And claim that the sea should have given him protection?
No- he said to himself as he lay on a shell,
Since I cannot remove it I shall try to improve it.
And the small grain of sand that had bothered him so…

Was a beautiful pearl all richly aglow.
Now the tale has a moral, for isn't it grand
What an oyster can do with a morsel of sand
What couldn't we do if we'd only begin with some of the things that get under our skin.

Inquiries

On the Mat: Irritation can take any number of forms in our yoga practice. We may feel it in a particular pose, in an interaction with a teacher, with the class as a whole, or even with one specific classmate. When we are swept up in agitation, it doesn't mean we have to leave or turn away. Rather, we stand to learn something new through the interaction if we simply sit with it, embracing our feelings and thoughts. In this way, we might find a glimmer of light in a practice that is frustrating or different from our expectations. Likewise, we may experience a moment of ease in a pose that is generating heat or discomfort in the body. What is the lesson embedded in each of these moments regarding ourselves and the way we live in the world? In every instance of irritation, we have an opportunity to welcome the possibility of culturing a pearl, becoming more aware of when and how we attempt to brush the obstruction aside, and acknowledging the times when we choose to coat it with the light of awareness. For this particular asana inquiry, explore your burgeoning relationship to arm-balancing asanas. Notice if arm balances are a source of irritation because you are overly fixated on the final pose even as you are making progress. Harvest this irritation to create something ever more brilliant and valuable that will aid you in expanding and enhancing your yoga. In addition, envision someone who is currently a source of frustration in your life and hold this person in your heart as you practice, making space for the pearl that might emerge from the irritation. Explore seated yoga mudra, down dog, three-legged dog twist, high lunge, chair, runner's stretch, core strengtheners, hands inside foot in knee-down lunge, plank, pigeon, side plank (*explore variations, one foot in tree or hand to big toe*), crane, eka hasta bhujasana, and dwi hasta bhujasana.

Off the Mat: Think of someone in your life who arouses feelings of irritation. Purposefully carve out time to be in this person's company, and dive into the inquiry of finding the pearl in the oyster. Stay mindful and aware of any annoyance that arises, and use it to seek out moments of wisdom and discovery. Over time, notice whether this particular relationship becomes easier to navigate.

Practices

I acknowledge any irritation showing up on my path and embrace it fully

Supportive Words
irritation, aggravation, frustration, abrasion, annoyance

Visualization
A strand of shimmering pearls.

Complementary Breath
bhastrika

Closing Ritual
journal contemplation
What is one example of irritation in your life at the moment? What might be the pearl that emerges from this frustration?

as channels for growth

I trust that by choosing to

I study my own internal triggers

engage with an aggravation, I will gradually create beauty

Stillness & Motion: {*inspired by Winter*}

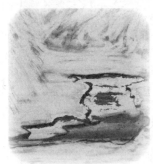

It is near the end of November, and darkness has settled more fully into the cycle of the day. Whenever I teach morning yoga at Kripalu, I wake up at four forty-five to walk my dog Knavin before arriving at work by half-past five. This morning, I paused to take in the soft luster of the morning sky, dark and dotted with twinkling pinpoints of light. What struck me most on our brisk walk was the stillness in the air. The birds, surrounding animals, and people of the neighborhood were all still asleep under the blanket of the dark sky. Yet even in the midst of the profound calm, I could sense the current of life still pulsing faintly in the background in the form of a shooting star, the sounds of a distant car, and the soft caress of the wind. This walk with Knavin inspired me to consider the relationship between stillness and motion. More specifically, I thought about how a pause always holds some activity and how, likewise, activity always finds a moment of pause. When we sleep, the body is immobilized, but life continues to pulse within. The breath ebbs and flows, the heart finds an eye blink of silence and then beats again, and the body continues its subtle functioning, cleansing and preparing for the day ahead.

When ice forms on the surface of a river or stream, the undercurrents still continue to flow beneath, exemplifying this partnership of stillness and motion. In other words, the notion of statue-like, frozen immobility is not really a fact of the natural world because life is always there, teeming even in the darkest and coldest realms of existence. Embedded in this recognition is an opportunity for rejuvenation and healing and, perhaps more importantly, permission to connect to our essential selves. The pulsation of being alive is like a constant dance, wherein there is always something transpiring inside of us or around us. When we get swept away by this dance, we lose our center and get mired in the fragmentation of our experience. How would life look, though, if we could cultivate inner stillness and rest while being present to the motion of the world continuing to shift and flux around us? Furthermore, how would our experience change if we were able to acknowledge this flux as a natural part of life, as opposed to constantly trying to force quiet and calm? String theory, which is often called the theory of everything, concurs with this idea that movement is essential and fundamental to the universe. In what is known as the standard model of particle physics, scientists proposed that the universe is made of steady, point-like particles. String theorists took this model a step further and asserted that there are tiny, vibrating strings in constant flux underneath these still particles[24]. Mindfulness practice and yoga are powerful conduits that aid us in realigning with these fundamental and natural movements of the cosmos and, consequently, our own lives.

At its inception, the practice of hatha yoga was designed to help the practitioner sit longer for meditation and thus cultivate this state of stillness. But even in meditation and yoga, the undercurrent of the universe is always with us. The practice of immobility in the body is in support of the willful and compassionate ability to be present with the creative motion of the mind. As such, stillness is not the process of forcing silence, but rather the journey of awakening to and flowing with the streams that continue to run beneath the quietude. Doug Keller says of Tantric meditation that "it makes meditation a creative act, it brings creativity into meditation, gives you permission to be creative…up till now meditation has largely been sit down, steady the breath, still the mind, and it's very hard to stay with it, kind of takes all the creativity out of the process, because in a sense you are trying to bring the mind which includes the creative mind to a halt. Tantrika philosophy is saying allow your mind its full creative play and in the experience of allowing your mind to play with visualization with reference to experiences, you'll start to intuit or feel the divine consciousness that is there in the play. So certainly meditation brings stillness, but it's the kinds of stillness an artist experiences in that moment before he finally, in a flash, conceives of what he wants to create…the spark of real meditation, where there is a flash of the fullness and full potential of consciousness[25]." Just as we observe it in nature and in our creative mind, recognizing the symbiotic relationship of stillness and motion in our lives can enable us to utilize each of these states more effectively as we investigate the ways they intermingle and serve one another. As Danna Faulds writes in *Still Point*: "…It vibrates with the music of life, dances in the wind, breaks forth from the trees into a clearing just as the sun rises, and settles into silence once again[26]."

Inquiries

On the Mat: Combine a faster flow with several extended holdings. During the flows, tap into the briefest moments of inaction even as your body continues to dance with the rhythm of the breath. Notice how the practice of yoga aids you in cultivating this skill of focus and calm while amidst the motion and turbulence of movement. In the moments of holding and stillness, watch the undercurrents of your creative mind and the subtle quivering of the body with intent, absorbing the sounds and movements into your experience. In tandem with this investigation, practice postures in which the lower part of the body is stable and still while the arms and torso are more fluid. In tree, first take the pose with stability, and feel the subtle pulse in the background.

After several breaths, animate your tree with expressive torso, arm, and hand movements to explore intuitive motion. Leave time at the end of practice to experience a meditation focused on flowing with the creative journey of your mind as opposed to one of rigid stillness. Investigate standing wind-relieving, wind-relieving, supine hand to big toe, eye of the needle, extended side angle, warrior one, fluid arms in warrior two, tai chi arms in goddess, fluid arms in chair, tree, and animated tree.

Off the Mat: Take a walk in nature. Pause every so often to notice the sources of movement, take note of the stillness, and sense how the two intermingle with one another.

Practices

Supportive Words
stillness: *calmness, inaction, quietude, pause*
motion: *action, flow, fluctuation, flux, stirring*

Visualization
The movement of water beneath the surface of a frozen lake.

Complementary Breath
ujjayi

Closing Ritual
As you prepare to emerge from relaxation, remain in stillness while slowly attuning your awareness to the subtle movement circulating in you and around you.

stillness and motion

I sense the moments of stillness amidst the flow of my practice

I feel the

I embrace the powerful symbiosis of

energy of flux in the moments of pause

the wheel of the year

holidays,
celebrations,
& sacred rituals

the wheel of the year

Rituals and celebrations have been an integral part of human existence for thousands of years. Holidays and special events bring people together in community and serve as opportunities for giving thanks in creative and playful ways. Many diverse spiritual traditions share similar rituals, highlighting common threads that weave their way through seemingly disparate pockets of humanity. At the same time, there are subtle yet significant differences that allow each culture to create wholly unique expressions of their specific beliefs and heritage. While the West has gradually become a vibrant melting pot comprised of people who have wonderfully diverse backgrounds, the resulting amalgamation of cultures has begun to dilute their respective celebrations and traditions over the past few generations. With an overemphasis on consumption and being entertained as opposed to generative creativity, many people have become disconnected with the deeper meaning of holidays and rituals. The following insights provide opportunities to re-familiarize ourselves with cultural celebrations and become newly inspired as we contemplate their offerings to present-day life. For an up-to-date listing of precisely when these holidays and rituals fall during a particular year, refer to *www.interfaithcalendar.org*.

Treasures of Spring:

Spring is a time of new light and new possibilities. The days grow longer as daylight expands its reach and the sun's rays become more potent. Green begins to infuse the surrounding landscape, invoking the qualities of heart energy, meditation, and peace with which it is associated. Spring is a time for planting seeds, watering the soil, and welcoming new growth and opportunity. This season of renewal is usually accompanied by a substantial amount of rain, which allows the earth to cleanse from the hibernation of winter and begin to restore movement, energy, and flow to the land.

With the return of the light, we too can awaken and grow as we attune to the burgeoning activity of the Earth. Spring beckons us towards greater self-expression and upward movement and serves as an opportune time for setting intentions in motion. As a result of longer days and plentiful rain, many nutrient-rich foods grow during this time of year, including dandelion greens, radishes, and spinach. These foods remind us that spring is an ideal time of year to engage in cleansing rituals to uplift the body and mind. In Chinese Five-Element Theory, the organs that most benefit from a spring cleanse are the liver and gallbladder. The liver is responsible for the formation and breakdown of blood, removing toxins and assimilating such minerals as zinc, copper, and iron, while the gallbladder stores and secretes bile, a substance that supports efficient and easy digestion. By nurturing these organs at the onset of the spring season, we can set the stage for their healthy functioning throughout the remainder of the year.

The Essence of Pesach: {inspired by Daniel Max}

Passover is the Jewish celebration in honor of the exodus of the Jews from Egypt and from slavery. It falls on the 14th day of Nisan in the Hebrew calendar, which typically corresponds to a date in March or April, and the celebrations last for seven days. One of the primary rituals of the holiday involves a special meal known as the Seder, which reunites family and friends to remember the past and rejoice in the present. The meal is characterized by a number of symbolic gestures and foods, beginning with a general blessing and lighting of candles to honor the sacred nature of the gathering. To start the feast, everyone drinks wine to acknowledge the power and potential inherent in the voyage of awareness, and then wash their hands at the table as a ritual of cleansing and new beginnings. Next, participants consume a bitter herb representing renewal, which is first dipped in salt water to acknowledge the tears that often accompany the journey of life. The matzoh, or unleavened bread, is then shared to symbolize our universal essence present in each moment. Although the meal incorporates many other rituals, the three that have always touched me most are the story of the exodus itself, the unprocessed matzoh, and the pause to embrace the bitterness.

The word Egypt in Hebrew translates as "narrow straits," and thus the exodus from Egypt is symbolic of the journey from a constricted state to a more expansive one. While we might feel enslaved by particular aspects of our lives, such as unhealthy relationships or destructive habits, this example prompts us to recognize that from constriction we are able to move into freedom. The key message here is that deep awakening is an ongoing process of moving toward a more expanded state rather than a journey toward a fixed point of ultimate liberation. When the Jews arrived in the Holy Land, they had to remain steadfast in their endeavor of continual expansion, even in spite of new challenges they faced. As we engage the various episodes of our lives, we can expect to ebb and flow between narrow states of being and more expansive ways of interacting with the world. In America, it is easy to claim that we are living in the "Land of the Free," and indeed we are blessed with many freedoms that citizens of other countries are denied. If we look deeper, though, we might notice the ways in which we create internal fortifications to block out certain people or aspects of life that cause us discomfort. Fear-based living resulting from media inundation, focus on the negative, imbalanced desires, and gross misalignment with nature are all common human patterns. When we retreat so deeply into the fabrications of our own beliefs, we end up spending the majority of our days in states of insecurity, unworthiness, fear, and powerlessness. As the Jews in the exodus story so clearly demonstrate, even when we recognize our inherent freedom, it is our responsibility to enact the journey of making it a reality in every instant of our lives. Ultimately, we empower our greatest sense of freedom when we recognize how we are being unconsciously enslaved and likewise how we are confining ourselves.

The concept that we are essentially unprocessed (as represented by the unleavened matzoh) holds great promise and possibility. As human beings, it can be easy to become captivated by the convenient, processed nature of the modern world, which can result in a feeling of enslavement at the subtlest level. In our minds, we tend to overly process life, ruminating on what we must consume next in order to create a temporary feeling of satisfaction. In the past, people lived closer to the earth and thus could clearly see and readily appreciate the interconnectedness of the planet and all of her living beings. Today, though, it is harder for us to link ourselves to the greater masterpiece of the natural environment. Although advances in technology are indeed remarkable and improve our quality of life, they are often taken to extremes. The matzoh reminds us that our nature is ultimately one of unprocessed beauty and simplicity; while we may sometimes get lost amidst the trappings of the world, this deeper essence is available to us at any time.

The bitter herb symbolizes the diversity of experience that characterizes the human path and reminds us that there is growth and learning even in our tears. Tasting its unusual flavor teaches us that experiencing diverse emotions is not a problem, and in fact is a common and normal part of human life. As we celebrate our own joy, we can still hold in our hearts those in the world who are struggling. We do this not as a means of deflating our own experience of happiness, but rather to hold space for others, trusting that the same kindness will be extended to us when we are in need of support. A second facet of bitter experiences is that they enable us to feel greater appreciation for the gifts of abundance we already possess.

In life, these three concepts intermingle with one another and manifest in different ways. When we reject the bitter facets of our experience, we can begin to feel immobilized and lose sight of our constantly fluctuating essential nature. Perceiving our lives as locked and vacant of possibility, we might lose sight of who we truly are. Through breath, movement, and mindfulness, we can reconnect to our divine nature, honor the tartness of life, and reaffirm our inherent freedom. As the Maharal of Prague wrote:

> We were always, in the depths of our hearts, completely free men and women. We were slaves on the outside, but free men and women in soul and spirit.

Inquiries

On the Mat: Focus on the simplicity of your practice, connecting to the unprocessed realms of breath and heart to access your deepest essence in each moment. Use a deep, stable ujjayi breath to evoke the organic nature that thrives in you as you. Be in the fullness of each movement as you affirm your ever-present freedom, and take time to honor the pungent moments that arise with the increasing intensity of your practice. Dance amidst inquiry of these three concepts of Passover as you recognize the remarkable alchemy of yoga for empowering, cleansing, and renewing your spirit. Explore knee-down lunge, hands inside foot in knee-down lunge, warriors one and two, reverse warrior, lateral angle, wide-angle standing forward fold, standing forward fold, chair, parsvotanasana, balancing half moon, pigeon, baby cradle, blissful baby, eye of the needle, seated forward fold, and cow face.

Off the Mat: Gather friends for a whole-foods meal, and serve a variety of dishes, incorporating flavors that are bland, bitter, and sweet. Encourage guests to exercise their personal freedom, choosing those dishes that appeal to them without feeling obliged to try everything.

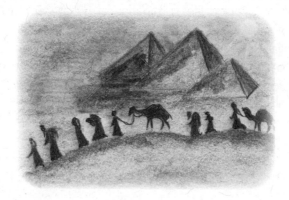

Practices

I notice the expansion available in each and every breath

Supportive Words
essence, innate nature, freedom, all embracing

Complementary Breath
ujjayi

Visualization
The Jews during their exodus from Egypt, walking through the desert with unleavened bread, determination, and hope.

Closing Ritual
journal contemplation

What is one area of your life you are choosing slavery? How might your essential nature support you in asserting your freedom?

I approach challenges as valuable

unprocessed parts of myself as they open and awaken

lessons on my path

I honor the

Mothering Powers: {*written by Anjali Budreski*}

During a visit home to Cape Cod, I was among the many women in my family who hosted a wedding shower for my new sister-in-law. Mothers, sisters, cousins, aunts, and women friends all squeezed into my Aunt Ann's home to celebrate Katie's rite of passage. It was wonderful to be with such a diverse group of female friends and relatives, who had combined their talents to prepare a party, cook wonderful food, and create a sacred space to honor my soon-to-be sister. During the festivities, I had an epiphany about my own mother. The different pieces of her life and diverse aspects of her personality suddenly became clearer to me; I thought about who she is and why she has chosen to live in a magical place, on a lake near the Atlantic Ocean. I also began to contemplate the qualities of my maternal and paternal grandmothers, where they had come from, and what they were like when I knew them as a child. Grandmother Agnes embodied zest for life, playfulness, humor, and a witty irreverence, while Grandmother Eva was an exceptional cook of Eastern European delicacies, strong and self-sufficient, fun-loving, and hard-working. My mother is unconditionally loving and nurturing, passionate about life, and deeply concerned about others' well-being. She is also incredibly open-minded, as demonstrated when she took me by the hand at a young age and opened my eyes to embracing a wide variety of spiritual perspectives.

Writer and shaman Frank Mac Eowen refers to these diverse qualities embodied by women as "Mothering Powers." Mothering powers can take many forms including the healer archetype of Mother Teresa, the protector energy of Julia "Butterfly" Hill (*who lived in and protected a tree named Luna for two full years*), the compassionate energy of teacher/nun Pema Chodron, the mystical poet qualities of St. Brigid, and the powerful warrior energies of Kali and Durga in Hindu mythology. Eowen reminds us that during the annual celebration of Mother's Day, we have an opportunity to acknowledge the greatness of Mother Earth in addition to that of our human mothers. Spring, particularly the time around Mother's Day, is a time when the earth literally gifts us with fields of flowers, fresh green leaves, and shoots of all kinds. Just as Mother Earth blossoms in diversity, so do our mothers take on the assorted qualities of protector, teacher, poet, and warrior. As we give flowers to our mothers, the earth gives flowers to us. How can we honor both? Every day we have an opportunity to connect to these mothering powers as they manifest on the stage of our planet. An old Scottish Highland saying states that within the heart of God is the heart of a mother, and yet our culture tends toward neglect of the feminine and over-emphasis of the masculine, which is profoundly evident in our abuse of the Earth and her resources. Slowly, women are becoming increasingly more caught up in the masculine world, and as a result are beginning to crave this reconnection to their mothering powers. It is vital, therefore, to nurture the relationship to the feminine in ourselves and recognize its importance in everyday interactions. When both men and women are able to connect to their feminine aspects and reclaim their empowered vulnerability, the result is deep healing for our communities and the planet as a whole. As Janet Ryan writes:

Goddess stands on the earth
She is the earth
And Bigger
She is sun and bigger
Universe and bigger
She is the essence that recieves
She surrenders and invites surrender
She yields
She holds and embraces
She accepts all things
She invites
She opens
To you
She offers herself
she is invisible
She is curve
She is round
She is sprial
She is dance
She is movement
She is rotation ·
She is center
She is silence
She is not there
She is waiting
She is listening
She accepts you
She is unconditional
She waits

A Woman[1]

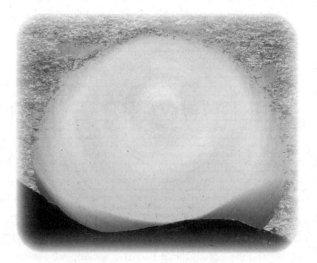

Inquiries

On the Mat: Invoke these beautiful mothering powers in their many forms. At the beginning of practice, hold your female ancestors close to your heart. Focus on the legs, thighs, and hips to embody the feminine or goddess energy in your postures and root deeply into your familial heritage. In more challenging poses, tap into the fierce protector energy of Julia "Butterfly" Hill, who stood firm to preserve a tree. While breathing in quiet poses like child, connect to your own mother as you soften and nurture yourself, physically embodying the archetype of the child. Throughout the practice, make space for restful moments to allow self-love and nurturing, and let the moments of effort cultivate gentle power, resolve, and courage. Think of the poses as offerings to your beloved mothers and grandmothers, and meditate on the image of Mother Nature in full bloom as she offers herself in the form of flowers, greens, and the first hints of springtime. At the end of practice, remain in fetal pose longer than usual, resting in the safe womb of your mother while sourcing the mothering energy in your own heart. Investigate standing forward fold, standing half moon, seated yoga mudra, baby cradle, seated wide-angle forward fold, bound angle, easy pose twist, marichyasana one, moon salute, and goddess.

Off the Mat: Write a letter to a cherished woman in your life, outlining the qualities about her you most appreciate and admire.

Practices

I breathe in the striking qualities of my own mother or grandmother. I connect to the power of the feminine that lives inside of me.

Supportive Words
mother, goddess, creator, advocate, caregiver

Visualization
A full, glowing grandmother moon reflecting the light of the sun with a soft glow and cycling in sync with the feminine.

Complementary Breath
kapalabhati

Closing Ritual
chant
Bhajamana Ma
praises to the great mother

I honor the gifts of Mother Earth

Remembrance: {inspired by Ann Greene}

Memorial Day is a time when we pause to intentionally honor and remember those who have passed. By recalling wonderful memories shared with loved ones, we can step back in time in the spirit of remembrance and also invite their presence into the present moment. Coincidently, Memorial Day is observed when spring flowers are beginning to bloom and the Earth is literally re-membering herself after the emptiness of winter. This natural cycle illuminates the value of pausing to inquire into the forgotten parts of ourselves. In infancy and childhood, we are ardent explorers of life, actively seeking to experience and understand as much as we possibly can. Although we do not necessarily verbalize this intention as children, it is readily apparent in the curiosity we embody on a daily basis. As we grow older and become more influenced by culture, we slowly lose sight of our inherent multidimensionality. Suddenly there is only one lens through which to see and interact with the world, and anything that contradicts this becomes a problem to be rooted out. Approached with this perspective, life echoes a serious tone, and the simplest treasures are lost in a whirlwind of "should" and "must". As we stray further from our inquisitive, explorative nature, our existence can develop qualities of constant bitterness and negativity. We become so enmeshed in this way of being that we are unable to see our own role in our unhappiness, and we easily blame our partners, kids, or external circumstances. The body is an intricate instrument that indeed mirrors the way we lead our lives. When we consistently make choices that take us out of alignment, the systems of the physical frame become less effective and begin to constrict, resulting in drying of synovial fluid *(which is essential in lubricating the joints)*, tightness in the muscles, *(which can lead to pain in the low back and legs)*, shallow breathing *(which impedes the optimal health of our cells)*, lowered immunity, and general discomfort.

The practice of yoga supports us in literally re-membering the diverse parts of the body *(and consequently the mental/emotional dimensions that correspond to them)* that have become disconnected from lack of attention. Moving in this skillful way aids the brain in reconnecting to the hundred billion nerve cells and neurons that gather and transmit electrochemical signals and thus support the body in everyday functioning. At one time, scientists believed that when certain brain cells were lost, they could never be replenished. Yet modern research has shown that the body always produces more cells, and that yoga can stimulate and support neural development. Daniel J. Siegel, MD writes, "The connections among the 100 billion neurons in the brain are continually carving out new pathways, which can support ongoing learning and can enrich our mental health well into our nineties[2]." Yoga serves us as a medium for becoming more mindful so that we can support the intelligence of the body in doing what it does best. By working to remember and enliven even just one part of our physical structure, we revitalize our entire internal circuitry. Through the process of mindful movement, especially that which crosses the midline, we can relieve aching in the physical body, sharpen the mind, and realign vital energy with the greater natural flow. Randy Miskesh, a martial arts teacher, writes, "The more you force your body to cross the midline plane, the more neural pathways your brain will create to handle the confusion of the movement. More pathways will translate to better defined movement, improved motor-skill development and increased cognitive capacity. Essentially, it is fitness training for your brain[3].

As the Pawnee/Osage/Omaha Native American Song teaches:

Remember, remember the circle of the sky
the stars and the brown eagle
the supernatural winds
breathing night and day
from the four directions.

Remember, remember the great life of the sun
breathing on the earth
it lies upon the earth
to bring out life upon the earth
life covering the earth.

Remember, remember
the sacredness of things,
running streams and dwellings
the young within the nest
a hearth for sacred fire
the holy flame of fire[3].

Inquiries

On the Mat: Recall and revisit aspects of your personality or a part of your body that once nourished you but has long been forgotten. Hold reconnection with this facet of yourself as your intention for this sadhana. Practice a wide variety of poses to nurture the relationship between mind and body, focusing on crossing the midline with poses like eagle, twists, and crisscross warm-ups. Incorporate several minutes of toe yoga (*toega*) into your warm-up sequence, as working to isolate movements of the toes helps reawaken long-lost connections to the extremities. Spend time contemplating parts of the body you don't think about on a daily basis. Investigate standing crane, tree, standing half moon, standing marichyasana, hand to big toe, eagle, balancing half moon, revolved balancing half moon, standing forward fold, seated forward bend, head to knee, ardha matsyendrasana, and revolved heron.

Off the Mat: Create a collage illustrating forgotten aspects of yourself. When it is complete, choose one thing you would like to invite back into your life.

Practices

Supportive Words
be aware of, elicit, recognize, recall, recollect, summon

Visualization
Earth remembering herself as spring fills in the empty spaces of winter with vibrant colors, thick new growth, and the warmth and light of the sun.

Complementary Breath
bramari

Closing Ritual
Find a picture of yourself when you were young. Spend a few moments taking in the energy and spirit of yourself as a young child, remembering your sweet essence.

Additional Spring Inquiries:

Purim (Jewish), Norouz (Persian/Zoroastrian New Year), Naw Ruz (Baha'l New Year), Holi (Hindu), Hola Mohalla (Sikh), Easter (Christian), New Year (Hindu), Ramayana (Hindu), Hanuman Jayanti (Hindu), Passover (Jewish), Beltane (Wicca), Yom HaSho'ah (Jewish), Yom Ha'Atzmaut (Jewish), Buddha Day (Buddhist), Ching Ming (Chinese), Sacred Heart of Jesus (Christian), Shavuot (Jewish), Guru Arjan Dev (Sikh).

Treasures of Summer:

Summer officially begins on the 21st of June and is the time of year when we experience extended daylight hours. The bright, lasting light provides added time for play, vitamin D for the body, and a wealth of flowers, fruits, and vegetables. This season of warmth is a time of growth and maturation, which can be witnessed in our gardens as well as throughout the natural environment. Flowers are in full bloom, vegetables and fruit are ripening on the vine, and grasses are in abundance.

According to Chinese medicine, summer is a season of fire, which correlates to both the heart and the small intestine. The fire of the heart is essential for healthy bodily function, as the heart is responsible for blood circulation and delivery of vital nutrients to every cell, organ, and system of the body. The fire of the small intestine is also vitally important, as it digests the food we eat, enabling absorption of essential vitamins and minerals to be used by the body. It literally extracts the beneficial elements from everything we ingest, fueling the body and providing immune support.

Beyond the physical plane, the heart's constant beat serves as a reminder of the gift of life and can thus attune us to the precious nature of our unique path. This spiritual center is also related to compassion, understanding, clear vision, and wholehearted service. Summer invites us to experience clarity, invoke our personal power, and seek out people and situations that support our highest calling. Indeed, the warmest months of the year provide us with added time to both formulate our own visions for the future and support others around us. Finally, the fiery qualities of summer are representative of outward, active masculine energies as well as creativity, passion, and motion. Consequently, this season can be a dynamic time for cultivating the seeds and intentions that were planted in spring.

Summer Solstice: {*written by Anjali Budreski*}

Although the days actually begin to shorten soon after the summer solstice in the northern Hemisphere, this time typically feels like the beginning of summer and is marked by the sun's long pause on the horizon. The word solstice has its roots in Latin and is comprised of the words "sol," which translates as sun, and "stitium", meaning to stop or pause. The summer and winter solstices each signify the beginning of one dramatic slice in the wheel of the year and the ending of another. An interesting paradox with regard to these two seasonal markers is that the winter solstice actually signals the return of the light *(yet the real cold has not even yet begun in most places)*, and the summer solstice marks its retreat *(while the hottest days are still to come)*. This is reflective of the idea that both birth and death are embedded in each of these auspicious times of year. At the height of summer, the journey back to winter's cold begins, serving as a powerful reminder of how precious this spell of green really is. In the garden, the solstice brings about great growth and fullness by virtue of the sun's vibrant rays. Even after the sun sets, the energy of the light lingers as our houses stay warm well into the evening. During this time of brightness, we are reminded of change, and the Earth literally hums with life; migrating birds return with their songs, tadpoles are born, crickets drone late into the evening, and wild scents and smells of all kinds blanket Mother Earth. It is not a quiet, inward time, but rather one of surging, social energy, with plants literally growing overnight and family and friends gathering to enjoy nature and celebrate during extended daylight hours. We gather for picnics, bonfires, potlucks, games, and camp-outs, mindful not to burn ourselves out but taking full advantage of each precious moment of the warm season.

At the summer solstice, we are reminded of the beauty of things in their wholeness. As we shed the heavy layers of winter and spring, our bodies open, ideas come into full blossom, and exuberance rules our minds and hearts. In tandem with nature's great pause, we are called upon to stop, take a deep breath, smell the flowers, and linger for a moment on this delicate, fleeting edge. We allow winter to fall away, welcoming the emergence of the new season in the same breath. The moment of pause is also one of rejuvenation; taking a deep breath, we literally come back to life as we awaken from our dormancy and free ourselves of old skins and burdens. During the pause of this solstice day, contemplate emerging qualities, relationships, or things in your life. What is fresh, vibrant, and colorful? What has finally come to fruition after many months of dreaming and planning? What is ready to be picked and harvested, and what still needs time to mature? Take time on the solstice to pause and give thanks. Slow down and savor as you reach out, connect, and allow yourself to be touched by the magic of the earth. Let the light of the warm sun penetrate your skin and the winds toss your hair as the summer pauses, matures, and then moves on. Mary Oliver beautifully describes in *The Summer Day* the fleeting nature of that which is before us as it moves on too soon, she asks the profound quesiton, "tell me, what is it you plan to do with your one wild and precious life?[5]"

Inquiries

On the Mat: In our practice, the pose at the height of each sadhana represents the solstice of yoga. With our energy at its peak, we can let our light shine in all of its brilliance as we revel in the available energy, beauty, and abundance of the moment. Take your time as you build towards the pinnacle of your practice. Enjoy the quick bursts of energy that surface as you build the experience, and invite moments of play, celebration, and pause at the height of each posture. Acknowledge the distinctive heat and energy of each asana, the light pouring through your being, and the body's natural cleansing of residual toxins. Savor the abundance of light as inspiration as you use the breath to fuel the fire of your internal landscape. Immerse yourself in vital energy through sun salutes, core strengtheners, plank, warrior one, two, and three, twisting warrior one, chair, twisting chair, side plank, twisting three-legged down dog, balancing half moon, revolved balancing half moon, scorpion dog, lateral angle, hands clasped in lateral angle, and revolved lateral angle.

Off the Mat: Take time to savor the sunset, or make a bonfire with friends and bathe in the firelight. Research the various solstice rituals of different cultures such as drumming, chanting, and dance, and bring these into your celebration.

Practices

I let the radiance of the summer sun pour into my heart.

In the pause between seasons.

the earth's abundance

Supportive Words
apex, crest, crown, peak, pinnacle

Visualization
The bright light of the sun bathing the earth, sending forth rays of warmth and light on the longest day of the year.

Complementary Breath
sitali
Cooling in the midst of peak intensity and heat.

Closing Ritual
chant
aum suryaya namaha

I dance, celebrate, and revel in the marvel of

embrace the promise of summer.

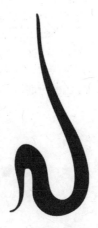

Lammas: {*inspired by Anjali Budreski*}

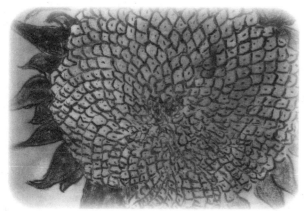

The Celtic festival of the harvest is named Lammas or Lughnasad, which literally means "loaf-mass" and celebrates this season when the fruits of what we have sown are ready to be gathered. This celebration takes its name from the time when grains form as a mass, ready to be harvested to make bread. Traditionally, this was a time for abundant fresh food and local festivities, which still exist in New England as harvest celebrations and fairs in many rural communities. Lammas day usually falls around the first or second of August. It marks the halfway point between the summer solstice and the fall equinox, when the days begin to grow noticeably shorter and the colors of the garden deepen into rich hues of orange, brown, and gold. At this time of year, the first fruits of our labors literally flourish on the vine as we become intoxicated with the sheer abundance offered up by garden and earth. Reflective of this activity in nature, Lammas is an ideal time to contemplate what is ripening in our life and what is already heavy with fruition, just waiting to be picked. As we contemplate the ripeness manifesting along our path, we can pause to remember that one tiny seed planted in the spring creates an entity containing hundreds more, each laden with immense promise. In my personal yoga practice, I had been working for a long while with the transition from upward-facing bow directly into camel by first lowering onto my knees. In spite of regular practice, I never felt fluid or fully confident as I awkwardly rolled only halfway up. In a workshop, though, I approached the posture again with a few technical refinements I had learned and sensed that it was at last ripe for the picking. This time, I rolled up with graceful ease, experiencing a precious moment in the spirit of Lammas; a huge smile emerged, and I paused to receive the offering of the pose.

In life, we have an opportunity to delight in real sweetness when we recognize and taste the fruit of our labor for the first time. Even when we consume familiar fruits and veggies, we can experience moments of awe as we revel in the distinctive qualities of food fresh from the harvest. In this same way, familiar experiences with different people or in new environments can be ripe with excitement and infused with new flavors. The Lammas festivities teach us to recognize when food is ripe for the picking, a skill that is also useful in life. As we develop dexterity in harvesting opportune moments, we can relish and bear witness to all of the love, effort, patience, and work that goes into manifesting a single intention. What has ripened in your life? What is ready to be harvested and shared? Every step of the way is imbued with magic, and all that is required of us is our attention, loyalty, and creativity. As we cultivate the garden of our life, we become highly skilled at recognizing the ripe moments worthy of celebration. As Lisa Masé shares:

Under yellow curling leaves
a garnet secret concealed.
Barely connected to thorny shrubbery,

sweet promise seduces me deeper
into the thicket until the next branch
dangles just out of reach
and I must retreat, almost satisfied.
Summer's day completes under dark skies
with one small miracle:
new stars[6].

Inquiries

On the Mat: In our practice, Lammas is the yoga of harvest and deepening. It is not only a posture in its fullness (*solstice*), but also the pause immediately following this expression, when the pose responds with its own ripening. When we fully embody the pose, holding it long enough to feel its weight and depth, we can then share resulting energetic harvest with others. Choose to cultivate certain poses in your practice, and recognize when an asana is ripe for the picking. Each time you successfully attempt a more difficult pose, enjoy the value of pausing and reveling in this experience of first harvest. Although repeating the asana a second time can still facilitate sweetness, it is indeed the first taste that tends to linger. Also explore Lammas just before savasana when

you feel a tangible sense of the work you have done, and bask in the juicy sweetness and fruition of cool-down poses. Relish these moments when your hard labor is done and you can delight in storing, preserving, and savoring the fruits of your sadhana. Experiment with standing yoga mudra, standing forward fold, standing wide-angle forward fold, pigeon, cow face, fire log, heron, seated forward fold, lateral angle, warrior two, hands inside foot in knee-down lunge, humble warrior, and hands clasped in lateral angle.

Off the Mat: Gather a group of friends to share a Lammas meal. Encourage them to bring local, organic food, and enjoy the ripe flavors and textures of the feast.

Practices

I recognize which aspects of my life need more time to develop

Supportive Words
appreciation, ripeness, savouring, sweetness

Visualization
Heavy fruit on the vine; a sunflower abundant with seeds; large squash blossoms, vibrant and full.

Complementary Breath
ujjayi
Focus on the ability of the breath to ripen and mature throughout the class.

Closing Ritual
Take time to fully savor the varieties of ripe fruit available locally at different times of year. Allow this to be an ongoing celebration of rich, delectable flavors.

Teacher's Note
Bring in a basketful of harvest goodies to share. Have students choose one item that resonates with the spirit of the harvest for them. Invite them to savor it personally or offer it to a friend.

fuel my inspiration and heart

I awaken to what is ripe

I honor the brief, sweet moments that

and ready to be harvested in my life

Additional Summer Inquiries:

Ulambana, Obon (Buddhist), Asalha Puja (Buddhist), Lammas (Christian), Lughnassad (Wicca), Raksha Bandhan (Hindu), Lailat Bara'ah (Islam), Krishna Janmashtami (Hindu), Ramadan (Islam), Ganesha Chaturthi (Hindu), Holy Cross Day (Christian), Moon Cake Festival (Chinese Taoist), Niman Kachina, sun & fire festivals (Hopi), Summer Solstice, Litha (Wicca), First Nations Day (Canadian Native People), Sacred Heart of Jesus (Catholic Christian), Feast Day of Saints Peter & Paul (Christian).

Treasures of Autumn:

In autumn, nature bears fruits to be enjoyed in the moment and also preserved for the colder months ahead. A seed was planted, then nourished in its growth, and now the intention has manifested itself at last. It is up to us to receive this gift and allow it to bolster our inner light as the dark season approaches. Autumn begins at the autumnal equinox, around September 22nd, and is a time to begin preparing for the coming season of rest and introspection. During this time, days grow noticeably shorter, and leaves change color as we progress towards the winter solstice in December. This time of year beckons us to establish balance between outward and inward activities as we bridge the natural extroversion of summer with the innate introversion of winter. Fall is a time of vibrant and profound change; as the leaves come into their full expression of color, we can literally bear witness to nature's dramatic transition. As such, it is also a potent season for tying up loose ends and completing projects that could become burdensome in the weightier months ahead.

Autumn is another opportune season for cleansing, this time to prepare body and mind for the colder months to come. In Chinese Five Element Theory, this season is linked to the lungs and large intestines. Through the mechanisms of the lungs, we take in something new with each inhale and eliminate what is not serving us as we exhale. We literally inspire and expire, alluding to the idea that each ending corresponds to a new beginning. The large intestine completes the last steps of digestion; this is where undigested waste is processed, stored, and then eliminated. The fall is a good time to set new practices in motion to support healthy functioning of the large intestine, like eating high fiber foods, taking probiotics, and doing agni sara dhauti *(belly pumping)*, all of which prime the large intestines for the heavier foods of winter. When fall arrives at our doorstep, it serves as a reminder to soften and let go, bask in the brilliant colors of life, and begin our preparations for what lies ahead.

Honoring our Ancestors: {inspired by the Wisdom of Ancesotrs}

When the sun begins to sink lower on the horizon and the leaves turn from bright reds to golds to eventual deep browns, it is time to celebrate Samhain (sow-in). Samhain is a Celtic festival of the New Year honoring the end of the harvest, remembering our ancestors, and acknowledging the advent of cold weather. This celebration is also known as Hallowmas, All Soul's Day, Day of the Dead, or, more recently, Halloween. On the medicine wheel of the year in the Native American tradition, this time is associated with the Bear Clan, as it is around this time that bears move into their dens to semi-hibernate until spring, when they emerge with their cubs. The tradition of giving sweet treats to children on this occasion serves a reminder of the continuing cycle of life and of the possibility that always exists, even amidst death and decay. In our culture, children love to dress up in costumes, which were traditionally seen as a means of aligning with the "spooky" spirits of the dead by becoming more like them. At this time of year, the gossamer veils between the worlds of seen and unseen become increasingly thin, and contact between the living and those who have passed becomes more palpable. As a result, ancestors and loved ones who have passed over can easily offer us guidance, strength, and aid. For this reason, Samhain can be a time of sourcing the stabilizing, supportive power of our own family roots, acknowledging all that our ancestors did for us and honoring the many gifts they passed down.

Heirloom traits are truly remarkable; they have thrived for generations, and even if we are not fully aware of our past, our lineage still lives in us through these characteristics. This personal history is carried in our cellular memory, and as such it serves as a thread connecting our individual identity with both those who preceded us and those who will arrive after our departure. When we take the time to honor and connect to our ancestors, we can access a deep sense of comfort and support. Through endeavoring to learn about those who came before us, we can enhance our understanding of who we truly are and how we came to be. What gifts from your ancestors do you continue to carry forward? One of the ways to pay homage to our family lineage is to create a memory altar and burn a candle there overnight to honor the light that has been passed down to us through our ancestral line.

As we practice yoga in our chosen tradition, we also link ourselves to a lineage of teachers who have come before us. Drawing upon their wisdom, we craft our own rituals for the practice, adopting certain principles and ideas while leaving others behind. Asana is an ever-expanding inquiry, and we learn to artfully meld inherited knowledge with new investigations and methods as our practice matures. The number of yoga postures and variations are endless, even more so as we create new forms through experimentation. Yet, each and every one of us has a group of "ancestral" poses—those that comprised our foundation when we first started the practice. In my own early experiences of yoga sadhana, I fell in love with a pose called seated yoga mudra. This posture embodies a sense of softness through the bowing of the head towards the earth, but at the same time it requires the body to stay active as the arms flow overhead. Yoga mudra allowed me to explore putting weight on my head, something that was completely foreign to my life before yoga. As the years progressed and my practice advanced, I forgot about seated yoga mudra and stopped incorporating it into my practice. One day many years later, I remembered the pose while playing around on the mat, and I flowed into it almost without thinking. Immediately, I felt the sense of comfort and familiarity associated with meeting an old friend or reigniting a forgotten conversation. Doing the pose was like offering my respects to a sacred ancestor who had shared her knowledge and helped me build confidence. By practicing our ancestral poses and honoring our lineage of teachers, we affirm our trust in their wisdom, offer gratitude for their grace, and sustain centuries-old connections. As Chinook writes in *Teach Us, and Show Us the Way*:

We call upon the earth, our planet home,
with its beautiful depths and soaring heights,
its vitality and abundance of life,
and together we ask that it

Teach us, and show us the Way.

We call upon the mountains, the Cascades and the Olympics,
the high green valleys and meadows filled with wild flowers,
the snows that never melt, the summits of intense silence,
and we ask that they

Teach us, and show us the Way.

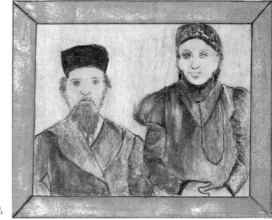

We call upon the waters that rim the earth, horizon to horizon,
that flow in our rivers and streams, that fall upon our gardens and fields,
and we ask that they

Teach us, and show us the Way.

We call upon the land which grows our food, the nurturing soil,
the fertile fields, the abundant gardens and orchards,
and we ask that they

Teach us, and show us the Way.

We call upon the forests, the great trees reaching strongly to the sky
with earth in their roots and the heavens in their branches,
the fir and the pine and the cedar,
and we ask them to

Teach us, and show us the Way.

We call upon the creatures of the fields and forests and the seas,
our brothers and sisters the wolves and deer, the eagle and dove,
the great whales and the dolphin,
the beautiful Orca and salmon who share our Northwest home,
and we ask them

Teach us, and show us the Way.

We call upon all those who have lived on this earth, our ancestors and our friends,
who dreamed the best for future generations, and upon whose lives our lives are built,
and with thanksgiving, we call upon them to

Teach us, and show us the Way.

And lastly, we call upon all that we hold most sacred,
the presence and power of the Great Spirit of love and truth which flows through all the Universe,
to be with us to

Teach us, and show us the Way.

Inquiries

On the Mat: Think about your ancestors both on and off the mat, and hold the image of one of these sacred elders in your heart. Revisit basic poses that would be considered ancestors in your particular tradition. Feel the effect of reconnecting to this heritage, and attune to the gifts these postures still have in store. Discover mountain, standing half moon, standing yoga mudra, warriors one and two, chair, sphinx, cobra, child, high lunge, knee-down lunge, runner's stretch, bridge, bound angle, easy pose twist, seated yoga mudra, and reclining twist.

Off the Mat: Get to know your ancestors by researching information about your grandparents' and great-grandparents' lives. Create a summary card for each of these loved ones, and contemplate what gifts they have passed down to you or write them a heartfelt letter. Share your findings with someone else in your family or a close friend as you savor the feeling of interconnectedness.

Practices

Supportive Words
ascendant, forefather, foremother, predecessor

Visualization
A beloved ancestor still present in spirit, guiding us when we ask for support.

Complementary Breath
dirgha
Focus on the foundational aspects of the three-part breath.

Closing Ritual
candle lighting:
After centering and setting the context, invite students to light a candle and place it on the altar in memory of a beloved ancestor, stating the person's name aloud and sharing one gift they left behind. At the end of practice, invite students to return to the altar to blow out their candles.

I feel the deep roots of my lineage stabilizing and nurturing my path

pass on to future generations

I will cultivate the treasures I acknowledge and remember loved ones who have passed

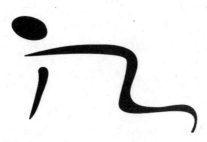

Thanksgiving: {*written by Anjali Budreski*}

Thanksgiving as a modern-day celebration has profound and potent meaning. Many families use this day together to connect with one another and share delicious food. In my family, we honor the day's focus on gratitude by taking a few moments for each person to share aloud something for which they are grateful. Despite the joy and humor of family and amazing home-cooked food, it is clear that what we call Thanksgiving today was not necessarily a thankful time for the Native peoples who inhabited this continent long before the settlers arrived. In elementary school, we were taught that the Natives and Pilgrims sat down to an abundant and harmonious feast, complete with turkey, squash, corn, and smiles all around. Although there was actually a feast shared by the Wampanoag native people (*who live in the Massachusetts Bay Area of Plymouth*) and the Colonists, the peace and camaraderie was very short-lived as the natives' land was invaded and tensions began to rise. The colonists brought scurvy and other debilitating diseases to the native people of Plymouth Colony, which spread like wildfire among the population. Since those early days of colonization, the indigenous culture has been all but wiped out, and the notions of abundance, giving thanks for our food, and connection to the greater circle of life have all but vanished as well. The original people of North America depended on the land for their survival, and they learned experientially through direct contact with nature. Consequently, they recognized that their lives were inextricably linked to the well-being of Mother Earth and the whole web of creation. There was and still remains among some native peoples a sense of attunement with everything and everyone on the planet, as evidenced by the skillfulness of memorizing and understanding all of the subtle details of the landscape such as rocks, roots, tracks, and natural signs. As a result of this bond with the land, the Native people of North America had deep appreciation for even the smallest elements of the natural world that enabled their survival.

In our fast-paced, divorced-from-nature, technologically-driven culture, we have largely abandoned this attunement. Many people don't even know or acknowledge where their food comes from. During my time working on a farm in southern Vermont, I was privileged to both educate others and learn about my own survival as a human being. I learned to drive a tractor, run a good-sized maple sugaring operation, plant and grow gardens, and harvest, preserve, and store foods for winter. I helped little white and black lambs make their way into the world, rescued a chicken with frostbite, and assisted in gutting and processing chickens for the freezer and our bellies. One of my most memorable days on the farm was the day we slaughtered about fifteen turkeys for all of us to take home for Thanksgiving. I wanted one of those turkeys I had raised, but I was less attracted to the idea of actually being the one to kill, gut, process, and cook her. I knew in my heart, though, that if I didn't have the courage to take part in ending her life, I did not want to eat her; I wanted to participate in the full cycle. I sat with my turkey on my lap as I awaited my turn, talking to her, thanking her, and holding her beautiful, warm body close to mine. Soon after, I ended her life with my own hands. Even now, I remember the intense blue of the sky as I walked home along the lower field and the profound gratitude I felt for the understanding that everything has a time and a purpose and that every beating heart is precious. On this particular Thanksgiving, I became part of the cycle of life, which included joy, beauty, pain, and loss all gathered into one crisp autumn afternoon on a farm in Vermont.

To be truly thankful is to acknowledge our connection to the greater web of life; it is to feel the sun warming our face after working in the bitter cold all day, to appreciate the animals that provide us with nourishment, to value fresh food, and to nurture the land, plants, and animals with great care and love. Inspired by Chief Seattle, Ted Perry writes: "All things are connected. This we know. The earth does not belong to man; man belongs to the earth. This we know. All things are connected like the blood which unites one family. All things are connected. Whatever befalls the earth befalls the sons of the earth. Man did not weave the web of life, he is merely a strand in it. Whatever he does to the web, he does to himself." These potent words remind us that being thankful means taking the time to stop and appreciate what we have. When we are connected and tuned into the abundance of our lives, thankfulness and gratitude naturally begin to arise in our hearts. In the beginning, this takes practice, but as we slow down and savor the gift of a juicy carrot, a hug from a friend, or a cool breeze on a hot day more of our life begins to be framed in the context of thankfulness. As Haven Trevino articulates:

Daily without toil
Mother Earth offers her bountiful
*   harvest.*
Life springs from every nook and
*   cranny,*
Feeds and animates all
Regardless of religion or reputation..

All we have
All we are
From All That Is
A gift[7].

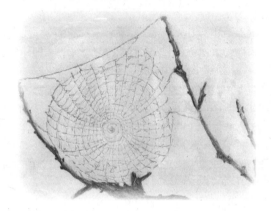

Inquiries

On the Mat: Use this time as a chance to attune your body and breath to its indigenous nature, and notice whether this engenders a sense of greater connection to yourself and to all of life. Cultivate thankfulness for your body, breath, mobility, community, and practice time, and notice whether this reawakens a sense of beauty in the everyday. Use silent mantra in every pose as a means of acknowledging what you are thankful for in life both on and off the mat. Alternate one posture focused on thankfulness for an aspect of your body with one focused on gratitude for something or someone in your life. Explore standing forward bend, standing splits, warrior one, two, and three, triangle, hand to big toe, humble warrior, knee-down lunge, runner's stretch, bound angle, head to knee, heron, baby cradle, reclining hero, seated forward fold, and trianga mukhaikapada pascimottanasana.

Off the Mat: For the three days before and after Thanksgiving, write down ten things for which you feel grateful upon waking in the morning and again right before sleep. Notice whether this inquiry shifts your experience of the holiday.

I live each day with a grateful heart and attract more of what I desire

connection to the web of life

Supportive Words
appreciation, gratefulness, gratitude

Visualization
A spider's web; if one strand shifts, the whole web is affected.

Complementary Breath
natural
Focus on the gift of soft, simple breath.

Closing Ritual
Stream-of-consciousness gratitude list.

Teacher's Note
Give students one minute to put pencil to paper and list what they are thankful for in a stream-of-consciousness writing exercise. Encourage them to simply write thoughts as they appear without trying to steer them or influence the outcome. After one minute, invite them read over their words and choose five things from their list to share. Form pairs or small groups, and allow a few minutes for exchange.

I acknowledge my   I open to the power of thankfulness with every cycle of breath

Additional Autumn Inquiries:

Autumnal Equinox, Mabon (Wicca), Rosh Hashanah (Jewish), Navaratri (Hindu), Dassera (Hindu), Sukkot (Jewish), All Hallows Eve (Christian), All Saints' Day (Christian), Samhain (Wicca/Neo Pagan), All Souls' Day (Christian), Diwali (Hindu, Sikh, Jain), Birthday of Guru Nanak Dev Sahib (Sikh), Day of Covenant (Baha'i).

Treasures of Winter:

During the colder season, our part of the world becomes dormant; many animals hibernate to conserve energy, and trees and plants rest and recharge for their inevitable return in the spring. Winter is a time for spending quality time with family and friends and also for becoming more sensitive to the inner landscape of our own thoughts, feelings, and emotions. The first day of winter falls on December 21st, and from this day forward, days gradually become lighter as the approach to the warmer season begins. In Chinese medicine, winter is related to the two organs associated with the element of water, the kidneys and the bladder. The kidneys are responsible for filtering the blood and aid in removing toxins from the body through urine. On an energetic level, they store life force and thus provide us with a constant yet invisible connection to the universal presence that surrounds us. The bladder's physical task is to store our urine while it awaits excretion, while it is considered the seat of sentiments on the emotional level. Through nurturing these organs during the colder months, we can facilitate internal cleansing as well as emotional clarity. By utilizing this season to huddle into the introspective realm of the heart, we enhance our ability to access the depths of our being at other times during the year.

Cherishing the Darkness: {*inspired by John Friend*}

For humans, vision is the primary guiding sense for interacting with the world at large. For this reason, we tend to feel an underlying sense of trepidation when darkness sets in, and yet the darkness can remind us of our more subtle capacities for perception and interaction. During the winter, the energies of introspection and inner growth become especially buoyant, corresponding to the absence of prolonged daylight. Even so, we find many ways to distract ourselves from this ripe opportunity for expansion. As we examine the functioning of the natural world, we can see that the darkness holds many treasures awaiting birth and discovery. The moon begins its cycle as a dark, muted shadow whose reflective glow returns in slivers as the nights progress. When seeds fall back to the earth in autumn, they are enveloped by the darkness of the soil for the cold months that follow. This time serves as an incubation period, allowing them to assimilate nutrients, accumulate energy, and eventually sprout. Only after they have nestled into the darkness of earth are they ready to blossom and contribute their offerings to the grander play of life. The same is evidenced by the life cycle of humans; we spend nine months in the complete darkness of our mother's womb where we absorb nourishment, develop in safety, and prepare to embark on the journey of embodied life. And every night for the remainder of our lives, we retreat into darkness for sleep, as this environment allows the body to relax, rebuild, and replenish. Although darkness is a vital facet of existence in these and many other ways, it is typically portrayed as daunting, scary, or even evil. If we adopt this antagonistic relationship to darkness, though, we might find ourselves increasingly disconnected from the natural rhythms of the world and living our lives with little time for pause as a result. Nature purposefully offers darkness as a respite for healing and rejuvenation; it is our challenge to embrace this restorative pause in all its forms, as it can greatly enhance numerous aspects of our lives. As Wendell Berry writes:

> To go in the dark with a light is to know the light.
> To know the dark, go dark. Go without sight,
> and find that the dark, too, blooms and sings,
> and is traveled by dark feet and dark wings[7.5].

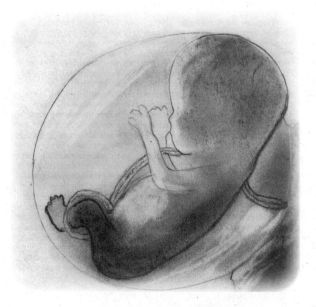

Inquiries

On the Mat: In yoga, there is often a tendency towards vigorous movement that generates sweat, heat, and inner light, yet the real treasures of our practice are often only accessed when we pause to retreat within. When we approach our practice from this alternate perspective, we can experience profound shifts as we access forms of nourishment that simply aren't available through a more active practice. Flow through a more slowly-paced sadhana, and allow ample time for moving towards your darker inner realms. Utilize forward folds, hip-openers, and soothing twists to infuse a sense of comfort into even the darkest areas. Focus on cultivating reverence for the darkness within as an internal temple inviting pause and retreat. Flow through the majority of the practice with your eyes fully closed, or utilize a soft gaze to mimic the effects of low light. Begin your practice in child's pose or fetal position to simulate time spent in the space of the womb. End your sadhana with a long, restful savasana, incorporating a restorative pose. Investigate standing forward fold, gate, humble warrior, standing yoga mudra, runner's stretch, bound angle, head to knee, baby cradle, seated wide-angle forward fold, pigeon, supine hand to big toe, one-legged cow face, seated forward fold, and seated forward fold with one leg in half lotus.

Off the Mat: Take time to be in darkness, either inside your home or out in nature. Pause to appreciate the softness, the quietude, and the subtlety of contrasts.

Practices

Like an embryo in the womb, I pause and receive the gifts of my surroundings.

Supportive Words
blackness, dimness, dusk, shadow, twilight

Visualization
A mother's womb, completely dark yet nurturing, safe, and life-giving.

Complementary Breath
analum valom
Focus on the introspection of the breath.

Closing Ritual
Pause in fetal position for five slow cycles of breath, fully sensing the darkness and rejuvenation of the womb.

nourish and replenish

I honor the healing that comes with rest, rejuvenation, and integration.

I affirm the darkness inside and its ability to

Shivaratri: {inspired by Kajal Dhabalia}

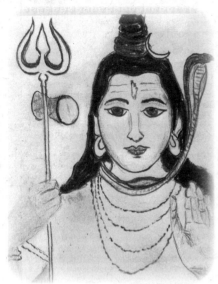

Shivaratri, or the "Night of Shiva," occurs every year in mid-February on the eve of the new moon. Legend has it that when the gods and demons churned the ocean of consciousness, a lethal poison capable of wiping out all of creation emerged from the water. Vishnu suggested that Shiva be summoned to consume the poison and thereby protect all beings from its toxicity. Shiva agreed and drank the deadly blue liquid, holding it in his throat by fastening a snake around his neck. As a result of the poison, his throat turned blue, but Shiva was not harmed. The divine doctors advised the gods to keep Shiva awake for a full night to allow the poisons to be cleansed from his body. The gods and goddesses responded with energetic dances, uplifting music, and ecstatic chanting until sunrise so that Shiva would not fall asleep. As day broke, the poison was neutralized; Shiva was safe, and the festivities came to an end. Each year in commemoration of this event, people all over India gather to celebrate, engaging in chanting and other revelry throughout the night to honor Shiva's heroic act. One of the rituals of the night involves gathering around the Shiva lingam (the phallus which serves as a representation of Shiva) and chanting, "Aum Namah Shivaya." The lingam, through its natural symbolism as well as its association with Shiva, represents the vast potential and possibility that lies within each and every one of us. Other pujas (rituals) performed throughout this evening of celebrations include: decorating the lingam with flowers and garlands, walking around the lingam three or seven times, and bathing it with water, milk, and honey before applying a sandalwood paste. People offer wood apple or bel (Aegle marmelos) leaves for cleansing, food for longevity, incense to symbolize wealth, flame to represent deep-seated knowledge, and betel leaves in gratitude for worldly pleasures[8].

Sadly, many of our modern-day rituals have become devoid of meaning and heart connection. As opposed to using rituals to mark time, we take part in activities that "kill time" and pacify surface boredom that is never fully alleviated. In the past, our ancestors spent more time interacting with community, partook in activities that activated all levels of their being, and stimulated their minds through a kinesthetic whole-body approach. In the past, ritual involved gathering in community, eating, dancing, playing music and constructing altars or other sacred venues. Shivaratri is a celebration that encourages us to stay up all night in order to awaken to the fullness, freedom, and gift of embodied life. By staying awake all night, we depart from routine and open to the possibility that one sleepless night approached with intent can actually energize us, honoring the importance of skillful participation in connecting to deeper aspects of ourselves. Furthermore, this night invites us to reclaim the kinds of rituals and celebrations that help us connect to our greater community, empower us see the light and beauty of nature, and simply make us feel alive. During the winter months, we can easily be lulled into the sleepiness, isolation, and lethargy of a slower season. Yet even on nights devoid moonlight when we find ourselves in complete darkness, there is potential for opening and awakening. As Danna Faulds writes, "Why wait for your awakening? The moment your eyes are open, seize the day[9]." As we engage this night of festivities in honor of sustained alertness, we can consider what parts of our life have fallen asleep. What offerings of life are we allowing to simply pass us by without seizing their potential? As demonstrated by the story of Shiva, the process of true awakening involves making unprecedented decisions and choosing to celebrate our lives while honoring those who help us stay alert.

Yoga is a ritual celebration in and of itself, as we utilize the practice to cultivate space for both physical and spiritual awakening, tapping into our own inherent potential for heeding the difficult calls of life. When body, mind, and emotions are nourished in the finite space of the mat, we are able to approach life off the mat with more kindness, creativity, and possibility. Ultimately, it is through our dedication to personal awakening that we develop appreciation for all of life, resulting in an eagerness to extend more of our energy outward. The inquiry of yoga is an ever-evolving, ongoing voyage into the essential self; the more we practice, the further we can extend to meet our own needs, as well as those of friends, loved ones, and peers who likewise support us, as an act of celebrating the wonder of life.

Inquiries

On the Mat: Keep your eyes open throughout the practice, and use energetic pranayama and vibrant music to foster an atmosphere conducive to waking. Experiment with chanting repeatedly to Shiva as you flow through your practice, and meditate on the idea of yoga as a sacred ritual and celebration that invites all parts of your being to thrive. Cultivate sacred space by lighting a candle, chanting, burning incense, offering water, rice, or sandalwood paste to an altar, or bringing in an element of nature that inspires you. Discover cow face arms, high lunge, knee-down lunge, warrior three, balancing half moon, standing splits, eagle, cobra, locust, bow, half frog, quad stretch in pigeon, mermaid, camel, and dancer.

Off the Mat: Gather a group of people and create your own ritual for celebrating awakening. Some ideas include: staying up late chanting mantras to Shiva, doing puja, dancing, or taking a hike in the brisk night air.

Practices

I open to the possibility of each day as a rich celebration   With dedication

Supportive Words
celebration, ceremony, ritual, rouse, stir, awaken

Visualization
Blue-throated Shiva staying awake to honor the celebration of life, song, dance, and joy.

Complementary Breath
kapalabhati & bhastrika

Closing Ritual
japa mala
Chant 108 rounds of Aum Namah Shivaya with or without beeds.

Additional Winter Inquiries:

Hanukkah (Jewish), Bodhi Day (Buddhist), Hajj (Islam), Winter Solstice/Yule (Christian, Wicca/Neo Pagan), Christmas (Christian), New Year's (Interfaith), Gantan-sai (Shinto), Muharram (Islam), Maghi (Sikh), World Religion Day (Baha'i), Tu B'shvat (Jewish), Mahayana New Year (Buddhist), Candlemas (Christian), Imbolc (Wicca), Ash Wednesday/Lent (Christian), Chinese New Year (Confucian, Daoist, Buddhist), Vasant Panchami (Hindu), St. Patrick's Day (Christian), Vernal Equinox, Ostara (Wicca), Mawlid an Nabi (Islam), Good Friday (Christian).

the details...

*"You can preach a better sermon with
your life than with your lips."*

-Oliver Goldsmith

Inquiry Index: *In Alphabetical Order*

The Gifts of Embodiment

Wisdom of Yoga

Hindu Gods & Goddesses

The Alchemy of Nature

The Wheel of the Year

Endnotes:

opening

[1] *Teachers*. Copyright © 2004 by Danna Faulds. Reprinted with premission of Danna Faulds.

introduction

[1] http://www.kripalu.org/pdfs/kyta_quotes.pdf
[2] http://www.yogahealsus.com/downloads/Yoga_Heals_Us_News_January_2006.pdf

the gifts of embodiment

[1] Byrd Baylor, *The Way to Start a Day*, p. 25-27
[2] Reprinted from *Call Me By My True Names: The Collected Poems of Thich Nhat Hanh* (1999) by Thich Nhat Hanh with permission of Parallax Press, Berkeley, California, www.parallax.org
[3] Dana Faulds, *Go In and In*, p. 2, reprinted with premission of Danna Faulds
[4] Douglas Brooks, *The Rasas*, Todd Norian Teacher Training, Lenox, MA, 11/2007
[5] http://webapps.uni-koeln.de/tamil/
[6] http://www.whereincity.com/medical/education/body-facts.php
[7] Frank Stewart, *Natural History of Natural Writing*, p. 209
[8] Coleman Barks, *The Essential Rumi*, The Guest House, p. 109
[9] John Cook, Steve Deger & Leslie Ann Gibson, *The Book of Positive Quotations*, p. 328
[10] Robert Fulghum, *All I Really Need to Know I Learned in Kindergarten*, p. 82
[11] Robert Fulghum, *All I Really Need to Know I Learned in Kindergarten*, p. 83
[12] Gray, Macy. "Sexual Revolution." Lyrics. ID. 2004
[13] http://www.pubmedcentral.nih.gov/articlerender.fcgi?artid=1174919
[14] © 2009 Lester Long, reprinted with permission of author
[15] Anusara Yoga Teacher Training Manual, p. 27
[16] http://www.gaia.com/quotes/topics/krishnamurti
[17] http://www.haaretz.com/hasen/spages/959332.html
[18] Douglas Brooks, Rajanaka Winter Retreat, Bristol, NY, 3/2007
[19] http://en.wikipedia.org/wiki/Darkness
[20] http://www.tibet.com/DL/10mar97.html
[21] http://en.wikipedia.org/wiki/Lekhah_Dodi
[22] http://www.earthministry.org/Congregations/UN_Sabbath.htm
[23] Thich Nhat Hanh, *Present Moment Wonderful Moment*, p. 3
[24] Douglas Brooks, Rajanaka Summer Retreat, Bristol, NY, 7/2008
[25] Jack Kornfield & Joseph Goldstein, *Seeking the Heart of Wisdom*, p. 50
[26] Haven Trevino, *The Tao of Healing*, meditation 28, © 1993, 1999 by Haven Trevino. Reprinted with permission of New World Library, Novato, CA. www.newworldlibrary.com
[27] http://news.bbc.co.uk/2/hi/science/nature/7201994.stm
[28] http://www.mro.org/zmm/teachings/daido/teisho46.php

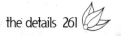

29 Coleman Barks, The Essential Rumi, p. 132-133, © 1997. Reprinted with permission of Coleman Barks

30 Eckhart Tolle, The Power of Now, chapter 8

31 Daniel Ladinsky, Henry S. Mindlin, H. Wilberforce Clarke, I Heard God Laughing, p. 89, © 1996. Reprinted with permission of Daniel Ladinsky.

32 Erich Schiffmann, Yoga: The Spirit and Practice of Moving into Stillness, p. 74

33 Elizabeth Roberts, Elias Amidon, Earth Prayers, p. 45, © Charlie Mehrhoff. Reprinted with permission of Charlie Mehrhoff

the wisdom of yoga

1   Douglas Brooks, The Secrets of the Three Cities, p. 4

2   Douglas Brooks, "Yogasutra of Patanjali," Matrika Yoga, Winter 2006, p. 24

3   Doug Keller, Heart of the Yogi, p. 121-122

4   http://webapps.uni-koeln.de/tamil/

5   http://www.space.com/scienceastronomy/star_count_030722.html

5.5 © 2009 Lisa Masé. Reprinted by permission.

6   Viktor Frankl, Man's Search for Meaning, p. 75

7   Jon Kabat-Zinn, Wherever You Go, There You Are, p.26

8   Douglas Renfrew Brooks, The Secret of the Three Cities, p. 272

9   http://thinkexist.com/quotation/have_patience_with_everything_that_remains/339301.html

10 Doug Keller, Heart of the Yogi, p. 116

11 Michael Leunig, The Prayer Tree, p. 1-2

12 Mary Oliver, Dream Work, Wild Geese, p. 14

13 Marianne Williamson, A Return to Love, p. 165

14 Yoga Journal, Sept. 2009, p. 94

15 Douglas Renfrew Brooks, Auspicious Wisdom, P. 115

16 The Fire Rises In Me, © Ivan M. Granger. Reprinted by permission of Ivan M. Granger.

17 Robert Gass, Chanting, Discovering Spirit in Sound, p. 37

18 http://www.yogabasics.com/learn/-unlocking-the-mystery-of-om.html

19 Robert Gass, Chanting, Discovering Spirit in Sound, p. 45

20 Esther Hicks, Abraham, Jerry Hicks, Louise L. Hay, The Amazing Power of Deliberate Intent, p. 93-94

21 http://www.yogajournal.com/lifestyle/724?page=2

22 Doug Keller, Heart of the Yogi, p. 192

23 Written for the presentation of The Collier Trophy to the Boeing Company, 1996
        From The House of Belonging , David Whyte & Many Rivers Press, Copyright 1996. Reprinted by permission.

24 http://www.experiencefestival.com/a/Sri_Sri_Ravishankar/id/221399 (true teacher)

25 Douglas Renfrew Brooks, Swami Durgananda, Paul E. Muller-Ortega, William K. Mahony, Constantina Rhodes Bailly,
        S.P. Sabharathnam, Meditation Revolution, p. 226 (true teacher)

26 Douglas Brooks, Rajanaka Winter Retreat, Bristol, NY, 3/2007

27 Coleman Barks, The Esential Rumi, Two Kinds of Intelligence, p. 178

28 Judyth Hill, Wage Peace, © Judyth Hill. Reprinted by permission of Judyth Hill.

28.5 Jalal al-Din Rumi; Reynold Alleyne Nicholson, The Mathnawí of Jalálu'ddín Rúmí, Part 6, p, 494

29 Danna Faulds, Go In and In, I Am All of This, p. 22

30 Hafiz, Daniel Ladinsky, The Gift: Poems by the Great Sufi Master, p. 281

31 Danna Faulds, Go In and In, First Leaf, p. 66

32 The Mother, Commentaries on Dhammapada, p. 18

33 Gary Snyder, The Practice of the Wild, p. 163-164, Copyright © 2003 by Gary Snyder from The Practice of the Wild: Essays. Reprinted by permission of Counterpoint

34 http://animals.howstuffworks.com/mammals/beaver-dam.htm

35 From Where Many Rivers Meet, copyright 1990, Many Rivers Press

36 YOGA magazine, September 1996.

36.5 Thich Nhat Hanh, Transformation and Healing: Sutra on the Four Establishments of Mindfulness p. 106-107

37 Doug Keller, Heart of the Yogi, p. 201

38 Jack Kornfield, A Path with Heart, p.102

39 Daniel Odier, The Yoga Spandakarika, p. 21

40 "proprioception." The American Heritage® Science Dictionary. Houghton Mifflin Company. 18 Feb. 2008. Dictionary.com http://dictionary.reference.com/browse/proprioception

41 Mary Oliver, New and Selected Poems, p. 23

42 Mary Oliver, New and Selected Poems, p. 174

43 Douglas Brooks, The Secret of the Three Cities, p. 62

44 Anodea Judith, Wheels of Life, p. 18

45 Anodea Judith, Wheels of Life, p. 23

46 http://www.experiencefestival.com/a/Petals/id/10289

47 Anodea Judith, Wheels of Life, p. 65

48 Anodea Judith, Wheels of Life, p. 55

49 http://www.kheper.net/topics/chakras/Muladhara.htm

50 Anodea Judith, Wheels of Life, p. 112

51 http://www.yogajournal.com/basics/898?page=3

52 Anodea Judith, Wheels of Life, p. 166

53 http://www.yogajournal.com/basics/898?page=4

54 Anodea Judith, Wheels of Life, p. 210

55 http://www.bbc.co.uk/science/humanbody/body/factfiles/heart/heart.shtml
'vizuddha' http://webapps.uni-koeln.de/tamil/

56 Anodea Judith, Wheels of Life, p. 258

57 http://webapps.uni-koeln.de/tamil/

58 Douglas Brooks, Siva Sutra Study, 7.1.3

59 Anodea Judith, Wheels of Life, p. 314

60 Anodea Judith, Wheels of Life, p. 334

61 Gratitude to Bhavani Lorraine Nelson for introducing me to chant

62 Anodea Judith, Wheels of Life, p. 366

63 Douglas Brooks, Summer Retreat, Bristol NY, 2009

64 Hafiz, Daniel Ladinsky, The Gift: Poems by the Great Sufi Master, p. 78

65 Anne Cushman, Metta in Motion, Yoga Journal, 11/03

66 Sharon Salzberg, Loving Kindness, p. 39

67 Sharon Salzberg, Loving Kindness, p. 119

the hindu gods & goddesses

1   A G Mitchell, Hindu Gods and Goddesses, p. v-viii
2   Eva Rudy Jansen, The Book of Hindu Imagery, p. 83
3   W.J. Wilkins, Hindu Gods and Goddesses, p. 99-100
4   Eva Rudy Jansen, The Book of Hindu Imagery, p. 87
5   W.J. Wilkins, Hindu Gods and Goddesses, p. 120
6   Eva Rudy Jansen, The Book of Hindu Imagery, p. 91
7   W.J. Wilkins, Hindu Gods and Goddesses, p. 170-197
8   http://webapps.uni-koeln.de/tamil/
9   Hafiz, © Daniel Ladinsky, The Gift: Poems by the Great Sufi Master, Reprinted with Permission of Daniel Ladinksy
10 Diane Bergstorm, Remind Me, WeMoon © 2008. Reprinted with Permission of Diane Bergstorm
11 Mitchel Bleier, "Ganapati," Matrika Yoga, Winter 2006, p. 71-79
12 Haven Trevino, Tao of Healing, meditation 36, © 1993, 1999 by Haven Trevino. Reprinted with permission of New World Library, Novato, CA. www.newworldlibrary.com
13 A G Mitchell, Hindu Gods and Goddesses, plate 43
14 Eva Rudy Jansen, The Book of Hindu Imagery, p. 127
15 http://webapps.uni-koeln.de/tamil/
16 W.J. Wilkins, Hindu Gods and Goddesses, p. 296-307
17 Dr. Madan Lal Goel, University of West Florida, The Sacred Feminine in Hinduism, p. 5 (http://www.uwf.edu/lgoel/ documents/ASacredFeminineinHinduism.pdf)
18 A G Mitchell, Hindu Gods and Goddesses, plate 46
19 Pradeep Kumar Gan, "The Lion: Mount of Goddess Durga", Orissa Review, 10/2004, p. 22-25
20 Haven Trevino, Tao of Healing, meditation 51, © 1993, 1999 by Haven Trevino. Reprinted with permission of New World Library, Novato, CA. www.newworldlibrary.com
21 http://webapps.uni-koeln.de/tamil/
22 Eva Rudy Jansen, The Book of Hindu Imagery, p. 89
23 http://www.fws.gov/birds/documents/MigrationofBirdsCircular.pdf
24 http://webapps.uni-koeln.de/tamil/
25 Eva Rudy Jansen, The Book of Hindu Imagery, p. 92
26 W.J. Wilkins, Hindu Gods and Goddesses, p. 127-133
27 Dr. Madan Lal Goel, University of West Florida, The Sacred Feminine in Hinduism, p. 5 (http://www.uwf.edu/lgoel/ documents/ASacredFeminineinHinduism.pdf)
28 For more specific information on this practice, refer to the book Ask and It Is Given by Jerry and Esther Hicks.
29 http://www.archive.org/stream/hindumythologyve00wilk/hindumythologyve00wilk_djvu.txt
30 W.J. Wilkins, Hindu Gods and Goddesses, p. 309-310
31 Douglas Brooks, Rajanaka Winter Retreat, Bristol, NY, 3/2007
32 David Whyte, from Where Many Rivers Meet, Many Rivers Press, © 1990

the alchemy of nature

1   Elizabeth Roberts and Elias Amidon, Earth Prayers, p. 200
2   Doug Keller, Refining the Breath, p. 133-137
3   Doug Keller, Refining the Breath, p. 133-137

[4] John Fire, Richard Erdoes, Lame Deer, p. 119

[5] http://mayoclinic.com/

[6] http://en.wikipedia.org/wiki/Graphical_timeline_of_human_evolution

[7] http://www.data360.org/dsg.aspx?Data_Set_Group_Id=757

[8] Living on Earth, Steve Curwood, PRI, 8-17-07

[9] Elizabeth Roberts & Elias Amidon, Earth Prayers, p. 134-135

[10] http://www.epa.gov/gmpo/edresources/soil.html

[11] Elizabeth Roberts & Elias Amidon, Earth Prayers, p. 136

[12] Douglas Brooks, The History of Yoga, Todd Norian Teacher Training, Becket, MA, 4/2006

[13] http://thinkexist.com/quotation/to_live_content_with_small_means-to_seek_elegance/12394.html

[14] http://en.wikipedia.org/wiki/Honey_bee

[15] Douglas Brooks, The Rasas, Todd Norian Teacher Training, Lenox, MA, 11/2007

[16] Douglas Brooks, The Rasas, Todd Norian Teacher Training, Lenox, MA, 11/2007

[17] http://www.idahoforests.org/salmonpn02.htm

[18] © Kirstin George. Reprinted by permission.

[18.5] Copyright © 1999 by Wendell Berry from /The Selected Poems of Wendell Berry/. Reprinted by permission of Counterpoint.

[19] John Welwood, Relationship as a Spiritual Cruicible, http://www.johnwelwood.com/articlesandinterviews.htm

[20] Richard LaMotte, Pure Sea Glass, p. 15

[21] http://orientalpearls.blogspot.com/2007_07_01_archive.html

[22] http://www.zalecorp.com/jewl/jewelry.aspx?pid=67

[23] http://www.thepearlmarket.com/pearlformed.htm

[24] http://www.superstringtheory.com

[25] Doug Keller, Tantra: Consciousness as Creative, 6/10/08, http://www.doyoga.com

[26] Danna Faulds, Go In and In, Still Point, p. 9

the wheel of the year

[1] © Janet Ryan. Reprinted with permission.

[2] http://www.kripalu.org/article/322/

[3] http://www.sejongtkd.org/training/Miskech/CrossingtheMidline.pdf

[4] New & selected essays By Denise Levertov p.171

[5] Mary Oliver, New and Selected Poems, The Summer Day p. 170

[6] © Lisa Masé. Reprinted with permission.

[7] Haven Trevino, Tao of Healing, meditation 34. © 1993, 1999 by Haven Trevino. Reprinted with permission of New World Library, Novato, CA. www.newworldlibrary.com

[7.5] Copyright © 1999 by Wendell Berry from /The Selected Poems of Wendell Berry/. Reprinted by permission of Counterpoint.

[8] http://www.indiancultureonline.com/details/Hindu/SHIVARATRI.html

[9] Danna Faulds, Go In and In, Awakening Now, p. 52

Expand Your View:

The following books were used as sources for both information and inspiration in writing *Nourishing the Teacher*. If you are interested in delving more fully into the ideas presented in this text, these are wonderful places to start. In the interest of conservation, please try to find these books used *(BetterWorld or Powell's)*, check them out of the library, or download them digitally.

Author(s)	Book(s)
Abraham & Esther Hicks	Ask and It Is Given
Amit Goswami	The Self-Aware Universe
Anodea Judith	Wheels of Life Eastern Body, Western Mind
Bruce Bowditch	The Yoga Practice Guide, *Dynamic sequencing for home practice and teachers*
Brian Greene	The Elegant Universe The Fabric of the Cosmos
Charles Phillips	Color for Life
Daniel Odier	Tantric Quest The Yoga Spandikarika Desire
Danna Faulds	Go In and In Prayers to the Infinite One Soul
Donna Farhi	The Breathing Book
Douglas Brooks	Rajanaka Heart (*not yet published at time of printing*) Poised for Grace, Annotations on the Bhagavad Gita from a Tantric View Auspicious Wisdom The Secret of the Three Cities: An Introduction to Hindu Sakta Tantrism
Douglas Brooks, Swami Durgananda, Paul Muller-Ortega, William Mahony, Constantina Bailly, S.P. Sabharathnam	Meditation Revolution: *A History and Theology of the Siddha Yoga Lineage*
Doug Keller	The Heart of the Yogi Refining the Breath Yoga as Therapy
Eva Rudy Jansen	The Book of Hindu Imagery
John Friend	Anusara® Yoga Teacher Training Manual

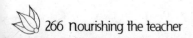

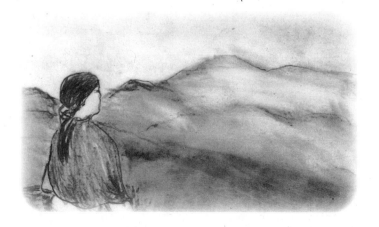

Pure Potential: *Create Your Own Inquiries & Contemplations*

Inquiry	Inspiration
Attention & Intention	Whatever we focus our attention on will grow. "Cultivate the vibe to make it come alive."
Authentic Nature	Cultivating the tools that aid us in staying true to our most authentic selves.
Blessing in Disguise	If approached skillfully, any crisis can become an opportunity for growth and healing.
Dedication	Acknowledging the importance of steadfastness and courage in manifesting our dreams.
Don't "Should" on Me	Examining the ways we place the unnecessary burden of "should" on ourselves and others.
Everyday Pilgrimage	Pilgrimages are usually thought of as grand expeditions to far away places, yet even the little journeys we make each day (to the supermarket, to work, out with friends) are sacred voyages imbued with magic and discovery.
Faith in a Seed	Because seeds are embedded in dark soil, we can't see their progress; we nurture and water them in the hope that our loving intention will sprout.
Honoring Silence	Cultivating the quiet spaces in the breath, between poses, and in life.
Integration Hour	Taking time to integrate and digest the many experiences of life provides us with balance and clarity as we move forward. Integration might take the form of journaling, art, co-listening, nature, or meditation.
Life-Quenching Tears	Even though we may resist releasing our tears, their moisture is like healing rain that replenishes even the most parched, barren places within.
Light & Shadow	Honoring the parts of ourselves which shine brightly as well as those hidden in shadow.
Limitless Possibilities	Living in the light of pure, untapped potential, following your dreams despite all odds and obstacles.
Vinyasa	This Sanskrit term is usually associated with fast moving, vigorous classes; yet the word also signifies order, conscious placement, arrangement, and attitude. These definitions provide us with new perspectives though which to explore this fluid practice, whether fast or slow.

Listening with Intent	*Truly taking time to pause and listen, not only with our ears but also with our bodies, senses, and intuition.*
Lunar Light	*Exploring our relationship to the various cycles of our lives as symbolized by the phases of the moon. Appreciating the cooling, reflective light of the moon and the many ways it nurtures us.*
Ordinary Beauty	*Delving more deeply to see the subtler, less apparent manifestations of beauty.*
Blessed Sanctuary	*The notion of how creating sacred space in the physical realm directly affects our emotional and spiritual landscape.*
Sacred Spiral	*Contemplate the ways in which life continuously twists and turns, as reflected through the widespread structure of the spiral in nature.*
The Asymmetrical Nature of the Universe	*Honoring the imperfections that make life interesting, unique, and whole. Our asymmetry makes us all the more beautiful.*
The Power of Patience	*Fostering the capacity to wait, breathe, and trust amidst eagerness and urgency*
Turning Apples into Cider	*Seeing the opportunity in the already present abundance, as we creatively participate to take the raw materials of life that beckon us and transform them into our own unique offering.*
Hidden Masks	*In many cultures, masks are used as a playful means of embodying different aspects of being. Utilize masks to explore the roles you currently play in your life and to investigate the characters you've always wanted to be. Notice any masks you hide behind that are impeding your highest potential.*
Central Channel	*Sushumna is the central nadi in the subtle anatomy of yoga, which runs along the axis of the spinal cord. As babies, our bodies grow outward from this central channel. In yoga, we continuously draw in towards this midline to nourish its functioning in the physical and subtle realms and to source strength.*
Affirming the Good	*It is easy to focus on the many ways challenge and difficulty infuse our lives and the world. Affirming the good invites us to look for the positive in each moment; rooted in this sense of affirmation, we can navigate our experience with greater clarity and skill.*
Bursts of Potential	*Fireflies are actually beetles that utilize a special organ to generate a radiant burst of light. They remind us that oftentimes a single burst of possibility can send us sailing off in the right direction.*

Beginner's Mind	*When we approach life with beginner's mind, we develop a spacious capacity for receiving and learning from the various facets of life. Yoga supports us in cultivating the skills needed to approach any situation with an open heart and a welcoming mind.*
Sonic Resonance	*Vibrational sounds comprise what we see and consider tangible. The sounds we encounter both internally and externally can alter our emotions, presence, and way of life. Yoga can help us cultivate a more skillful relationship to the sonic universe.*
Experiments in Love	*What would shift if we embraced love as an experiment instead of something to acquire? What would happen if we took time to investigate and determine what love truly means for us? We can contemplate love as an offering to ourselves, to those who frustrate us, and to those who happen to be our family.*
Sweet Resistance	*When we encounter resistance on our path, our first inclination is to move away from the discomfort. Instead of walking away, we have the option to dive in and explore what this feeling is all about. Is it a genuine preference we choose to honor, or is it one that is ultimately blocking the flow of energy?*

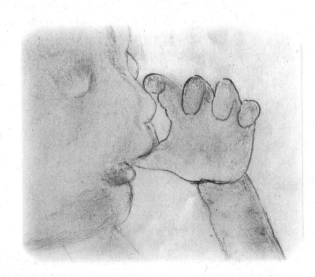

The Team: *From the Ground Up*

Danny Arguetty, Anjali Budreski, Kelli Adams, Bella Arguetty, and Cody Drasser

Where are you from?

DA: *At times I think another planet, which is technically true in a certain sense. My motherland is Israel, but I have had the privilege of living in many other places that have enriched the story of my life.*

AB: *The place of salt marsh & herring, winding North River, Atlantic salt, inky black and blue waters, coastal dreams, Eastern sunrise, white pines and beeches, lady slippers, Emerald Isles landscapes, Eastern European mountains, farmers, doctors, healers, and love.*

KA: *The edges of places, apparently…first a small, southern mill town in Virginia a stone's throw from North Carolina, and then a tiny Japanese farm hamlet that hugs the border between Fukuoka and Oita Prefectures, and now Providence, Rhode Island, which is just shy of Massachusetts.*

BA: *I am from a very problematic part of the Universe, but it is beautiful at the same time: The Middle East - Israel.*

CD: *Long Island, NY. Currently living in the Berkshire Mountains, working and teaching yoga at Kripalu Center for Yoga & Health.*

What is your favorite leafy green vegetable?

DA: *Rainbow chard, hands down.*
AB: *Kale with caramelized onions.*
KA: *Danny's rainbow chard, hands down.*
BA: *Arugula with tomatoes, garlic, and olive oil.*
CD: *Spinach with olive oil, garlic, and a little turmeric and Bragg's.*

What is your favorite yoga posture right now?

DA: *Parsvakonasana-hands bound.*
AB: *Gomukhasana*
KA: *Savasana*
CD: *Parsva Bakasana*

How has yoga shifted your life?

DA: *Yoga has instilled in me an expansive vision that is layered with deep trust, possibility, and the desire to savor every moment of my life. Through this skillful inquiry, I find that I am more compassionate, clear, and excited in co-creating the reality that is before me. Most of all, I am grateful for yoga's emphasis on the power and necessity of community, which reminds me that I don't have to do it all on my own, and that in supporting others to thrive, I am uplifted twofold.*

AB: *Yoga brought me home to myself; it continues to amaze me, every day. It helped me to melt into the beauty of who*

I am, breath by breath, and relax into the home of my heart. Yoga has helped me bridge my life and my work; there is no separation. Moving into yoga poses connects me to the unfathomable beauty and layers of my being, and it is my passion to guide others in doing the same.

KA: *Yoga has beckoned me to live with eyes (and ears, and mind, and heart...) wide open. It has enabled me to truly understand that the essence of life resides in process and journey as opposed to end results or destinations. Through my practice, I have cultivated profound trust in my capacity for creativity and manifesting abundance. Yoga has also empowered me to recognize the vitality and possibility inherent in darkness as well as light.*

CD: *Seeing myself more clearly — giving equal space to those parts of me that I wish were not there as well as welcoming those aspects of myself that I admire. Also, the ability to notice and control my energy level and how it affects my perspective on the world and my place within it.*

Your friends love you because?

DA: *I am silly, opinionated, blunt, compassionate, and get things done.*
AB: *I am willing to be with their joy as well as their pain, I am a total goofball sometimes, and the Anjali laugh makes them laugh.*
KA: *I laugh easily, live courageously, and love with the whole of my being. And because I'm a pixie.*
BA: *I am honest and generous.*
CD: *I am clearly and unmistakably me in every way.*

What is your nature scene?

DA: *From growing up in concrete central, I have come along way. I adore walks in the forest, time spent hiking, basking in the sun, ocean waves, and snowy days.*

AB: *I live in a little valley in a little city called Montpelier (the smallest capital in the country and the only one without a McDonald's). Nature is everywhere...my scene is comprised of walks on high country roads, deer and wild turkeys, moon and stars over Montpelier, brilliant leaves in autumn, and cold, clear, pebbled rivers in summer; it is sub-zero winter nights with crunchy snow under my boots and hot, humid summer ones on the front porch swing. The top of Camel's Hump or White Rocks is balm for my soul.*

KA: *The soft glow of sunrise on a vast, deserted beach*

BA: *In the late afternoon, I see the sunset from my room's window; as the sky becomes red, I feel a moment of peace.*

CD: *Morning, silence, a wooded path, and the earth waking up all around me. Sitting quietly on the beach watching the ocean. A cold winter evening, outside while the wind whips around me and the moon shines brightly on everything.*

How do you make art?

DA: *More and more, I find that areas of my life I never viewed as creative become threads of the tapestry I weave day in and day out. These areas include the practices of: teaching yoga, cooking, collage, graphic design, altar rituals, design of living space, and writing.*

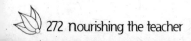

AB: *Poetry, journaling, wrapping gifts, stacking stones in the forest, decorating luscious treats that come out of my oven, watercolor, yoga, and dance.*

KA: *Most recently, I craft a luscious, smoothed surface of wet clay and use my body and my yoga practice to imprint it with movement and energy.*

BA: *Everything is art: my work (costume and set design), my teaching, and my free time painting. I love to create all the time.*

CD: *Beginning with color or simple forms, I build up from there with layers of paint, paper and ink, or other various media. Sometimes I move in the direction of a concrete visual idea and expand upon that notion, and sometimes I allow the layering process to reveal whatever wishes to emerge without too much thought behind it…essentially allowing the energy of the piece to fuel and drive itself. I scrape away and destroy little pieces of the imagery to reveal layers underneath, and then build up again from there. I building and erase, construct and destroy. I have fun, stepping out of the way and relaxing around the attachment connected to wanting a particular outcome in my work. I have a few different styles, as well—collage, illustration, paint, etc.*

How do you thrive?

DA: *By…remembering possibility, doing my practice, spending time with family and friends, eating tasty food, dancing, being in nature, honoring the darkness, exploring conscious relationships, chanting, and listening to music.*

AB: *I could not live without beautiful friends, fresh air and wild spaces, organic local food, home sanctuary, beauty, simplicity, quiet, solitude and the love of community. Smiling yoga students, challenge, change, travel, and play!*

KA: *By taking time to prepare delicious and healthful foods, moving and stretching both body and mind through yoga and dance, immersing myself in the studio, taking leisurely walks, enjoying live music, making time for solitude, reveling in life with friends and family, and remembering to breathe deeply and savor the moment.*

BA: *Taking long walks at night with Hanan, mornings without time pressure, eating good and healthy food, going to the theatre almost every week, and of course doing my art.*

CD: *Enough sleep, nourishing meals, a yoga practice that strengthens me and restores my body, mind, and spirit, sharing yoga with others, ample space for myself to journey inward and then reach out to connect to those I love, long walks to nowhere, creating space in my life to create art, and music, music, music!*

What's one vice you want to share with the world?

DA: *Sometimes I become an overbearing, drill sergeant of a control freak*
AB: *Deep Fried delicacies; cider donuts, sweet potato fries with garlic aioli, potato chips, latkes…and root beer.*
KA: *chocolate and my mom's biscuits.*
BA: *Sometimes I'm too stubborn.*
CD: *Coffee!*

What is one thing that people are surprised to learn about you?

DA: *That I am gay…ok, that's not a surprise. That English is my second language and I learned most of it in six months at the age of nine.*
AB: *How big of a Red Sox fan I am!*
KA: *That I speak Japanese fluently.*
BA: *That I don't eat dairy.*
CD: *That I love scary, violent, gory movies.*

What Scares You?

DA: *Waking up in the morning without purpose.*
AB: *Fast-moving rivers, gas station bathrooms, and war.*
KA: *Limited thinking and nuclear weapons.*
BA: *Sickness and cockroaches.*
CD: *Growing old alone.*

What have you learned working on this book?

DA: *That everything I do in life reflects and deepens my connection to who I already am, illuminating my fragmented yet interwoven nature. I got to know all the various Dannys, including the dedicated, neurotic, control freak, creative, depleted, energized, surrendered, steadfast, unworthy, worthy, scared, and excited ones. Most of all, I learned that I can't do it on my own, and that having a team of brilliant people is priceless.*

AB: *I've learned to do what I think I cannot do, to work hard, be a source of strength and support, and know my limits; it's hard to write a book, and it requires patience, dedication, and tapas!*

KA: *I've learned that semicolons are extremely useful, that true friendship can sustain any amount of pressure with grace and ease, and that writing a book is a process of mammoth proportions, complete with inconceivable challenges and unparalleled rewards.*

BA: *Usually my oil paintings take a couple of months or even a year because I use the layered system of the old masters. However, I found out that black and white drawings like those for the book are much more fun to do because I can see the results immediately.*

CD: *Patience. Allowing others to express their views on my work and how it will fit into their vision of the completed piece.*

If you had to sum it all up in one word it would be?

DA: *Participation*
AB: *Trust*
KA: *Space*
BA: *Great joy.*
CD: *…Sigh*

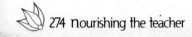

Next Steps: *Trainings & Support*

In our endeavor of sharing yoga, we are gifted with abundant possibility for growth and expansion of our knowledge, skills, and heart space. If you wish to engage in further study of Tantric Yoga Philosophy, yoga asana, dynamic language, and techniques for weaving inspirational, heart-opening themes into your classes, please stay in touch.

For current workshops and trainings dates, visit www.nourishyourlight.com

For teaching resources, green-living ideas, an inspirational newsletter, and more
visit www.nourishingtheteacher.com

Regarding specific questions or to arrange a Nourishing the Teacher training or workshop in your area, please contact me at danny@nourishyourlight.com.

Let go of perfection,
there are no mistakes,
only learning.
Accept where you are,
embrace your resistance,
and be open to growth through experience.
Honor your humanity
and learn from all teachers.

-Anonymous

Notes:

Notes:

Notes:

Notes:

Notes:

Notes:

Notes:

Notes:

Notes:

Notes:

Notes:

Notes:

Notes: